Cases and Concepts
for the new MRCGP

2nd Edition

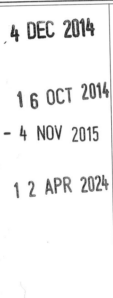

Cases and Concepts
for the new MRCGP

2nd Edition

Clinical Skills Assessment and Case-based Discussion

P. Naidoo
MBChB, MRCGP, DRCOG, DFFP, Dip Occ Med, MSc
GP in Oxfordshire

Includes contributions from

C. Monkley
MBBS, DRCOG, MSc (Sports Medicine), MRCGP, FFSEM (UK)
GP in the Defence Medical Services – for the CSA cases

A. Davy
MBBS, BSc, MRCGP, DRCOG
GP in the Defence Medical Services – for the CbD cases

NEWMRCGP

Scion

Second edition © Scion Publishing Ltd, 2009

First edition published 2008 (ISBN 978 1 904842 53 8); Reprinted 2011, 2012

A CIP catalogue record for this book is available from the British Library.

ISBN 978 1 904842 67 5

Scion Publishing Limited
Bloxham Mill, Barford Road, Bloxham, Oxfordshire OX15 4FF
www.scionpublishing.com

Important Note from the Publisher
The information contained within this book was obtained by Scion Publishing Limited from sources believed by us to be reliable. However, while every effort has been made to ensure its accuracy, no responsibility for loss or injury whatsoever occasioned to any person acting or refraining from action as a result of information contained herein can be accepted by the authors or publishers.

The reader should remember that medicine is a constantly evolving science and while the authors and publishers have ensured that all dosages, applications and practices are based on current indications, there may be specific practices which differ between communities. You should always follow the guidelines laid down by the manufacturers of specific products and the relevant authorities in the country in which you are practising.

Typeset by Phoenix Photosetting, Chatham, Kent, UK
Printed by TJ International Ltd, Padstow, Cornwall

CONTENTS

PREFACE TO SECOND EDITION

The aim of this book is to help candidates prepare for the Clinical Skills Assessment (CSA) and Case-based Discussion (CbD) components of the new MRCGP exam by making explicit 'what' to do and 'how' to do it to achieve success.

'What' is needed in CSA and CbD is the ability to:
- gather and assess medical information
- make structured, evidence-based and flexible decisions
- communicate with patients in a way that moves the consultation forward in an ethical and responsible manner

'How' this is demonstrated to examiners is by:
- asking the right questions, at the right time, in the right way
- performing the right examination correctly
- communicating the right things in the right way to patients and colleagues

This book tries to teach candidates how to demonstrate their competence in an exam by showing them how two general practitioners approached the presentations of their patients:
- the questions they asked to get to the crux of the problem
- the examinations they chose to conduct
- the decisions they made
- how they communicated with their patients

By breaking down each case in this way, this book provides a structured approach for candidates to aid them in their exam preparation.

Unlike its companion guide, *Consultation Skills for the new MRCGP*, which primarily focuses on teaching consulting skills, our primary aim in this book is to mentally model for candidates an ordered, step-wise approach to data gathering, analysis, management and communication. In some cases, additional medical information is provided to clarify the management decisions. While the book does not aim to be completely comprehensive in its coverage of medicine or examination techniques, this second edition does include over 200 questions and answers to help candidates revise the background factual information. Candidates are also signposted to useful, usually internet-based, sources of information for aiding their medical revision.

We hope that this book is useful to you in developing a step-wise approach to CSA and CbD.

Dr P Naidoo and Dr C Monkley
November, 2008

ACKNOWLEDGMENTS

I would like to thank Dr Clive Monkley for his contribution to the Clinical Skills Assessment cases, and Dr Andrew Davy for his contribution to the Case-based Discussion cases.

Thank you to Dr Sarah Butterfield and Dr Samantha Wild for their helpful comments and critiques.

Thank you to my good friend Dr Dougie Wyper, for improving my social life. Life would be a lot less interesting without you.

Finally, a reminder to my husband Anton – you owe me a farm in Africa, at the foot of the Drakensberg Mountains.

Dedication

This book is dedicated to my father for his love and encouragement – thank you dad.

ABBREVIATIONS

BDD	body dysmorphic disorder
BMA	British Medical Association
BMJ	*British Medical Journal*
CAM	complementary and alternative medicine
CBT	cognitive behavioural therapy
CG	clinical governance
CHD	coronary heart disease
CHI	Commission for Health Improvement
CHRE	Council for Healthcare Regulatory Excellence
CME	continuing medical education
CPD	Continuing Professional Development
CPP	Committee on Professional Performance
DENs	doctors' educational needs
DVLA	Driver and Vehicle Licensing Agency
EC	emergency contraception
EBM	evidence-based medicine
GMC	General Medical Council
GP	general practitioner
GPwSI	GP with special interests
GUM	genito-urinary medicine
HFEA	Human Fertilization and Embryology Authority
IUD	intra-uterine device
IVF	*in vitro* fertilization
JC	journal club
LCR	ligase chain reaction
LMP	last menstrual period
MAAG	Medical Audit Advisory Group
MCA	Medical Council on Alcohol
MDU	medical defence union
MI	myocardial infarction
MS	multiple sclerosis
MUS	medically unexplained symptoms
NAPCE	National Association of Primary Care Educators
NCAA	National Clinical Assessment Authority
NEJM	*New England Journal of Medicine*
NHS	National Health Service
NICE	National Institute for Health and Clinical Excellence
NNT	number needed to treat
NPSA	National Patient Safety Agency
NRT	nicotine replacement therapy
OCD	obsessive compulsive disorder
OM	otitis media
OPD	outpatients department

PCC	Professional Conduct Committee
PCOS	polycystic ovary syndrome
PCR	polymerase chain reaction
PCT	primary care trust
PDP	personal development plan
PHCT	Primary Health Care Trust
PID	pelvic inflammatory disease
PM	practice manager
PTSD	post-traumatic stress disorder
PUNs	patients' unmet needs
RA	rheumatoid arthritis
RCGP	Royal College of General Practitioners
RCPCH	Royal College of Paediatrics and Child Health
RCT	randomized controlled trial
SEA	significant event audit
STD	sexually transmitted disease
TIA	transient ischaemic attack
TOP	termination of pregnancy
UTI	urinary tract infection

An introduction to clinical skills assessment (CSA)

This introductory chapter discusses:
- the structure of CSA
- the marking of CSA
- assessment within the nMRCGP:
  - curricular objectives: six domains and three essential features
- assessment within CSA:
  - blueprints for writing cases
  - blueprints for selecting cases
- preparing for the CSA
- how best to use this book to prepare

The structure of CSA

The CSA is one of the three components of the nMRCGP assessment. The other two components are the applied knowledge test (AKT), and workplace based assessment (WPBA). The Royal College of General Practitioners (RCGP) will make CSA available from October 2007. Thereafter, the assessment will be available during a 3 or 4 week period in sessions in February, May and October each year. It will take place in one location, initially in Croydon, and in later years in a purpose-built centre in London.

The CSA is not primarily a test of knowledge or examination techniques. It is an assessment of a doctor's ability to *integrate* and *apply* clinical, professional, communication and practical skills appropriate for general practice, 'to produce a consultation that is meaningful to both patient and doctor and which moves the patient forward towards a justifiable management of their presenting problem' (Hawthorne, 2007 – on the RCGP website).

What happens on exam day

- On the day of the examination, at the examination venue, each candidate will be given a consulting room.
- The candidate will be briefed to treat the examination session as if he were a locum doctor.
- The candidate is to interact with the patient and not the examiner, who will remain a silent observer.
- The candidate's surgery has thirteen booked patients who enter his consulting room when the buzzer sounds.
- At the end of ten minutes, the buzzer sounds to signal the departure of the patient.
- There will be a two minute gap between consultations.

- Twelve patients are true examination cases on which the candidate is assessed. One is a 'trial station' in which new clinical scenarios are trialled. The candidiate will not know which is the trial case.
- There will be a short break in the middle of surgery.

The marking of CSA

The patients, played by trained actors, will move from room to room, together with the examiner for that case. The examiners are all general practitioners who are selected and trained in assessment by the RCGP. Each examiner will mark the same case all day, thus providing standardized marking. Each case is marked in three domains, all have equal weighting:
- data gathering, examination and clinical assessment skills
- clinical management skills
- interpersonal skills

The performance will be graded as Clear Pass, Marginal Pass, Marginal Fail or Clear Fail. The candidate is then given an overall grade.

In assessment speak, the four grades, from Clear Pass to Clear Fail, are called grid descriptors – they describe the standards, knowledge and skills found at each grade. The pass mark is set as the standard required to practice independently as a licensed GP. The marking sheet contains positive indicators and negative indicators of practice, which inform the examiner's global judgement of the candidate's performance.

The examiner does not tick boxes, as in the old MRCGP video marking sheet, and the pass is not determined by number of ticks the candidate scores in each case. This is what makes CSA a competency-based assessment – the candidate passes if he meets the criteria for competence, to the standard required to practice independently as a licensed GP. This is not a norm-referenced assessment in which a pre-determined number of the highest ranking candidates pass. Theoretically, if all the candidates meet the marking criteria to the pre-set standard required for passing, then all of them should pass.

Therefore, to prepare for CSA, it is useful to understand what is being assessed by the nMRCGP, and by the CSA in particular.

Assessment within the nMRCGP

- Assessment is about making a judgement as to whether trainees have fulfilled the training objectives. The assessor should be able to say, 'By the end of this training, the trainee should be able to…'.
- To make this judgement, the assessor needs to measure the trainee's progress against defined criteria.
- Therefore, to understand assessment within the nMRCGP, we need to be familiar with its 'training objectives', and to understand the 'criteria against which trainees are measured'.

The nMRCGP objectives

The nMRCGP objectives are described within the curriculum for speciality training for general practice. By the end of speciality training for general practice, trainees should have:

> 'the wide-ranging knowledge, clinical skills and communication skills required by doctors who will specialise in general practice, to ensure the delivery of high quality standards of patient care in the NHS' (RCGP, 2007).

Exactly what constitutes the knowledge, clinical skills and communication skills is described further in the GP curriculum, a rather large body of work. A summary of the GP curriculum is available as a core statement, within which six domains of core competencies and three essential features of patient-centred care are described. These constitute 'criteria against which trainees are measured'.

The six domains (D1 – D6) and three essential features (EF1 – EF3)

D1. Primary care management – is about having the ability to recognize and manage common medical conditions in primary care. Trainees demonstrate the ability to deal with multiple complaints and co-morbidity.

D2. Person centred care – is about appreciating the patient as a unique person in a unique context, taking into account patient preferences and expectations at every step in the consultation. Trainees demonstrate the use of recognized communication techniques to gain understanding of the patient's illness experience and develop a shared approach to managing problems.

D3. Specific problem solving skills – is about adopting a problem-based approach to practice in which uncertainty may have to be tolerated; time used as part of the diagnostic process; and incremental investigation undertaken. Trainees demonstrate proficiency in performing physical examination, and in using diagnostic and therapeutic instruments. The consultation itself is used as a diagnostic or therapeutic instrument; for example, the patient's health beliefs are explored and later incorporated into the doctor's explanation.

D4. A comprehensive approach – is about addressing multiple complaints and co-morbidity; using an evidence-based approach; and minimising the impact of the patient's symptoms on his wellbeing by taking into account his personality, family, daily life, economic circumstances, and physical and social surroundings. Trainees demonstrate the ability to promote self-care and empower patients.

D5. Community orientation – is about understanding the potentials and limitations of the communities in which doctors' work. Trainees demonstrate an ethical approach to rationing and a responsible approach to influencing health policy.

D6. A holistic approach – is about integrating the physical, psychological and social components of health problems in making diagnoses and planning management. Trainees demonstrate an understanding of the bio-psycho-social elements of illness and a willingness to use a wide range of interventions.

EF1. Contextual aspects – is about understanding the doctor's context, the environment (community, culture, environment and regulatory frameworks) within which he works. Trainees demonstrate an understanding of the impact care given to an individual patient has on the practice's resources (staff, equipment) and acts within financial and legal frameworks.

EF2. Attitudinal aspects – is about the doctor's capabilities, values, feelings and ethics. Trainees demonstrate ethical practice with respect for equality and diversity issues and in line with the accepted codes of professional conduct.

EF3. Scientific aspects – is about adopting an evidence-based and critical approach to practice to continually improve quality. Trainees demonstrate familiarity with the concepts of scientific research, statistics, and critical appraisal, and apply their learning to improve the quality of their practice.

Assessment within CSA

The objective of the nMRCGP is to develop practitioners with wide-ranging knowledge, clinical skills and communication skills which, in assessment speak, are called the intended learning outcomes. The intended learning outcomes form the blueprint of the CSA. The RCGP published the blueprint for the CSA on its website. The table below is adapted from the RCGP web publication and shows the clinical, professional, communication and/or practical skills required of each criterion (A –F).

Blueprint area – criteria	Descriptors of the criteria
A. Data gathering and interpretation	Gathering of data for clinical judgment, choice of examination, investigations and their interpretations
B. Management	Recognition and management of common medical conditions in primary care. Demonstrates flexible and structured approach to decision making
C. Co-morbidity and health promotion	Demonstrating ability to deal with multiple complaints and co-morbidity and to promote a shared approach to managing problems
D. Person-centred approach	Use of recognized communication techniques that enhances understanding of a patient's illness and promotes a shared approach to managing problems
E. Professional attitude	Practising ethically with respect for equality and diversity in line with accepted codes of professional conduct
F. Technical skills	Demonstrating proficiency in performing physical examinations and using diagnostic and therapeutic instruments

Each CSA case must be constructed to test criteria A to F. How is this done? Marks are awarded for:

- Efficient and targeted **data gathering** – the ability to take a targeted history and perform a focussed physical examination. Candidates are expected to be knowledgeable and skillful in their examination techniques and in the appropriate use of medical instruments. Marks are awarded for the fluency with which procedures are performed.
- Formulating **clinical management** in line with current accepted British general practice.
- **Interpersonal skills** – the candidate shows an ability to engage patients in the consultation, using recognized interpersonal skills, such as enquiring about the patient's health beliefs and incorporating these into the explanation given to the patient. Some cases also assess the candidate's ability to value patients' contributions, and to respect their autonomy and decision-making.

The overall mark given to the case will depend on the candidate's ability to combine the two areas of clinical consulting with interpersonal skills.

In very simple terms, data gathering is about *how* you get to the 'nub' of the presenting problem; clinical management is about *what* you do to move the problem forward; and interpersonal skills is about *how* you go about doing it.

Each case is written to focus on a particular 'nub'. The marking schedule, using positive and negative indicators, reflects this nub. For example, Case 30 in this book is written about a patient with multiple sclerosis who presents with balance problems. You may want to read this case before proceeding. The marking schedule is provided below:

Generic indicators for targeted assessment domains	Descriptors – positive and negative
A. Data gathering, technical and assessment skills: - Gathering of data for clinical judgement, choice of examination, investigations and their interpretations - Demonstrating proficiency in performing physical examinations and using diagnostic and therapeutic instruments Maps on the blueprint to: - Data gathering and interpretation (A) - Technical skills (F)	Positive indicators: - establishes exactly what is meant by 'my balance is shot' - finds out details of home stresses and how these affect today's presentation - performs a targeted neurological examination so that any significant pathology responsible for 'a drunken gait' is unlikely to be missed Negative indicators: - makes assumptions regarding what is meant by balance difficulties – for example, assumes this is vertigo

Generic indicators for targeted assessment domains	Descriptors – positive and negative
	• fails to identify the contribution of stress to poor sleep, which aggravates the balance problem • appears disorganized or unsystematic in performing the targeted neurological examination
B. Clinical management skills • Recognition and management of common medical conditions in primary care; demonstrates flexible and structured approach to decision making • Demonstrating ability to deal with multiple complaints and co-morbidity and to promote a shared approach to managing problems Maps on the blueprint to: • Management (B) • Co-morbidity and health promotion (C)	Positive indicators: • shows an understanding of natural history of MS, including relapses and remissions • discusses strategies to address home stresses, restore confidence and maintain long-term mobility • discusses the need for sickness certification and weighs up its pros and cons with the patient Negative indicators: • fails to consider that balance difficulties could be a presentation of an MS relapse • fails to take into account the social stresses, therefore fails to outline appropriate coping strategies • by failing to openly consider or discuss the sick note, does not take steps to establish a doctor–patient relationship or to improve future health-seeking behaviour
C. Interpersonal skills • Use of recognized communication techniques that enhances understanding of a patient's illness and promotes a shared approach to managing problems • Practising ethically with respect for equality and diversity in line with accepted codes of professional conduct	Positive indicators: • shows empathy when exploring the possible physical, psychological and social issues affecting her presentation today • involves the patient in identifying strategies for dealing with 'stress at home' • when conducting the examination, appears professional, and is sensitive to the patient's feelings

Maps on the blueprint to:	Negative indicators:
• Person-centred approach (D) • Professional attitude (E)	• fails to empathize with how the patient's life is affected by the problem • fails to construct a shared management plan incorporating strategies for dealing with 'stress at home' • when conducting the examination, appears unprofessional, or hurts or embarrasses the patient

Assessors also want to assess breadth of knowledge – they want cases to sample patients of different ages, and diseases of various systems. Hence, a case selection blueprint (see table below) is used so that the twelve examination cases in each CSA diet are sampled from across the grid.

CSA – case selection blueprint	Primary nature of cases					
Primary system or area of disease	Acute illness	Chronic illness	Undifferentiated illness	Psychological and social	Preventative/ lifestyle	Other
Cardiovascular						
Respiratory						
Neurological/ psychiatric						
Musculoskeletal						
Endocrine/ oncology						
Eye/ENT/skin						
Men/women/ sexual health						
Renal/urological						
Gastrointestinal						
Infectious diseases						
Etc						

Preparing for CSA

Do the job
The CSA cases are all written by GPs active in the UK NHS and reflect real-life presentations. Therefore, candidates with some experience in NHS general practice should not have difficulty with the exam. The RCGP recommends that candidates first complete at least 6 months of UK NHS general practice before sitting the exam.

Read the website
Candidates are advised to read the Curriculum Statements from the RCGP website. Each curriculum statement has a section on common and important conditions and cases are quite likely to be based on one of these.

Analyse your video consultations
Candidates are advised to video their own consultations, watch them with a colleague, and analyse them for the clinical approach and interpersonal skills displayed.

Practise clinical examinations
Candidates are advised to practise the focussed examinations that are most likely to be tested, such as assessment of a limb, chest or abdomen. Some examinations, such as intimate examinations on a role player, or examinations that might cause discomfort if repeated are less likely to be tested. Candidates are advised to be familiar and confident with medical equipment, such as otoscopes.

Interpret data
Candidates are advised to practise to become familiar with the letters GPs receive from secondary care, and test results such as ECGs, spirometry, blood tests, urinalysis, skin scrapings, and swabs. Candidates need to ensure that they can interpret results correctly and explain them to a patient.

The CSA cases in this book include cases that require candidates to practise physical examination and interpret test results.

How best to use this book to prepare

This book is divided into three parts:
- the clinical skills assessment section
- the case-based discussion section
- the concepts section

The **CSA section** will pose a typical CSA scenario.
- If further information, such as blood results or a hospital discharge summary, is needed for the consultation, this will be indicated as 'see Appendix at the end of the case.'
- Under **targeted history taking**, will provide a list of questions that could be asked to the patient to gather relevant data.

- Under **data gathering**, provides the information elicited from the patient if the relevant questions are asked. Question one from the targeted history gets answer one under data gathering.
- Under **targeted examination**, will provide a list of focussed examinations that could be performed to gather relevant data.
- Under **clinical management**, suggests ways in which a mutually agreed plan can be negotiated with the patient to produce a consultation that moves the patient forward towards a justifiable management of their presenting problem.
- Under **interpersonal skills**, provides positive indicators, or negative indicators, or both, of communication skills, ethical practice and/or professional conduct. Indicators of positive practice are provided most often, in line with current educational norms. Examples of negative indicators are provided only to illustrate the concept.
- Under **additional information**, provides some additional, usually theoretical information candidates may find useful to reach a deeper understanding of the issues dealt with in the case.
- The case usually concludes with signposting to the primary sources of information. The literature changes at a rapid pace, and web sources are usually a good source of updated information. Where possible, useful websites are listed.

The **case-based discussion** section is discussed in detail under the chapter *An introduction to case-based discussion* – see page 179.

The **concepts** section:

- explores the background knowledge and skills that are required for the interpersonal skills section of CSA in greater detail. The *Consultation models* chapter is particularly useful.
- discusses common themes that run through most questions within case-based discussions. The concepts chapters provide generic background information that could be useful when preparing for CbD.

Additional information

Grand'Maison P (1993) Canadian experience with structured clinical examinations. *Canadian Medical Association Journal*, **148**: 1573–1576.
This article describes the development and use of the structured clinical examination to assess medical students and graduates in Quebec over the past 25 years. Also described is the input from Canadian medical educators. The review of the Canadian experience discusses simulated-standardized patients, objective-structured clinical examinations and the use of such examinations for licensure and certification.

Malik S (2006) An OSCE actress. *BMJ Career Focus*, **332**: 110.
Ms Malik describes her experience as an OCSE actress, how she was briefed to play the case, and what examiners asked of her regarding the candidates. She also gives her tips on how candidates should prepare:

'I would suggest that if you can sense the acting patient is not happy with the situation then you should ask: "Is there anything I've said that is confusing or not clear or that you want explained again?' Another tip is to have a mental checklist of questions prepared and if you find yourself in an awkward situation, go back to where you left off in the list.'

Relevant literature

Simpson RG (2007) Preparing for practice: nMRCGP and the Clinical Skills Assessment. *Update,* **75**: 36–37.

Royal College of General Practitioners nMRCGP website – http://www.rcgp.org.uk/nmrcgp_/nmrcgp.aspx , particularly:

- http://www.rcgp.org.uk/nmrcgp_/nmrcgp/csa/csa_cases.aspx?theme=print for a document on CSA prepared by Hawthorne (May 2007)
- for the GP curriculum – the core statement: http://www.rcgp-curriculum.org.uk/PDF/curr_1_Curriculum_Statement_Being_a_GP.pdf
- for in-depth reading of learning outcomes for general practice: http://www.rcgp.org.uk/pdf/curriculum_Guide_for_Learners_and_Teachers .pdf

Case 1 – Back pain

Miss AT is a 25 year old woman who presents asking for a letter saying she needs a new chair at work. She gives an eight month history of intermittent back pain, but it has been worse in the last two months. In the last week, the back pain has been worse as the day progresses. She also complains of 'dead legs' which feel heavy and weak.

Targeted history taking

- What job does she do?
- Where is the pain? Elicit intensity, radiation, aggravating and relieving factors.
- Enquire about what she means by 'heavy and weak' legs, taking care to exclude nerve compression symptoms.
- Exclude cauda equine symptoms: perineal paraesthesia, bladder and bowel dysfunction.
- Does the pain disturb her sleep?
- What activities does the pain inhibit or limit?
- What treatments has she tried already?
- What are her expectations of this consultation: a note for the company, physiotherapy, a discussion on analgesia?
- What is her general health like – does she have asthma or indigestion?

Data gathering

Listed below is the additional information elicited from the patient with appropriate questioning.
- Allison works in telesales.
- Further questioning on 'heavy and weak legs' elicits a history of pain extending into the buttocks only, with no actual loss of power or altered sensation in the legs.
- The history sounds like mechanical back pain and there are no features to suggest more serious pathology.
- She is in good health, systemically well and sleep is undisturbed. She does not have morning stiffness.
- She lives alone in a 2nd floor flat and has to walk up the stairs with her shopping.
- She is active and does weekly tai chi.
- She has had one previous episode of back pain three years ago after back-packing. This improved with yoga and Pilates.
- She does not like tablets and prefers alternative medicines.

Targeted examination

- Expose the back – there is no scoliosis or kyphosis of the spine.
- She points to pain 'like a band' around her lower back.
- Palpation of spinous processes and paravertebral muscles does not elicit any tenderness.
- She is able to reach her lower shins but not her ankles. Extension and lateral flexion are not reduced. Watch her face during movements and when she moves about the room.
- Straight leg raising and femoral stretch tests are normal.

Clinical management

- Discuss the natural history and aetiology of mechanical back pain.
- Reassure the patient that the pain usually improves within six weeks. Unless her symptoms deteriorate within six weeks, further investigation such as imaging is not required.
- Address the patient's ideas: she may believe that her back is aggravated or provoked by her chair. You may be able to link this to a discussion on posture, and advise her on good posture.
- Encourage Miss AT to continue with tai chi provided it does not make her symptoms worse; encourage activity and avoid long periods of prolonged sitting at work.
- Address the patient's concerns and expectations: the issue here may not be the incorrect chair; it may be prolonged periods of sitting at work. Therefore, instead of a letter, perhaps she could consult her Occupational Health department or her Health and Safety officer to have a work-place assessment. A new chair may not be the whole answer – she made need reconfiguration of her workstation.
- Discuss whether she is happy to continue with posture exercises or whether she would like analgesia or a referral to physiotherapy.

Interpersonal skills

Good communication with the patient explores:
- her agenda (to improve her back pain)
- health beliefs (chair, posture, tai chi, etc.)
- preferences (natural remedies and advice of avoiding prolonged periods of sitting at work)

Therefore, it results in an agreed management plan.

Additional information

From: **Koes BW**, *et al.* (2006) Diagnosis and treatment of low back pain. *BMJ*, **332**: 1430–1434.

'Red flags'
- Onset age < 20 or > 55 years
- Non-mechanical pain (unrelated to time or activity)
- Thoracic pain
- Previous history of carcinoma, steroids, HIV
- Feeling unwell
- Weight loss
- Widespread neurological symptoms
- Structural spinal deformity

Indicators for nerve root problems
- Unilateral leg pain > low back pain
- Radiates to foot or toes
- Numbness and paraesthesia in same distribution
- Straight leg raising test induces more leg pain
- Localized neurology (limited to one nerve root)

Treatment
- Reassure patients (favourable prognosis)
- Advise patients to stay active
- Prescribe medication if necessary (preferably at fixed time intervals):
  - paracetamol
  - non-steroidal anti-inflammatory drugs
  - consider muscle relaxants or opioids
- Discourage bed rest
- Consider spinal manipulation for pain relief
- Do not advise back-specific exercises

Test your knowledge

Answer true (T) or false (F) for each of the following statements.
1. Back pain is the second commonest cause of long-term sickness absence
2. Straight leg raising (SLR) is a sensitive (0.88–1) and specific (0.84–0.95) test for diagnosing nerve root compression
3. Bilateral neurological symptoms and signs, saddle paraesthesia and urinary frequency are features of cauda equina syndrome
4. In L3/4 compression, the knee reflex may be impaired
5. In a patient >50 years, severe unremitting night pain which gets worse on standing is suggestive of cancer

Case 2 – Injectable contraception

Mrs HW is a 23 year old woman who presents saying that the practice nurse whom she saw yesterday advised her to see the doctor for her depo-provera to be prescribed. See Appendix for summary details.

Targeted history taking

- Why has the nurse referred her?
- Why is she late for her depo?
- Is she happy on the depo or is she experiencing side effects?
- Is she aware of alternative contraception, including long-acting contraception such as implants and IUDs?
- What are her expectations of this consultation: for the depo to be given or for contraception options to be discussed?
- Does she have risk factors for osteoporosis such as a past history of eating disorders (anorexia or bulimia), does she smoke, does she drink alcohol, does she have a family history of osteoporosis, does she have a balanced, calcium-rich diet and does she undertake regular weight-bearing exercise?
- If she smokes, has she considered stopping?
- What is her general health like – is she on medication, including over-the-counter medication such as St John's Wort, which could interact with hormonal contraception?
- What is her occupation and does it affect her choice of contraception?

Data gathering

Listed below is the additional information elicited from the patient with appropriate questioning:
- The nurse said she was too late for her (the nurse) to give the depo. It needed to be prescribed by a doctor.
- Mrs HW works as an air hostess for Virgin. She is late because she swapped shifts with a colleague and was in Australia when her depo was due.
- Over the last two years, she has not had difficulties with depo. She has been amenorrheic for 18 months and with her busy job, prefers not having periods.
- She had discussed implanon and IUDs with the practice nurse but a colleague had experienced irregular bleeding on implanon and her older sister had had an ectopic pregnancy with an IUD *in situ*. For the moment, she is happy on depo.
- She is willing to discuss the risks of an IUD with you and to read further on the Mirena IUS but for today, she would like to have the depo-provera injection please.

- She is in good health and is not taking any medication except for the occasional supermarket own-brand sleep aid, a herbal product.
- She does not have any risk factors for osteoporosis except she smokes 10 cigarettes a day. She is not ready to give up smoking just yet because she enjoys smoking and says it helps her cope with her busy schedule.
- She is active and runs 3 miles two or three times per week.
- She finds taking pills difficult with her current flying schedule.

Targeted examination

- Although not strictly necessary, it may be good practice to measure her blood pressure and weigh her.

Clinical management

- The Family Planning and NICE guidelines now advise that depo can be given up to 14 weeks since last administered, i.e. up to two weeks late.
- Mrs HW can be given depo today, without the need for a pregnancy test.
- She does not have to use extra precautions (condoms) if the depo is given today. In the unlikely event that she is pregnant, and depo is given, the hormone is not known to have any adverse, long-term effects on the fetus.
- Address the patient's ideas: Mrs HW may be happy with her amenorrhea without realising that the oestrogen suppression resulting in the amenorrhea is also responsible for a transient decrease in her bone mass density. There is little evidence to suggest that she needs to have bone scans or oestrodiol blood levels measured as it is extremely likely that her bone mass will increase once her periods restart.
- Address the patient's expectations: she expects to be given the depo today and it can be given. However, she needs to be aware that there is an extremely small chance that she could be pregnant – would she be happy to take the risk of having hormones knowing that this small chance of pregnancy existed?
- Discuss whether she would like to know about alternative methods of contraception. At this later consultation, you could address her ideas on implants and IUDs in greater detail. Perhaps, instead of relying on anecdotal evidence alone, she could read the Family Planning leaflets or website, and come back in a week or two to discuss alternatives either with yourself or one of the family planning-trained practice nurses.
- Mention local initiatives (such as the practice's smoking cessation clinic) and advise her to make an appointment to discuss options once she has a firm intention to quit.

Interpersonal skills

Good communication with the patient:
- explores her agenda and preferences (getting the depo today)

- explores her health beliefs (amenorrhea is a good thing)
- communicates the risks and benefits of depo in simple language, enabling the patient to weigh the information and come to a decision that suits her best

Therefore, the doctor's inclusive and cooperative approach results in a management decision that enhances the patient's autonomy.

Additional information

NICE (2005) Long-acting reversible contraception. See: http://www.nice.org.uk/CG030.
- Women attending up to 2 weeks late for repeat injection of DMPA may be given the injection without the need for additional contraceptives.
- Women who wish to continue DMPA use beyond 2 years should have their individual clinical situations reviewed, the balance between the benefits and potential risks discussed, and be supported in their choice of whether or not to continue.
- Healthcare professionals should be aware that if pregnancy occurs during DMPA use there is no evidence of congenital malformation to the fetus.
- Because of the possible effect on bone mineral density, care should be taken in recommending DMPA to adolescents, but it may be given if other methods are not suitable or acceptable.
- Injectable contraceptives are more cost effective than the combined oral contraceptive pill even at 1 year of use.

Appendix: Patient summary

Name	HW
Date of birth (Age)	23
Social and Family History	Married, one child
Past medical history	TOP, age 18
Current medication	Depo-provera – last issued 13 weeks ago
Values screen	Done 13 months ago
Height	167 cm
Weight	75 kg
BP	106/67

Notes from nurse consultation yesterday

Mrs HW has used depo-provera contraception since the birth of her son 2 years ago. Unfortunately, she presents to me at 13 weeks and according to the nurse protocols, she is too late for the depo to be given. Appointment made with doctor: '*Thank you for seeing Mrs HW who is happy on depo. Unfortunately, she is too late to me to administer depo, as per practice protocols. If you are happy to prescribe the depo, I will give the patient the injection directly after your consultation.*'

Test your knowledge

Answer true (T) or false (F) for each of the following statements.
1. In patients with sickle-cell disease, depo-provera (DMPA) reduces the number of crises
2. At 12 months, 75% of women on DMPA are amenorrheic
3. If concerned about prolonged amenorrhea in long-term DMPA users, bone densitometry should be reserved for women with low serum estradiol
4. The efficacy of DMPA is not affected by enzyme-inducers
5. If erratic bleeding develops on DMPA, one option is to give a second injection of DMPA early, that is, between 4 and 12 weeks after the initial dose

Case 3 – Blacked out

Ms KL is a 26 year old lady. She presents today informing you that she 'blacked out' at a friend's house 2 days ago and that her friend says she 'twitched a bit'. She is frightened because she has never had anything like this happen to her before and also because she is getting married in 5 months and does not want a medical problem hanging over her. See Appendix for further details.

Targeted history taking

- Clarify what she means by 'blacked out'.
- Clarify the circumstances – had she been standing a long time, dehydrated or hungry, hot or anxious?
- Any symptoms suggesting a cardiac cause?
- Was she exercising?
- What are her memories immediately preceding the event? Look for symptoms suggesting a vasovagal faint, any cardiac symptoms, an aura or déjà vu suggesting a seizure.
- Clarify what her friend meant by twitching. Was this a rhythmic sustained jerking suggesting a seizure or the isolated twitching and jerking often seen if a patient does not fall flat to the ground after a vasovagal attack?
- Did her friend mention what colour she was? Was she pale or cyanosed?
- What can she remember when she came round? Is Ms KL describing a post-ictal state?
- Had she been incontinent or bitten her tongue?
- Enquire about her physical health and whether she has any other symptoms.
- Could she be pregnant?
- Any relevant past history? Any other 'funny turns'?
- Does she drive? Does she work?
- Does she smoke? Is she drinking more alcohol or smoking more than previously?
- What does she hope to gain from this consultation – an examination, an explanation, reassurance, or further investigation?

Data gathering

Listed below is the additional information elicited from the patient with appropriate questioning.
- She had been shopping with her friend most of the day looking at bridal dresses. They had only just arrived back at her friend's flat and, as they had missed lunch, her friend was making them a mug of tea.
- They were standing talking in the kitchen when Ms KL suddenly felt hot and dizzy. She remembers that her friend's voice sounded very distant.

- She had no palpitations, chest pain or dyspnoea.
- She then remembers coming round on the floor with her friend talking to her. She felt sick and clammy.
- Her friend helped her to the bedroom and she lay down on the bed, but soon felt fine and got up.
- She had not been incontinent but had bitten the tip of her tongue.
- Her friend told her that she noticed she was going very pale and then she slid down the wall and sat slumped on the floor. Her head and arms twitched and jerked a few times. Her friend laid her flat and she came round in a few seconds.
- She has felt well recently.
- She has never had anything like this before and has had no serious illnesses in the past.
- She likes to keep fit and has been going to the gym more frequently to try and tone up for her wedding.
- She smoke 10 cigarettes a day and drinks at weekends.
- Her period is due. She has not forgotten to take her contraceptive pill.
- She drives. She works in a local building society.

Targeted examination

- You should perform a targeted examination looking for signs of cardiac disease and a brief neurological examination.
- Check pulse, heart sounds and BP lying and standing.
- Cranial nerves, fundi and reflexes.
- *In this case examination is entirely normal.*

Clinical management

- Discuss examination findings.
- Reassure Ms KL that although the episode was very frightening, she is likely to have had a vasovagal faint.
- Discuss natural history of condition.
- Discuss possible contributing factors.
- Address patient's concerns: consider investigations – FBC, U&Es and glucose. Consider whether a pregnancy test is indicated.
- Arrange for Ms KL to have an ECG (NICE guidelines).
- Discuss what to do if she has any other 'funny turns'.

Interpersonal skills

Good communication skills are essential to:
- get a clear description of the event
- give Ms KL a clear understandable explanation
- reassure Ms KL that more serious causes of collapse are unlikely

You are able to reassure and gain Ms KL's trust by:
- a careful history
- a focussed examination
- agreeing a shared management plan including whether blood tests are to be performed
- discussing what to do if she has another attack

This is a common dilemma in primary care. A careful history is essential here. The examination is to exclude cardiac causes and to reassure the patient that you have taken her symptoms seriously. An ECG should be arranged, but other investigations are unlikely to be abnormal and again are done largely to reassure the patient.

Additional information

Stone J, *et al*. (2005) Systematic review of misdiagnosis of conversion symptoms and "hysteria". *BMJ*, **331**: 989.
- Some patients in whom a diagnosis of "conversion" symptoms later turn out to have a disease explaining their unexplained paralysis, seizures, or sensory symptoms – 4% misdiagnosis rate.
- Many of the rediagnosed conditions such as epilepsy and movement disorders rely predominantly on a clinical diagnosis.
- Up to a quarter of patients with epilepsy have other conditions, most commonly syncope.
- In one study, 8% of patients with a diagnosis of multiple sclerosis were later found to have conversion disorder, illustrating that misdiagnosis can also happen in the opposite direction.

Bergfeldt L. (2003) Differential diagnosis of cardiogenic syncope and seizure disorders. *Heart*, **89**: 353–358.

Syncope is a symptom, defined as a transient, self-limited loss of consciousness with a relatively rapid onset and usually leading to falling; the subsequent recovery is spontaneous, complete, and usually prompt. The underlying mechanism is a transient global cerebral hypoperfusion. Involuntary movements, often referred to as myoclonic jerks, may accompany syncope due to cardiovascular causes.

Seizure is synonymous with *an epileptic fit*, which is the manifestation of a paroxysmal discharge of abnormal rhythms in some part of the brain. A diagnosis of epilepsy may lead to significant psychosocial consequences – delaying the diagnosis probably results in a lot less harm than making a false positive diagnosis.

Relevant literature

NICE (2004) The epilepsies: the diagnosis and management of the epilepsies in adults and children in primary and secondary care. See: http://guidance.nice.org.uk/CG20/niceguidance/pdf/English.

Appendix: Patient summary

Name	KL
Date of birth (Age)	26
Social and Family History	Single
Past medical history	TOP 4 years ago
Recent reports	None
Current medication	Microgynon
Investigations	None

Test your knowledge

Please fill in the missing words.

A patient is said to have status epilepticus if more than one seizure occurs without regaining (1) ...., or if the fitting continues for over (2) .... minutes. If the patient fits for more than five minutes, give (3) .... mg of diazepam rectally. Although unlicensed, buccal (4) .... may be used within a locally agreed protocol. A third option is intravenous (5) .... but this drug needs to be kept refrigerated.

Case 4 – Menorrhagia

Mrs AB is a 45 year old woman who presents asking for advice on whether she should proceed with her gynaecological surgery for menorrhagia. She has not had any vaginal (PV) bleeding for the last seven weeks. Despite attending the gynaecology outpatients department (OPD) two weeks ago, there is no outpatient letter in her notes as yet. See Appendix for details

Targeted history taking

- What did the gynaecology consultant advise at the time of her appointment? Why did he/she advise this?
- Is there any reason for the seven weeks of amenorrhea – was she given any medication or has she been on hormone tablets?
- What are her concerns regarding the seven weeks of amenorrhea?
- What job does she do and is this affected by her current symptoms?
- Does she have any ideas regarding her treatment options and what are her preferences? What treatments has she tried already or what treatments is she not keen on?
- What are her expectations of this consultation: advice on the surgery, reassurance regarding the safety of the surgery, a discussion on alternative treatment options?
- Is she using contraception?
- What is her general health like – does she suffer from migraines, gallstones or does she have a past history of DVT?
- Does she have a family history of early menopause, breast/gynaecological cancer, or cardiac disease?

Data gathering

Listed below is the additional information elicited from the patient with appropriate questioning.
- Mrs AB is a first year, mature student nurse. She appears to be exploring her treatment options and wants to gain an understanding of what is happening to her. She does not appear to be anxious or depressed.
- The gynaecology consultant said that the pelvic ultrasound showed a polyp, which he was unsuccessful in removing in the OPD. Hence, she was listed for an endometrial resection under GA. Mrs AB is not keen on having a GA but will have the operation if it is really needed.
- Since the birth of her son six years ago, she has had heavy periods. Initially, the time between the periods was shorter (21 days) but over the last two years, her cycle has been more erratic with the time between periods anything

from 21 to 35 days. This is the first time she has not had a period for seven weeks.

- She is experiencing flushing, sometimes up to three times each day. She feels very warm at night and her sleep is interrupted. She experiences mood swings with periodic low moods. Trivial events at work and at home upset her. Once upset, she is tearful and sensitive for the entire day and can't shake it off. Usually, she is slightly anxious about things – doing well with her studies, juggling home life with her new studies, but she enjoys these challenges. Her family is very supportive but concerned about her mood swings. There have not been any specific problems at home or work as yet.
- The proposed scheduling of the operation would not cause problems at home or work.
- She does not think that she is pregnant; she uses barrier contraception and is careful.
- Mrs AB does not want a Mirena IUS; this was discussed with her usual GP and the gynaecology consultant. She wants your advice on the endometrial resection – she thinks she is peri-menopausal and if her periods are stopping, should she go ahead with the surgery?
- She also wants some advice on treatments for the menopause. She says she prefers natural remedies but would like to read about HRT in greater detail.
- Mrs AB is in good general health; uses condoms reliably and is not on long-term medication. She does not have a history of gall-stones, migraines or DVT.
- She does not have a significant family history.

Targeted examination

- Does Mrs AB appear to be tearful, anxious, or depressed? Unless her demeanour and interaction suggest an underlying mood disorder, a formal mental state examination may not be needed.

Clinical management

- Address the patient's ideas – that seven weeks of amenorrhea may mean that she is unlikely to get further heavy bleeding, and her concern that the operation may now be redundant.
- Fulfil her expectations for advice: give advice about the polyp.
- Despite the seven week history of amenorrhea, histological evaluation of the polyp is needed, either by endometrial resection or by hysteroscopy.
- Regarding the endometrial section, you could say that this procedure is both diagnostic (the entire endometrium is available for histological evaluation) and therapeutic (as a treatment for menorrhagia).
- In contrast, hysteroscopy with endometrial biopsy would be diagnostic only.
- An IUS can be inserted at the time of endometrial resection or hysteroscopy: this treats the menorrhagia and also gives endometrial protection if

oestrogen-only HRT is used. Oestrogen-only HRT may have a lower risk of breast cancer than oral combination HRT.

- Address subsidiary concerns (about the menopause) and expectations (advice about the risks and benefits of HRT).
- If, based on her personal and family history, Mrs AB reported any significant contra-indications to HRT, you could advise her of this and not pursue the HRT option any further. Since she does not, you could now signpost her to good sources of information on HRT, such as www.besttreatments. co.uk/btuk/conditions/5295.html.

Interpersonal skills

Good communication with the patient:
- demonstrates a respect for her curiosity as a nursing student
- demonstrates a respect for the limitations of hospital systems within which consultant colleagues work. It would be easy to make disparaging comments about the relative lateness of the discharge letter.
- shows responsiveness to the patient's preferences, feelings and expectations for further information on surgery and HRT
- communicates the relevant information in a manner that is understandable to the patient, without slipping into jargon and without patronizing the patient

Therefore, it results in addressing the patient's expectations appropriately.

Additional information

Pitkin J. (2007) Dysfunctional uterine bleeding. *BMJ*, **334**: 1110–1111.
- Irregular heavy bleeding in women in their late 40s is often attributed to starting the menopause, but still needs investigation. Endometrial carcinoma can occur in the late 40s. About 6% of endometrial cancers can occur with heavy regular bleeds.
- Confirm that menorrhagia has been present for several menstrual cycles.
- **Investigation:** a full blood count is needed; endocrine investigations such as thyroid function tests are not routinely necessary. An endometrial biopsy is not required in the initial assessment of menorrhagia.
- **Treatment:** tranexamic acid and mefenamic acid are effective treatments for reducing heavy menstrual blood loss, even in women who have an intrauterine contraceptive device *in situ*. Combined oral contraceptives, a progestogen-releasing intrauterine device, or other long-acting progestogens can reduce menstrual blood loss.

Appendix: New patient summary

Name	AB
Date of birth (Age)	45
Social and Family History	Married, three children
Past medical history	Post-natal depression twelve years ago
Current medication	Mefenamic acid as required
	Ferrous sulphate 1 to 2 tablets twice daily
Blood tests	Blood tests done eight months ago
Hb	10.9g% (13–17)
MCV	86 (83–105)
BMI	25.6
BP	117/60
cervical smear	normal

Test your knowledge

Please fill in the missing words, choosing from the list below. Some words may be used more than once, others not at all.

danazol	NSAIDs	combined oral contraception
anti-fibrinolytics	progestogens	progestogen-containing IUD

The most effective non-surgical treatment for menorrhagia is (1) …………..
(2) …………., such as tranexamic acid 1g qds, can reduce bleeding by up to 70%.
(3) …………. can also reduce bleeding by 30 to 70%, however, use is limited by side-effects such as acne, oedema and irreversible voice changes, hence, it is not recommended by NICE. (4) …………. and (5) …………. (the latter is also useful for dysmenorrhea), should be commenced on day one of the cycle and used until heavy blood loss stops.

Case 5 – Knee injury

TR is the 17 year old son of a local dentist and attends with his mother. He attends a boarding school and limps into your surgery with his mother and informs you that he hurt his knee playing squash a week ago. His knee feels funny and has 'stuck' a couple of times. See Appendix for details.

Targeted history taking

- Clarify the mechanism of injury.
- Where did TR feel pain initially? Has the pain changed or moved?
- Has his knee been swollen? If so, when did the swelling appear and how long did it remain swollen?
- What does he mean when he says he knee has 'stuck'? Is he describing locking? Has his knee given way?
- Has he had any bruising around the knee?
- What is his knee function like at present? How far can he walk? Does pain disturb sleep?
- Any previous problems with his knee? Any other lower limb or back problems?
- What sports does he play and at what level?
- What has he done or tried to help the situation?
- What does he hope to gain from this consultation – an examination, further investigation, or referral to hospital?

Data gathering

Listed below is the additional information elicited from the patient with appropriate questioning.

- He lunged to make a shot, twisting his knee under him so that he landed on his left side.
- He felt pain around the medial side of his knee immediately and it has remained in the same place. He describes his pain as a constant ache deep inside his knee. It disturbs his sleep when he rolls over in bed. His pain is worse when he turns round or twists his knee.
- He was not aware of any swelling in his knee immediately, but by the time he was back home his knee looked a bit swollen. The swelling has gone down, but he thinks it is a bit puffy still.
- When he tries to get up, his knee sometimes hurts and he cannot straighten it. However, if he bends his knee a couple of times it seems to clear and he is then able to straighten it. He has noticed this happens sometimes when he rolls over in bed or if he turns round quickly. He has had no giving way.
- He was not bruised.

- He has had no major injuries in the past and his general health is excellent.
- He plays in his school's second team in rugby, hockey and cricket. He is very worried that he has done some serious damage to his knee and will be unable to get into the first teams next year, his last at school.
- Apart from an ice pack initially and then resting his knee, he has had no treatment. If any treatment were necessary they would prefer to be seen privately as they have private health insurance.

Targeted examination

- A targeted examination of TR's knee should be performed.
- He should be informed that it will be necessary to remove his trousers. If he is not wearing shorts, you should consider asking whether he is happy for his mother to see him in his underwear or whether he would like to be examined with her not present.
- Examination of his knee should specifically look for:
  - the presence of an effusion
  - any bruising around the knee
  - range of movement – is there any loss of full flexion or extension suggesting a block?
  - any problems with patella – position/alignment, tenderness, crepitus?
  - any laxity of collateral ligaments or cruciates
  - joint line tenderness, bony tenderness around the knee or patella
  - abnormal meniscal test, if he will tolerate this
- Gait – *in this case – he is limping, he has a small effusion, no ligamentous laxity, tender medial joint line and he is unable to tolerate a McMurray test due to pain.*

Clinical management

- Discuss the likely diagnosis from the history and examination.
- Discuss natural history of condition.
- Confirm that referral is indicated, and so he will need to see an orthopaedic surgeon.
- Confirm that they would like a private referral.
- Discuss his fears including recovery and future sporting capacity.

Interpersonal skills

Good communication skills enabled:
- clear history to be obtained
- reassurance following a focussed examination
- exploration of his fears and sporting expectations
- patient's agenda to be explored: private referral
- sensitive treatment of the confidentiality issue

Relevant literature

For an excellent website detailing the examination of the knee, with video-clips, see http://medicine.ucsd.edu/clinicalmed/Joints.html.

Appendix: Patient summary

Name	TR
Date of birth (Age)	17
Social and Family History	Schoolboy
Past medical history	Not available
Recent reports	Not registered with your practice
Current medication	Not available
Investigations	No information

Test your knowledge

Answer true (T) or false (F) for each of the following statements.
1. The 'Ottawa Knee Rule' states that an X-ray should be performed if the patient has tenderness at the head of the fibula
2. The 'Ottawa Knee Rule' states that an X-ray should be performed if, after the knee injury, the patient is unable to take four steps on each leg
3. Breast-stroke swimming and exercise-bike cycling should be avoided in patients with patello-femoral pain as these activities can provoke anterior knee pain
4. The 'Ottawa Ankle Rule' is better at eliminating patients who do not need an X-ray (high specificity) than identifying those who have a fracture (low sensitivity)
5. Refer patients with a suspected acute rupture of the Achilles as an emergency, ideally to be seen within 24 hours

Case 6 – Pins and needles in hands

Mrs PL is a 58 year old who consults you complaining of intermittent pain and pins and needles in her hands. See Appendix for further information on this patient.

Targeted history taking

- Where does she experience the pain and pins and needles?
- When does she experience the symptoms?
- For how long has she experienced these symptoms?
- Enquire about her physical health and whether she has any other symptoms. Specifically – any symptoms of thyroid disease, diabetes or arthritis. Check what medication she is taking – paraesthesia side effects (e.g. phenytoin) or Raynaud's (e.g. beta-blockers).
- Any history of injuries or neck problems?
- Enquire about work and leisure activities – any repetitive gripping, squeezing, vibration, keyboard use, racket sports?
- Does she smoke or drink?
- What has she done or tried to help the situation?
- What are her expectations of this consultation– an explanation, medication, further investigation, treatment or referral?

Data gathering

Listed below is the additional information elicited from the patient with appropriate questioning.

- She gets tingling in her thumb and index finger, and a vague ache in the hand, extending up into the forearm.
- She gets this intermittently during the day, but it is particularly troublesome at night – she has been woken up most nights by it in the past month.
- She has been getting this for the past 8 months, but it has got a lot worse in the past month.
- She feels well. She is unable to lose weight, feels the cold and feels that she has slowed up.
- She has no history of trauma or injuries. She has no neck pain.
- She gave up smoking 10 years ago and rarely drinks.
- She has tried some herbal water retention tablets from the supermarket but they did not seem to help.
- She would like a diagnosis and some tablets to get rid of the problem.

Targeted examination

- General assessment:
  - evidence of obesity
  - systemic disease – RA
  - evidence of hypothyroidism
  - check urine if any suggestion of diabetes mellitus
- Examine her cervical spine:
  - flexion
  - extension
  - rotation to left and right
  - side flexion to left and right
- Examine her elbow:
  - flexion
  - extension
  - pronation and supination
- Examine her wrists:
  - swelling
  - palmar and dorsi flexion
  - radial and ulnar deviation
- Examine her hands:
  - wasting of thenar muscles, check power of thumb abductors
  - check sensation in median nerve distribution in hand
  - slide finger across palm noting any increase in resistance (from lack of sweating) and temperature rise (vasodilatation)
- Special tests:
  - Tinel
  - Phalen
- *In this case examination of Mrs PL reveals an overweight lady with dry skin. She has reduced wrist palmar flexion, some wasting of the thenar muscles, and positive Tinel and Phalen signs:* (see photographs over the page).

Clinical management

- Discuss examination findings – she appears to have Carpal Tunnel Syndrome (CTS) and some suggestion of hypothyroidism.
- Discuss natural history of these conditions – hypothyroidism is associated with CTS and she may need to have an operation, especially as there is evidence of muscle wasting.
- Address patient's expectations – Mrs PL may need tests to confirm the CTS (e.g. electrophysiology) before the condition can be treated, and hence her symptoms relieved; she will need blood tests to see if she has hypothyroidism; and she would like tablets to treat her symptoms.
- Explore Mrs PL's feelings about having an operation.

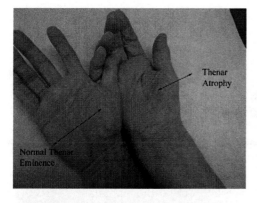

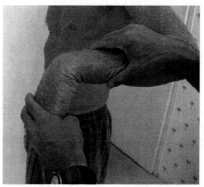

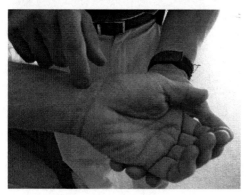

Top left: thenar atrophy;
top right: Phelan test;
bottom: Tinel test.

- Agree management plan which may incorporate:
  - weight loss
  - avoiding prolonged periods of time with wrist flexed or extended
  - wrist splint
  - corticosteroid injection
  - investigation prior to surgery
  - tests for hypothyroidism

Interpersonal skills

Good communication with the patient:
- enables clarification of symptoms and identification of two possible co-existent diagnoses
- reassures patient following a focussed examination
- reassures patient that she has two treatable conditions, even though one (hypothyroidism) was unexpected
- explores patient's agenda: her desire for diagnosis and drug treatment
- explores patient's health beliefs: tablets will get rid of her symptoms
- safety-net: what she can do to help her symptoms and when she should return to you for review of blood test results

Additional information

Atroshi I, *et al.* (2006) Outcomes of endoscopic surgery compared with open surgery for carpal tunnel syndrome among employed patients: randomised controlled trial. *BMJ*, **332**: 1473.

- CTS is a common medical cause of work absence; nearly half of all cases have an annual work absence of more than 30 days.
- Surgery is often required.
- Open and endoscopic surgery are equally effective in relieving symptoms.
- Endoscopic surgery is associated with slightly less pain than open surgery up to three months after operation.
- The cost benefits of endoscopic surgery are uncertain due to the marginal differences.

Relevant literature

See also related *BMJ* editorial:
Graham B. (2006) The diagnosis and treatment of carpal tunnel syndrome. *BMJ*, **332**: 1463–1464.
For patient information on hypothyroidism, see:
   British Thyroid Foundation (www.btf-thyroid.org/).
The following US site has extensive information: http://www.thyroid.about.com/.
For a detailed description and video clips on how to perform a physical examination for CTS, see: http://medicine.ucsd.edu/clinicalmed/Joints3.html.

Appendix: Patient summary

Name	PL
Date of birth (Age)	58
Social and Family History	Married, 3 children. Housewife.
Past medical history	Laparoscopic cholecystectomy 13 years ago
	Asthma
	Stress incontinence 5 years ago – responded to physiotherapy
Recent reports	Healthcheck 1 year ago – see investigations below
Current medication	None
Investigations	1 year ago:
BMI	33.2
BP	134/86
Urine	NAD

Test your knowledge

Please fill in the missing words, choosing from the list below. Each word may be used more than once.

sixty   abductor pollicis longus   ninety
abductor pollicis brevis   median   ulna
radial

The (1) .... nerve innervates opponens pollicis and (2) .... Shaking of the hand to alleviate symptoms (the 'flick test) is reported to have a sensitivity and specificity of (3) .... %. To perform Phalen's test, flex the wrist for (4) .... seconds and check if pain or paraesthesiae occur in the palmar aspect of the (5) .... 3½ digits. To elicit Tinel's sign, tap lightly over the (6) .... nerve at the wrist.

Case 7 – Smoking cessation

Mr DB is a 22 year old man who presents saying the nurse asked him to see you for advice about stopping smoking; he hadn't come back to his smoking cessation/nicotine replacement therapy (NRT) appointment with her three months ago.

Targeted history taking

- Why did he not continue with his NRT programme?
- How much does he smoke and under what circumstances?
- At what age did he start smoking?
- Do any others at home or at work smoke?
- What is motivating him to stop smoking?
- Did he have any problems with the NRT?
- What treatments, besides NRT, has he tried already?
- Is he aware of treatments other than NRT to help him stop smoking?
- Does he have any other health problems – obesity, diabetes, hypertension, hypercholesterolaemia?
- What are his expectations of this consultation: a further script for NRT, signposting to other smoking cessation services locally, advice?

Data gathering

Listed below is the additional information elicited from the patient with appropriate questioning.

- He was unable to see the practice nurse for further patches because he had to attend his grandmother's funeral in Cardiff. He was upset after her death and was not in the right frame of mind to continue with his smoking cessation programme. However, she died of COPD and he now feels motivated to try again.
- He smokes between 15 and 20 cigarettes per day. When he is very busy, he smokes much less. At work and when socialising with friends, he smokes every 30 to 60 minutes.
- He started smoking at age 14, and puts this down to peer pressure.
- Both his parents smoke, but his girlfriend, with whom he shares a flat, is a non-smoker and he has to go outside to smoke.
- He wants to stop smoking because his girlfriend hates it and because his grandmother died of smoking-related lung disease.
- He had some strange dreams on the patches but this might be due to worrying about his grandmother who was in hospital at the time.
- He bought over-the-counter gum but hated the taste of it and it didn't help.
- He has thought about hypnotherapy. His girlfriend had hypnotherapy for flying phobia but his friends think it is a waste of money for smokers.

- He has no other medical problems.
- He would like a script for NRT patches and wants to know your opinion on hypnotherapy for smoking cessation.

Targeted examination

As he does not have a significant history of co-morbidity, an examination is not necessary.

Clinical management

- Explain that the practice nurse was correct to refer him to see a doctor as current guidance from NICE says that if an attempt to stop smoking is unsuccessful, the NHS should not normally fund a further attempt within six months.
- However, despite the NICE guidance, you believe him to be motivated and committed and feel that it is appropriate to fund a further attempt.
- You briefly outline his treatment options and discuss his preferences: NRT (patches, gums, inhalators, nasal spray, lozenges, micro-tabs), bupropion (Zyban), varenicline (Champix) or alternative therapies (hypnotherapy and acupuncture). Be prepared to discuss the advantages and disadvantages of these different methods.
- In answer to his query about hypnotherapy, you could say that while some people find it helpful, there is no hard scientific evidence, so it is difficult to quote success rates. The NHS does not fund hypnotherapy.
- Alternative therapies may be of use to boost people's confidence and help them relax while quitting.
- When he indicates his preference for patches, you should discuss whether his dreams were related to the patches and consider whether he should start on lower strength patches (14 mg) or remove the higher dose patches at bedtime.

Interpersonal skills

Good communication with the patient:
- explores his agenda (giving up smoking to keep his girlfriend happy and to improve his long term health)
- explores and supports his health beliefs (that smoking is damaging to your health, and that alternative therapies may help)
- explores and assesses his motivation by paying close attention to his verbal and non-verbal cues
- explores his preferences (NHS-funded NRT)

By being flexible in interpretation of the NICE guidance and current NHS funding constraints, the doctor shows responsiveness to the patient's preferences and demonstrates his commitment to working in partnership with the patient.

Additional information

Aveyard P, West R. (2007) Managing smoking cessation. *BMJ*, **335**: 37–41.

- 78 attempts at smoking cessation per 100 smokers per year occur in the UK, with many smokers making several attempts in a year.
- Only 2–3% actually stop permanently each year. The most important factor leading to failure of attempts to stop is nicotine dependence.
- Effective treatments include varenicline, bupropion, nortriptyline, and nicotine replacement.
- What doctors say and do about smoking in consultations influences their patients, especially if they adopt a patient-centred approach, which is to ask the patient about their smoking, acknowledging that they may have tried to stop many times in the past, and discuss the options that exist to support a quit attempt.
- Varenicline is a newly licensed partial agonist acting on the $\alpha_4\beta_2$ nicotinic receptor. Studies show that varenicline is both more effective than placebo and probably more effective than nicotine replacement, but further comparative studies are needed.

Test your knowledge

- **A** Nicotinell patch (21 mg/24 hours patch) daily for two to three weeks
- **B** Bupropion (150 mg once a day) for 6 days, increasing to 150 mg twice a day, prescribed to last 3–4 weeks after the quit date
- **C** Nicotinell patch (14 mg/24 hours patch) daily prescribed to be able to last until 2 weeks after the quit date
- **D** NRT gum: chew one piece of 4 mg gum slowly for about 30 minutes when there is an urge to smoke; reduce gradually over 3 months; when daily use is 1–2 pieces of gum, stop
- **E** Nicotinell patch (14 mg/16 hours patch) daily for two weeks
- **F** NRT gum: chew one piece of 6 mg gum slowly for about 30 minutes when there is an urge to smoke; reduce gradually over 3 months; when daily use is 1–2 pieces of gum, stop
- **G** Bupropion (150 mg once a day) for one week, increasing to 150 mg twice a day for the next three weeks.

Regarding smoking cessation advice, for each patient described below select the single most appropriate advice using options A–G above. Each option may be used once, more than once, or not at all.

1. A 30 year old woman, currently breastfeeding, saw the local smoking cessation advisor for help. She currently smokes 10–15 cigarettes per day. Her quit day is the day after next.
2. A 35 year old man wishes to use NRT gum to help him kick his 30 per day habit. You advise him to …

3. A 42 year old woman, with a past history of bulimia, wishes to give up her 20–25 cigarettes per day habit. She does not wish to use NRT gum. An appropriate prescription may be …

4. A 55 year old ex-professional boxer developed local skin irritation when he used NRT patches two years ago. He tried over the counter NRT gum but does not like the taste. He would like to give up his smoking habit of 15 cigarettes per day. His medication includes cocodamol and ibuprofen for intermittent lower back pain.

5. A 19 year old girl requests Zyban. Provided there are no contra-indications, an appropriate prescription may be …

Case 8 – Termination of pregnancy

Mrs EJ is a 23 year old woman who presents requesting a termination of pregnancy (TOP). She has recently registered at your practice and her old notes have not yet arrived.

Targeted history taking

- How does she know she is pregnant?
- Has she experienced failure of her regular contraception?
- When was her last menstrual period (LMP)? Are her periods usually regular?
- What are home circumstances like at the moment?
- On what grounds does she want a termination?
- Has she considered the options?
- How does her husband feel about her TOP request?
- Would having a termination impact on her home and work situation?
- Has she had a TOP before?
- What are her expectations of this consultation: a confirmation of her suspicions that she may be pregnant, a referral to the TOP service, advice on her options, or contraception advice for the future?
- Does she have any general health problems, or is she on any medication that would make surgical or medical TOP unsafe?
- What does she already know about TOPs?
- If there any logistical difficulties in arranging a TOP with the local hospital, could she travel further to an out-sourced TOP service, such as Marie Stopes?

Data gathering

Listed below is the additional information elicited from the patient with appropriate questioning.

- Mrs EJ did two home pregnancy tests, once last week when her period was a few days late and one yesterday. Both were positive.
- She thinks that she missed taking a few microgynon pills at the time of her recent house move.
- Based on the dates she gives you, you calculate that she is five weeks pregnant. Her periods are usually very regular.
- Things at home have been hectic: she recently moved to the area from Chepstow when her husband's army unit was posted locally. Her husband is a 21 year old soldier and he has left, at short notice, on an overseas deployment two weeks ago. He is due back in two months.
- She telephoned her husband and they both agree that they would currently find looking after another baby emotionally and financially difficult. Her

husband got into debt with internet gambling, for which he sought help from the Army social services. He and Mrs EJ have been advised on a financial plan.

- She does not think that giving the baby up for adoption is a consideration and is adamant that she wants a TOP.
- Given her current financial difficulties, she is worried about taking time off work from her new job. She started working part-time in a supermarket last week and is still in the probation period. If she has to be admitted to hospital, she doesn't know how she will tell her manager and how she will pay for child-care. Her children are in nursery, using the nursery voucher scheme, while she works her Wednesday morning shift.
- She had not had a TOP before nor has she spoken to anyone about the procedure.
- She is in good health. Her two pregnancies were uneventful. Except for microgynon, she is not on medication.
- She believes she will need an operation under GA and may need up to two weeks to recover.
- Travelling to an out-sourced centre would be difficult because of child-care arrangements. Her family live in Northern Ireland. She has not yet made friends locally. She does not want to tell anybody about her decision to have a TOP.

Targeted examination

- Based on her LMP, calculate the date of her pregnancy.
- Once you establish from your history that she definitely wants a referral for a TOP, you may want to provide a BP reading in your referral reading.
- If she looks obese, you may want to weigh and measure her, to provide a BMI measurement in the referral letter.

Clinical management

- Address the patient's ideas: she believes that she needs a TOP, which she understands to be an operation under GA with a two-week convalescence. Speak to her about medical TOPs. Explain how the local TOP services are organized.
- Mrs EJ has two specific concerns: arranging time off from work and paying for additional child-care.
- You may advise Mrs EJ to tell her employers that she is having a one-off, emergency treatment – this may help to allay their possible concerns about sickness absence. You could offer to provide a sick note, if the hospital does not provide one, if she feels unable to return to work within a week of her TOP. What is written on the sick note could be carefully worded so as not to break her confidentiality. If Mrs EJ does not want to take sickness absence, she could try swapping shifts with a colleague to free up some time around the date of her hospital appointment.

- It may be better to defer the discussion on child-care arrangements until firm dates for the TOP are in place.
- Address Mrs EJ's expectations: she expects a referral to the hospital for a TOP. If the doctor feels unable to personally refer the patient for a TOP because of his or her own personal beliefs, then the doctor should explain this to the patient and make alternative arrangements for the patient's timely referral. It is reasonable to assume that Mrs EJ also expects to be treated with sensitivity and kindness, and for her confidentiality to be respected.

Interpersonal skills

Good communication with the patient explores the impact of her unwanted pregnancy on her life. This enables the doctor to obtain information about her social circumstances and helps the doctor to contextualise the problem. A willingness to listen and understand may prevent the doctor from allowing his own views, values or prejudices to inappropriately influence the patient's decision-making. Therefore, by showing responsiveness to the patient's preferences, feelings and expectations, the doctor and patient work in partnership to develop a shared management plan.

Additional information

Savulescu J. (2006) Conscientious objection in medicine. *BMJ*, **332**: 294–297.
The author writes, 'A doctors' conscience has little place in the delivery of modern medical care… If people are not prepared to offer legally permitted, efficient, and beneficial care to a patient because it conflicts with their values, they should not be doctors.'

Savulescu argues that a service which depends on the values of the treating doctor, results in patients shopping among doctors to receive services to which they are entitled. This introduces inefficiency and wastes resources. The less informed patients may fail to receive a service to which they are entitled – this inequity is unjustifiable.

In 1990, the Human Fertilisation and Embryology Act in the United Kingdom modified the limits:
- for 'social termination' to 24 weeks
- to prevent 'grave permanent injury to the physical or mental health of the pregnant woman' – there is no upper limit
- when there is 'substantial risk of serious handicap' – there is no upper limit
- Concern has been expressed about what constitutes a substantial risk and a serious handicap.

Relevant literature

For RCOG guidelines on termination, see:
   http://www.rcog.org.uk/resources/Public/pdf/abortion_summary.pdf.

Test your knowledge

Answer true (T) or false (F) for each of the following statements.
1. In a typical abortion service, up to 20% of women require in-patient care
2. A least one-third of British women will have had a TOP by the time they reach the age of 45 years
3. With surgical TOP, the risk of cervical trauma is less than 1 per 100
4. Post-abortion infection, including PID, occurs in up to 10% of cases
5. Intra-uterine contraception can be inserted immediately following a second trimester TOP
6. Following a TOP, the incidence of placenta praevia and infertility are increased by approximately 5%

Case 9 – Sore throat

Mr AP is a 22 year old man who has had a sore throat and headache for two and a half weeks and he is not feeling better. See Appendix for details.

Targeted history taking

- Clarify symptoms – is he complaining of a sore throat and a headache, or just a general discomfort?
- How did his symptoms start? Have they changed at all?
- Has he been febrile or had any other symptoms? Does he feel ill?
- What treatments have been tried already?
- How is it affecting him at home and at work?
- What is his general health like? Has he had lots of infections and does he struggle to fight them off?
- Why is he consulting now?
- What are his expectations – an explanation, medication, further investigation, or advice regarding work?
- Does he have any specific concerns?

Data gathering

Listed below is the additional information elicited from the patient with appropriate questioning.
- He has felt generally run down and achy, particularly getting vague headaches that get worse as the day goes on and in the evenings.
- At first he had a sore throat and felt a bit 'fluey' but that soon settled.
- He has never been feverish.
- He has tried throat lozenges but they did not help. He has taken paracetamol when he gets in from work.
- He is coping OK at work, but feels tired in the mornings and, as his job is very physical, he is worn out when he comes home. This means he cannot help his wife with their 3 month old baby who is waking a lot at night. He tells you that his wife had a difficult birth and could not do much for herself initially. He would like to help his wife more now, but just feels too tired. He feels that he should be helping her as she copes on her own all day. He feels guilty about this and really wants to feel better so he can help.
- He feels run down but not ill. He feels too tired to fight off the bug.
- His wife has suggested he may need antibiotics to help him fight off whatever is making him feel so run down. He is not sure if you can help him or if he just needs a bit more time to fight the bug off.

- His wife had glandular fever a couple of years ago, before they got married, but she was really unwell and he is not concerned that he has anything serious like that.

Targeted examination

- Appearance – does he look ill, jaundiced, or anaemic? Is there any evidence of weight loss?
- Take his temperature. Check whether he has any rashes and palpable lymph nodes.
- Examination of his throat – any erythema, palatal petechiae, mucosal lesions, enlarged tonsils, or exudate?
- Examine his abdomen for enlarged liver or spleen. Consider examining his urine if there is a history of recurrent infections.
- *In this case – he looks tired, but examination findings are otherwise normal.*

Clinical management

- Discuss examination findings and reassure him that you can find no sign of serious illness.
- Discuss the natural history of sore throats.
- Address Mr AP's ideas: indications for antibiotics and why they are not indicated in this case.
- Address his concerns: why he is run down and not recovering from a minor infection.
- Discuss the need for any investigations.
- Discuss how he is coping with a physical job and helping with a young baby while feeling run down. You could discuss whether he might benefit by taking a few days off work (self-certify) to get some rest.
- Enquire about his wife – is she getting support from the health visitor? Does she need more support?
- Discuss how they are coping at home with a baby.
- Is his baby registered and getting appropriate preventive care?

Interpersonal skills

Good communication with the patient:
- explores possible physical, psychological and social issues
- reassures Mr AP following exploration of his symptoms and social circumstances, supported by a focussed examination
- negotiates use of time as a therapeutic tool
- addresses social factors – supporting his wife and young baby
- explores Mr AP's agenda – need for antibiotics; guilt about being too tired to help his wife
- safety-netting: when to return, is his wife receiving the support she needs, is there a cause for the baby waking frequently?

Additional information

Sore throat is a common problem and raises issues such as antibiotic prescribing and patient expectations. By asking about social and occupational factors, it became apparent that tiredness was the likely cause of Mr AP's symptoms. By enquiring about his wife and family, the doctor has demonstrated an holistic approach. The consultation concluded with the doctor giving no prescription or sick note, but Mr AP self-certified for a couple of days.

You may want to consider other ways this case could have developed:

- Mr AP may have married his girlfriend because she was pregnant and is regretting his decision now the baby has arrived
- Mr AP had several trips to the GUM Clinic and keeps getting minor infections – he is now concerned he has HIV

Relevant literature

Sullivan F, Wyatt JC. (2005) Why is this patient here today? *BMJ*, **331**: 678–680.
Part of ABC of health informatics series, this article looks at the process of defining the reason for a patient's attendance. It provides useful tips and thoughts applicable to the CSA component.

Appendix: Patient summary

Name	AP
Date of birth (Age)	22
Social and Family History	Car mechanic. Married.
Past medical history	None
Recent reports	Last seen 3 years ago with urethral discharge and was referred to the GUM Clinic.
Current medication	None
Investigations	None

Test your knowledge

Answer true (T) or false (F) for each of the following statements.

1. Bacterial sore throat is more severe and lasts, on average, 48 hours longer than viral sore throat
2. NSAIDs are the drugs of choice for analgesia in sore throat
3. In clinically severe cases, if penicillin is prescribed, the appropriate dosage, as used in the majority of research studies, is penicillin V 500 mg, four times daily for 10 days
4. The incidence of rheumatic fever in the UK is extremely low and, to prevent its resurgence, clinically severe cases should routinely be treated with penicillin
5. Antibiotic therapy has been shown to alleviate symptoms even in sore throats not caused by bacteria

Case 10 – Struggling to cope with a baby

Mrs AP is a 21 year old mother of a 3 month old baby. She informs you that her mother has told her to see you. Mrs AP feels she is 'struggling to cope' and that her life is 'terrible'. See Appendix for further details.

Targeted history taking

- Clarify what she means by 'struggling to cope' and 'terrible' preferably with examples.
- How long has she felt like this?
- Enquire about her physical health and whether she has any other symptoms.
- Assess whether she is looking after herself – is she eating normally?
- Does she smoke? Is she drinking more alcohol or smoking more than previously?
- Was her pregnancy planned? How was the delivery – were there any complications?
- Assess whether she is depressed at the moment and ascertain whether she had any mental health problems in the past.
- What has she done or tried to help the situation?
- Explore what help is available to her. Can her mother or her husband's family help? Does she have any friends? Does she belong to a young mothers' group? Is the health visitor aware of how she is feeling?
- What does her husband think about how she is coping? Has he offered any suggestions?
- Try to get an idea of what her daily routine is like.
- Consider getting her to give a score for the quality of her life at the moment and compare it to a year ago.
- What was her life like before she had her baby? What hobbies does she have, what does she like to do to relax?
- What is the relationship like with her husband at the moment?
- Is she still breast-feeding? Try to assess her feelings towards her baby – is she bonding well?
- What does she hope to gain from this consultation – advice, reassurance, support, or signposting to other services?

Data gathering

Listed below is the additional information elicited from the patient with appropriate questioning.
- Mrs AP informs you that her baby cries all the time and that she feels that all she does is run around after the baby and her husband.

- She first started feeling like this when her husband returned to work two weeks after the birth. Since then, her feelings have gradually been getting worse.
- Apart from feeling tired and at the end of her tether, she is physically well.
- She is eating regular meals.
- She gave up smoking and has not had any alcohol since she discovered she was pregnant.
- The pregnancy was planned. She had a difficult forceps delivery after a long labour at the end of which she was exhausted.
- She has no major symptoms of depression and scores 5/27 on the PHQ-9 scale. She has had no mental health problems in the past.
- She does not know what she can do to help the situation. She talks to her mother on the telephone a lot.
- Her mother lives over 100 miles away and cannot come to help her at all due to work commitments. Her husband is fostered so has no available family. They have a few friends, but none has any children. She went to a mother and baby group once, but was put off by the other mothers there. She does not like the health visitor – she feels like she is 'snooping on her'.
- She thinks her husband is worried about her getting so tired. He offers to help a lot, but she feels that she should be able to cope and that it is unfair to ask him because he is working hard to support them all and to save money to buy a house. He has not been very well recently but still tries to do odd things around the flat to help her. She thinks he feels they both need to get out for a break, but she thinks this would be wasting his hard-earned money when they have a lot of expenses and are trying to save.
- She is still breast-feeding because 'everyone says it is the best thing to do'. She has no bad feelings about her difficult delivery and seems to be devoted to her baby.
- She hates every day; they all feel the same. The baby wakes them at 5 am for a feed and goes back to sleep at around 6 am. Her husband gets up at 6.30 am and leaves for work at 7.30 am; he brings her a cup of tea in bed, but she usually goes back to sleep before she drinks it. Her baby wakes at 8 am for another feed, after which she has a bit of breakfast while washing up and loading the baby clothes into the washing machine. She then tries to clean their flat, but cannot use the vacuum cleaner in case it wakes the baby. She then tries to have a quick shower before the baby wakes for her next feed. She tries to shop for food for their evening meal every afternoon because it gets her out of the flat, but the baby often cries all the way home because he is due for another feed. She then has to prepare dinner and get the baby bathed before her husband gets home at around 7 pm. They have to wait to eat until after he has played with the baby for a while – although she thinks he sometimes gets him 'over-excited so he won't feed properly and then takes ages to get off to sleep'. She then has a meal with her husband; they watch television for a while and then go to bed at around 9.30 pm.
- She says every day ranks as 2/10, previously she would have scored 6/10 on bad days and 9/10 on good days.

- She used to enjoy going to a dance group before she became pregnant. Her friends have asked when she will be rejoining but she says she cannot now she has a baby. She and her husband had a good social life before the baby; they knew things would be different, but she never thought all the fun would go out of her life.
- She is not sure what she hopes to get from the consultation. 'I wish you could just wave a wand and make me happy again.'

Targeted examination

- You should assess whether Mrs AP is depressed or not, including an assessment scale.
- Apart from assessing whether Mrs AP is anaemic, there is probably no need for a physical examination
- *In this case the patient looks tired but is not pale. You do not feel she is clinically depressed.*

Clinical management

- You have various options, but your primary aim should be to enable Mrs AP to gain insight into her problem.
- Reassure her that she does not appear to have any physical problem causing her symptoms.
- Reassure her that a lot of first-time mothers find adjusting to their new lifestyle very difficult.
- Explore with her and try to help her identify the factors in her lifestyle that may be contributing to her symptoms, and then to identify what changes she can make to start to improve the quality of her life. Sometimes getting the patient to concentrate on small changes is easier than big changes – she could have a leisurely bath or shower while her husband is playing with the baby, for instance.
- Reassure her that health professionals, including yourself and the health visitor, are there to support and not judge or check up on her.
- Encourage her to get support and information from her health visitor about other mother-and-baby groups and baby-sitting circles. Offer to arrange for the health visitor to visit her at home.
- Try to help her understand why her husband is encouraging her to go out, e.g. supporting her, thanking or rewarding her, and trying to maintain their relationship.

Interpersonal skills

This case hinges around gathering information in a systematic manner to exclude depression and identify lifestyle factors contributing to the patient's symptoms –

minimal physical examination is required to achieve this in the allotted time. Good communication skills both verbal and non-verbal are more important.

Good communication with the patient:
- explores possible physical, psychological and social issues
- reassures the patient
- explores what offers of help are available
- explores her expectations of being a new mother

Good communication enables the patient to:
- gain insight into the factors contributing to her problem
- identify simple achievable steps to improve her life
- identify offers of help and support
- maintain her relationship with her husband

Additional information

This patient is the wife of Mr AP in Case 9. You might like to re-read his case and consider whether you would have approached it differently if you were aware of his wife's case first.

Dennis C-L. (2005) Psychosocial and psychological interventions for prevention of postnatal depression: systematic review. *BMJ*, **331**: 15.
- Postnatal depression affects about 13% (1 in 8) of all new mothers.
- Psychosocial and psychological variables contribute to increased risk.
- No measure is available that has acceptable predictive validity to accurately identify women who will later develop postnatal depression.
- Many psychosocial or psychological interventions tested so far in trials do not effectively prevent postnatal depression.

Patel R, Murphy D, Peters T for ALSPAC (2005) Operative delivery and postnatal depression: a cohort study. *BMJ*, **330**: 879.
- Depression in the postnatal period affects 8–15% of women (similar to background rate).
- Postnatal depression is similar to depression occurring at other times in life.
- Depression is associated with negative sequelae.
- There are possible adverse long-term effects on child development.
- The Edinburgh postnatal depression scale was developed as a screening tool to detect women with postnatal depression. A score of ≥13 is highly predictive of postnatal depression in a UK population and warrants further clinical assessment. It has a sensitivity of 88% and a specificity of 92.5%.
- Elective caesarean section gives no protection against postnatal depression.
- Emergency caesarean section or assisted vaginal delivery patients can be reassured that these procedures are not associated with increased risk of postnatal depression.

Appendix: Patient summary

Name	AP
Date of birth (Age)	21
Social and Family History	Married, 3 month old baby
Past medical history	Difficult forceps delivery.
Recent reports	One of your partners visited her at home 1 week after delivery and recorded: *'Still uncomfortable but happy. No worries.'* Entry from health visitor 2 weeks ago from Baby Clinic: *'Baby growing well, following 75th centile. Doing well with breast-feeding, encouraged to keep up the good work! Well cared for baby, good bonding.'* Letter from hospital arrived last week: *'Seen 6 weeks postnatally. No problems, breast-feeding well. She can stop her iron supplements now. No further appointments.'*
Current medication	Was on ferrous sulphate 200 mg b.d. until her postnatal examination at the hospital
Investigations	Postnatal
Hb	11.8
Edinburgh scale score	8 at 4 weeks postnatal

Test your knowledge

Answer true (T) or false (F) for each of the following statements.
1. At present, the evidence supports routine screening for postnatal depression
2. The UK National Screening Committee recommends the Edinburgh Postnatal Depression Scale (EPDS) as a checklist, not a screening tool
3. In mothers suffering postnatal depression, weekly nondirective counselling by health visitors for eight weeks has no effect on the recovery rate
4. Tricyclic antidepressants, with the exception of doxepin, appear unsafe in lactation
5. Fluoxetine is as effective as cognitive behaviour therapy in reducing postnatal depression

Case 11 – Painful shoulder

Mrs CK is a 42 year old teacher. She presents complaining of pain in her left shoulder. See Appendix for details.

Targeted history taking

- Clarify her pain symptoms: site, spread, acute or chronic onset, any trauma, exacerbating or relieving factors, duration; any neurological symptoms?
- How long has she had this problem?
- Any problems with other joints? Any history of trauma?
- Enquire about her physical health and whether she has any other symptoms – especially fevers, weight loss, rash, respiratory problems.
- Enquire about her lifestyle and whether her symptoms are affecting this – occupation, sport and hobbies.
- What has she done or tried to help the situation?
- What does she hope to gain from this consultation – an examination, an explanation, medication, further investigation, treatment or physiotherapy referral?

Data gathering

Listed below is the additional information elicited from the patient with appropriate questioning.

- Her pain came on after a weekend decorating. She has a dull ache around her shoulder with sharp twinges on certain movements, particularly putting on a seat belt or coat.
- She has no neurological symptoms.
- She has had the problem for three weeks and it is not getting better, if anything her shoulder is getting stiffer.
- She has no other joint problems. No history of trauma.
- She enjoys good health.
- She is an art teacher and coaches the school netball team. She is keen on badminton but has been unable to play due to her shoulder pain – she is left handed. She is having some problems at work due to her restricted use of her dominant arm.
- She has taken some ibuprofen which has relieved the constant dull aching, but there has been no improvement in her shoulder movement or the sharp twinges. She has also had a sports massage but this did not help either.
- She hopes you will refer her for physiotherapy as she is very frightened she is developing a frozen shoulder.

Targeted examination

- Adequate exposure of her shoulder and neck are required.
- Inspect: general contours, attitude of shoulder, muscle wasting, swelling.
- Examine her cervical spine movements: extension, flexion, rotation to left and right, side flexion to left and right.
- Examine her shoulder movements: active movements – elevation through flexion, elevation through abduction (looking for painful arc), internal and external rotation; resisted – abduction, adduction, internal and external rotation, elbow flexion, elbow extension.
- Palpation: effusion, warmth, localized tenderness.
- *In this case, abnormal findings are: pain on resisted abduction and a painful arc (70–120°) on active abduction, no loss of external rotation.*

Clinical management

- Discuss examination findings.
- Discuss natural history of condition: painful arc and frozen shoulder.
- Reassurance.
- Address Mrs CK's ideas and expectations: physiotherapy may help.
- Address patient's concerns: no evidence of frozen shoulder.
- Agree management plan:
  - ○ analgesia (paracetamol with intermittent NSAIDs)
  - ○ encourage activity
  - ○ physiotherapy referral
  - ○ injection
  - ○ provide written information (e.g. ARC patient leaflet)

Interpersonal skills

Good communication with the patient:
- explores possible physical, psychological and social issues
- reassures patient following a focussed examination
- addresses social factors
- explores patient's agenda
- explores patient's health beliefs

Additional information

Mitchell C, Adebajo A, Hay E, and Car A. (2005) Shoulder pain: diagnosis and management in primary care. *BMJ*, **331**: 1124–1128.
- Shoulder pain is the third most common cause of musculoskeletal consultations in primary care.

- Occupational, physical and psychosocial factors are all important.
- Recurrence and chronicity are common.
- The four commonest causes of shoulder pain in primary care are:
  ○ rotator cuff disorders
  ○ glenohumeral disorders
  ○ acromioclavicular joint disorders
  ○ referred neck pain
  Combinations of these in the same patient are common.
- Management in primary care is very similar for all four categories:
  ○ analgesia
  ○ motivate and encourage rehabilitation
  ○ evidence for physiotherapy and steroid injections is relatively weak, but steroid injections may help pain in the short term
- Investigations are not usually indicated in primary care.
- Indications for referral include:
  ○ significant pain and disability for more than 6 months despite appropriate conservative management
  ○ history of shoulder instability
  ○ acute, severe post-traumatic acromioclavicular pain
  ○ red flag criteria
- Red flag criteria:
  ○ history of, or suspicion of, cancer
  ○ possible unreduced dislocation
  ○ trauma plus acute disabling pain plus significant weakness suggesting acute rotator cuff tear
  ○ possible neurological lesion

Relevant literature

For guidelines on diagnosis and initial management of shoulder problems see:
  http://www.oxfordshoulderandelbowclinic.org.uk.
Online learning module: Frozen shoulder (adhesive capsulitis). *BMJ* Learning
  (http://www.bmjlearning.com)
Educational leaflet for GPs, linked with patient information leaflet: Arthritis Research
  Campaign. *In Practice Series 4.* Hazleman, *Shoulder problems in general practice.*
For an excellent guide on how to conduct an examination of the shoulder, including
  video-clips, see: http://medicine.ucsd.edu/clinicalmed/Joints2.html.

Test your knowledge

Answer true (T) or false (F) for each of the following statements.

1. Pain in the mid-range of shoulder abduction suggests acromioclavicular arthritis
2. Pain at the end of shoulder abduction suggests a rotator cuff injury
3. Asking the patient to clasp his fingers behind his neck tests external rotation in abduction
4. When testing passive movement, a true assessment of scapulo-thoracic abduction involves pressing firmly on top of the shoulder with one hand while moving the patient's arm with the other hand
5. To test serratus anterior (long thoracic nerve, C3, 4, 5), ask the patient to push forcefully against a wall with both hands
6. If the right scapula stands out prominently when the patient pushes forcefully against a wall with both hands, this suggests a problem with the right serratus anterior (long thoracic nerve, C5, 6, 7)
7. Power in the pectoral muscle is tested by asking the patient to move his hand sideways to point to the ceiling, against resistance

Case 12 – Forearm in plaster cast

CJ is a 19 year old man who has been added on to the end of your full evening surgery as an extra. He walks in with his left arm in a plaster cast and in a sling and informs you that he fell over playing football three days ago and sustained an undisplaced fracture of the distal radius. The consultant in the Trauma Clinic has given him a sick note for 4 weeks, but he does not want to be off work.

Targeted history taking

There are five tasks here.
1. To determine why he does not want to take time off work when he has been advised to do so:
   - enquire why he does not want to be off work
2. To determine what his job entails:
   - ask what his job is
   - determine what functions he is actually required to do at work
3. To determine his degree of disability and hence assess whether he can perform his job:
   - determine his pain level and pattern
   - determine his current functional level – how much is he able to do for himself at home? Can he do the tasks required of him at work?
   - is he taking any medication? Is he taking any analgesia that may compromise his safety at work or his ability to work?
   - how does he get to work?
4. To try not to undermine the hospital consultant
   - clarify why he was advised not to work
5. To discover why he requested an urgent appointment
   - confirm that he did ask for an urgent appointment
   - explore his reasons for doing so
   - what are his expectations of this consultation: advice regarding work, a letter for work, signposting to appropriate services or medication?

Data gathering

Listed below is the additional information elicited from the patient with appropriate questioning.
   - He has only recently started working in the office of a small local business. He will not be eligible for much sick pay. His mother has MS and has been unable to work recently due to a flare up. She does not claim any benefits and so money is quite tight, especially as they are now having to employ a cleaner.

- He is responsible for filing and basic office duties. He does have to do some data-inputting, but his manager has said there are other things he can get on with if he cannot do this. He coped without any problems yesterday. He does not operate any machines other than a photocopier.
- His wrist aches, but he is coping with this. The hospital gave him co-codamol 30/500. He took some when he got back from casualty, but they made him nauseous and so he has not taken any since. He then informs you that he tried one of his mother's 'MS cigarettes' and this helped his pain.
- He walks to work. He does not drive.
- He believes the hospital advised him not to work as a matter of routine. They did not ask about his job or personal circumstances.
- He asked if he could be seen as soon as possible because he was unsure if he could go to work and ignore the hospital sick note.
- He hopes you will tell him he can continue to go to work.

Targeted examination

- There are no real issues requiring an examination here.
- You could check that there are no problems relating to his plaster cast – swelling, circulation and sensation.

Clinical management

There are four areas that you should consider covering:
1. Whether he can work:
   - discuss the natural history of the condition
   - reassure him that there are no obvious reasons why he should not work – he has an uncomplicated fracture and his employer is happy to support him working one-handed
   - as he is worried about any repercussions if he works when he has been given a sick note, you can provide him with a sick note confirming that he is fit to work with limited use of one hand
2. Cannabis:
   - you might like to explore whether this was an isolated use of cannabis, or whether he has a regular habit. If so, does he take any drugs? You could discuss the law relating to the use and possession of cannabis in an open, non-judgemental manner. You may decide to clarify how his mother obtains it if she has restricted mobility – has CJ been buying it for her?
3. His mother:
   - you should check whether his mother is entitled to any benefits and if so, whether she is claiming these. You might suggest they contact Citizens Advice Bureau, Social Services or MS support groups/charities for advice.
4. Requesting an urgent appointment:
   - you should decide whether you think it is appropriate to discuss requesting an urgent appointment for this problem.

Interpersonal skills

Good communication skills enable you to:
- assess whether his belief that he is able to work is correct
- be seen to support his health beliefs and positive desire to work
- explore the psychological and social issues in this case – the financial strain that he and his mother are living under
- offer constructive and moral support and guide them towards other agencies that may be able to give financial or physical support
- explore his cannabis use and demonstrate an awareness of ethical issues relating to cannabis use
- demonstrate an understanding of the social impact of illness and injury
- demonstrate judgement on whether to confront a patient who has made what may appear to be an unmerited request for an urgent appointment
- maintain patient confidence in the hospital consultant by taking a non-judgemental decision after obtaining an occupational health history

Additional information

Initially this appears to be a simple case, but it soon develops into a more complicated one. There are several directions in which it could develop in an examination situation which you might like to consider, for example:
- CJ disclosing a regular cannabis habit
- depression relating to looking after a mother who is progressively deteriorating
- the problems of being a carer

Mental Health of Carers. (2002) HMSO, London.
- Survey of health and well-being of carers in 2001, particularly looking at the impact of their caring responsibilities and support on mental health.
- Female carers were more likely to have neurotic symptoms than male carers (21% compared to 12%).
- Of carers who were working, 79% reported that being a carer had almost no effect on their job, 15% had a little impact, and 6% reported considerable problems.
- 53% of carers reported that being a carer caused them to be worried a little of the time, while 18% reported that they worried a lot of the time.
- 33% of carers said that caring made them depressed a little of the time.
- 48% reported that caring made them tired, but only 8% reported that caring had had a direct effect on their physical health.

Website aimed at professionals working with carers, see: http://www.carers.gov.uk.

Relevant literature

For interesting reading on the defence of 'medical necessity' for the use of cannabis to relieve symptoms of disease, pain or the side effects of other drugs, see: http://www.schmoo.co.uk/thclub/legal.htm.

Appendix: Patient summary

Name	CJ
Date of birth (Age)	19
Social and Family History	Lives with mother
Past medical history	Nothing of note
Recent reports	Last seen 6 months ago with D&V
Current medication	None
Investigations	None

Test your knowledge

Answer true (T) or false (F) for each of the following statements.
1. Heavy cannabis use does not cause short-term memory impairment
2. Heavy cannabis use reduces the ability to perform complex tasks
3. Euphoria and altered perception of passing time are symptoms of withdrawal from long-term cannabis use
4. If a patient experiences anxiety, nausea and hand tremor on reduction of heavy prolonged alcohol use, alcohol withdrawal is diagnosed
5. Historically, delirium tremens has had a death rate of about 5%
6. Cognitive behaviour therapy and motivational interviewing are less effective than twelve-step programmes for people with alcohol dependence

Case 13 – Haematuria

Mr AS, age 43, had an insurance medical one month ago. This picked up an isolated finding of microscopic heamaturia (2+); BP 132/86. The practice nurse arranged two further urine tests over the next two weeks. Both these showed isolated microscopic haematuria (2+ and 3+), no proteinuria. Mr AS is coming to see you to discuss these results.

Targeted history taking

- Has Mr AS experienced any urinary symptoms: frequency, dysuria, urgency, or any outflow obstruction symptoms such as a sensation of incomplete emptying, weak stream, straining, or nocturia?
- Has he ever experienced macroscopic haematuria?
- Has he passed frothy urine, had a sore throat recently or felt unwell with fever or weight loss?
- Has he had kidney stones in the past?
- What job does he do? Is he exposed to chemicals, dyes, solvents or petrochemicals that increase his risk of developing uro-genital cancer? Does he smoke?
- Does he have a past medical history of uro-genital problems? What is his general health like?
- What are his expectations of this consultation: completion of his insurance form, a referral for further investigation, a discussion with you?

Data gathering

Listed below is the additional information elicited from the patient with appropriate questioning.

- Mr AS is completely asymptomatic.
- He has never experienced any macroscopic haematuria. A few years ago, he ate some beetroot that turned his urine red.
- He has not passed frothy urine. He has not been ill or had a sore throat recently. He has not been febrile nor has he lost weight.
- One of his work colleagues had kidney stones. He has never had anything like that and having seen the discomfort his colleague suffered, he takes care not to dehydrate.
- He works as a salesman for the local Peugeot dealership. This has a forecourt with petrol pumps and a workshop, but he has never been employed in the petro-chemical industry. He uses glues and solvents to make and paint model aeroplanes, his hobby since adolescence. He gave up smoking ten years ago and prior to that smoked socially, never heavily.
- He has always worked in sales, usually car sales.

- He had a bilateral vasectomy 8 years ago. Eighteen months ago, while on holiday in Kenya, he had an episode of scrotal pain, which the local doctor thought was epididymitis. He got better after a course of antibiotics. He can't remember the name of the antibiotics, but they did give him diarrhoea.
- He would prefer not to have an examination because both he and his partner have had a good look and there is nothing to find. He looked up the symptoms of prostate disease on the internet and does not have any symptoms, so he does not feel an examination is warranted. He does not have a family history of prostate problems.
- He would like you to complete his insurance form stating that he is in good health. He does not believe there is anything wrong with him – he feels well.

Targeted examination

- Perform an abdominal examination to exclude the presence of masses.
- Recheck his BP.
- When you ask Mr AS for permission to perform a uro-genital examination (of the foreskin, penis and prostate), he declines saying that his partner, a surgical nurse at the local hospital, examined his genital area and did not find anything significant.

Clinical management

- Respect Mr AS's decision not to have a uro-genital examination. Try to maintain rapport by listening to him and acknowledging his values.
- Explain that patients with asymptomatic microscopic haematuria need further investigation to exclude kidney disease, kidney stones and uro-genital cancers, which while quite rare in his age group, would be quite important to catch at an early stage.
- Use an analogy to reinforce the need for investigation, such as BP or late on-set diabetes may be asymptomatic and are only really found with tests and investigations.
- Explain that while you respect his wish not to be examined further, you would really prefer to refer him to exclude potentially serious illness.
- Referral would be to the local urologist for an ultrasound scan of his kidneys, a KUB and quite likely, a flexible cystoscopy.
- You do not think that he has a cancer, hence referral on the two week wait is not needed.
- Regarding the insurance form, you are obliged to fill in the fact that haematuria has been detected on three occasions. You could advise him that his insurance quotations or premiums are likely to reduce once the investigations rule out uro-genital malignancy and if he and the insurance company are agreeable, you could complete the form once the investigations are complete.

Interpersonal skills

Good communication with the patient:
- provides the patient with sufficient information to make an informed decision
- respects the patient's preferences
- establishes rapport with the patient and is able to maintain this rapport while putting forth an evidence-based treatment plan

Therefore, it results in the doctor working with the patient to formulate an agreed management plan, which respects the patient's views, but ensures that either appropriate or essential treatment is given.

Additional information

Jones R, *et al*. (2007) Alarm symptoms in early diagnosis of cancer in primary care: cohort study using General Practice Research Database. *BMJ*, **334**: 1040.
- Haematuria, microscopic and macroscopic, with or without pain, accounts for approximately four consultations per thousand patients per year in primary care in the UK.
- The presence of painless, macroscopic haematuria is widely regarded as a red flag symptom suggesting the presence of a urinary tract neoplasm.
- For haematuria, the risk of a cancer being diagnosed is greatly increased in the first three to six months after presentation, particularly in younger patients, middle-aged men and older women.
- Haematuria that is unexplained by urinary tract infection should be investigated by careful physical examination, fibreoptic cystoscopy, and imaging of the upper renal tract.

From http://www.gmc-uk.org/guidance/current/library/intimate_examinations.asp:

'Obtain the patient's permission before the examination and be prepared to discontinue the examination if the patient asks you to. You should record that permission has been obtained.'

Relevant literature

For the International prostate symptom score (IPSS), see:
    http://www.gp-training.net/protocol/docs/ipss.doc.

Test your knowledge

Answer true (T) or false (F) for each of the following statements.
1. In men treated for a lower urinary tract infection, arrange for a mid-stream urine (MSU) before, and fourteen days after finishing, antibiotics

2. In men with a lower urinary tract infection, an ultrasound scan (USS) and abdominal X-ray of the urinary tract detect fewer cases of underlying pathology compared to intravenous pyelograms (IVPs)
3. 25% of patients with small renal stones (<5 mm) pass the stones spontaneously
4. Investigate patients with renal stone disease by checking serum calcium and uric acid and a 24-hour urinary calcium
5. Patients with calcium renal stones are advised to avoid spinach and tea
6. Patients with oxalate renal stones are advised to reduce their dairy intake

Case 14 – Erectile dysfunction

Mr TB is 64 year old estate agent who usually sees the senior partner. As the senior partner is on holiday, Mr TB comes to you for a repeat prescription of his anti-hypertensives (bendroflumethiazide 2.5 mg and atenolol 50 mg). You notice that he is overdue his annual check with the practice nurse. During the consultation, he mentions that he has difficulty with erections.

Targeted history taking

- For how long has he been hypertensive?
- Is he experiencing problems with his current medication?
- Does his BP or treatment impact on his home or work life?
- Has your senior partner discussed changing his medication (in accordance with current NICE guidance)?
- Does he have any other cardiovascular risk factors – diabetes, hyperlipidaemia, smoking, family history, obesity, inactive lifestyle or symptoms of peripheral vascular disease?
- Clarify what difficulty he is having with erections – initiating or maintaining?
- For how long has he had the problem? Has it developed gradually or is it of sudden onset?
- What is his relationship with his partner like?
- How much alcohol does he drink?
- Is he taking other medication, including herbal remedies?
- Exclude depression and anxiety.
- What are his expectations of this consultation: a repeat prescription and a BP check; a second opinion on his health; or investigation and treatment of his erectile problem?

Data gathering

Listed below is the additional information elicited from the patient with appropriate questioning.
- He has been hypertensive for 15 years and has been well controlled on his current medication since diagnosis.
- He has not experienced any problems with the medication.
- He believes that his BP is well controlled and reports no adverse impact of the hypertension or the tablets on his home and work life.
- The senior partner, with whom he gets on well, did discuss the new NICE guidelines with him but as he has been well controlled on his current medication, they agreed not to change the tablets.

- At his last annual check, no additional cardiovascular risk factors were identified. He intends to attend for his routine nurse appointment once he retires next month.
- He says that gradually, over the past two years, he has had difficulty maintaining erections such that over the last three months, he and his wife have been unable to have sex.
- His wife is not happy with the current situation as they previously enjoyed a full and active sex life. He is happily married. He is looking forward to retiring. He and his wife intend to play more golf and holiday in Spain where he has a second home.
- He drinks a couple of glasses of wine each night.
- Besides his BP medication, he is not taking any other tablets.
- He is not depressed or anxious.
- He wants to know if he could get a prescription for Viagra on the NHS.

Targeted examination

- General assessment – if he looks overweight, consider weighing him and calculating his BMI.
- Measure his BP – *the BP reading is 132/86.*
- Ask for permission to examine his genitalia for anatomical abnormalities such as hypospadias or Peyronie's, and to exclude testicular atrophy. *He produces a card saying that genital and prostatic examinations are normal.*

Clinical management

- Explain that while his BP is well controlled on his current medication, either one or both of his anti-hypertensive tablets may be contributing to his erectile dysfunction.
- However, there are other possible causes of erectile dysfunction such as cardiovascular disease, diabetes, heavy drinking, or psychogenic factors.
- The gradual onset of his erectile dysfunction suggests an organic cause, including possible drug side effect.
- Reassure him that, on examination, there was no evidence of testicular or prostatic problems; hence further investigations (testosterone, PSA, prolactin, and liver function tests) are not indicated at this stage.
- His options include:
  - ○ first, stopping atenolol and being reviewed in a month; the advantage of this option is that you would assess whether the erectile dysfunctile is a side effect of the medication
  - ○ secondly, changing his BP medication. Before you change his medication, you may want him to have blood tests done with the practice nurse. Advise him that to change his blood pressure medication safely, you will need to know the results of his blood tests. Therefore you will give him a repeat script of his current medication to tide him over until after his practice

nurse appointment. He will need to have fasting glucose, cholesterol, urea and electrolytes (pre ACE-I), both to exclude possible causes of erectile dysfunction and to initiate his new BP tablets safely.

○ thirdly, clarify whether he is asking you for your opinion and wishes to return to the senior partner for a definitive treatment plan.

○ fourthly, if he says he would definitely like a script for Viagra today, you could give a private prescription. However, the problem has not been investigated completely and Viagra, while not contraindicated in his circumstances, may not be entirely useful if his erectile dysfunction is a drug side effect. On the information available at this consultation, he would not be eligible for NHS treatment. However, should further tests uncover other problems, NHS-funded treatment might be possible.

Interpersonal skills

Good communication with the patient explores:
- his agenda (repeat prescription, exploration of his erectile dysfunction problem)
- health beliefs (Viagra treats erectile dysfunction)

By discussing issues openly and without embarrassment, the doctor will help the patient feel comfortable. By providing the patient with treatment options, the doctor shares management decisions, thus empowering the patient. The treatment options, as outlined above, do not criticise the senior partner's management and do not undermine his on-going care of the patient.

Additional information

McMahon CN, Smith CJ, and Shabsigh R (2006) Treating erectile dysfunction when PDE5 inhibitors fail. *BMJ*, **332**: 589–592.

Many men have underlying comorbidities that are risk factors for erectile dysfunction: diabetes, hypertension, cardiovascular disease, depression, prostatic hypertrophy, smoking, drug treatment, a sedentary lifestyle, drug and alcohol misuse. Control of these risk factors is essential:
- to treat erectile dysfunction in the first instance, and
- secondly, to improve erectile function and the patient's response to treatment. One study showed that modifying associated risk factors before sildenafil was started improved the overall success rate to 82%.

30–35% of men do not respond to oral phosphodiesterase type 5 (PDE5) inhibitors – sildenafil (Viagra; Pfizer), tadalafil (Cialis; Lilly), and vardenafil (Levitra; Bayer).

In non-responsive patients, the response may be improved by:
- educating patients on the correct use of the drug
- optimizing the dose
- daily dosing of the drug (rather than on-demand)
- improving co-morbid conditions

- treating hypogonadal men with testosterone
- combining PDE5 inhibitors with other classes of drug
- using alternative treatments, such as injecting drugs intracavernosally, psychosexual therapy, vacuum constriction devices, or penile prostheses

81% of patients initially took sildenafil incorrectly. Therefore, initial education should focus on:

- adequate sexual stimulation, ideally with a partner, is required
- correct dosing with respect to food and alcohol
- timing of the dose: tadalafil should ideally be taken several hours before sexual activity
- number of required doses: although most men will respond after one or two doses, some men may need six to eight doses before an optimal response occurs

Test your knowledge

For each of the following statements on prescription charges, answer true (T) or false (F).

1. GPs provide Hepatitis A immunisation for holiday travel free of charge to their NHS patients
2. GPs provide typhoid immunisation for holiday travel free of charge to their NHS patients
3. GPs provide Meningitis A and C immunisation for holiday travel free of charge to their NHS patients
4. Medication for malaria prophylaxis may be reimbursed under the NHS, as per Department of Health guidance, FHSL(95)7
5. Patients <18 years and >65 years of age are eligible for free NHS prescriptions
6. A diet-controlled diabetic is not eligible for free NHS prescriptions
7. A woman who delivered a baby in the last 12 months is eligible for free NHS prescriptions

Case 15 – Hypothyroidism

Mr DF is a 41 year old man who presents with tiredness. He was diagnosed with hypothyroidism 5 months ago and has been taking thyroxine 75 µg daily. His TSH from a month ago was 3.99 (0.35–5.5). He presents asking if he should increase his thyroxine dose.

Targeted history taking

- What does he mean by tiredness? Is he describing mental or physical fatigue, lethargy or general malaise?
- For how long has he been tired?
- When is he tired?
- When does he take his medication? Is he compliant?
- Why was he put on this dose of thyroxine?
- Does he have other symptoms of hypothyroidism, such as weight gain, constipation, hoarse voice, or dry skin and hair?
- What job does he do?
- Could there be other reasons for his tiredness, such as poor quality and quantity of sleep, changes at home or at work, stress?
- What are his expectations of this consultation: an exploration of the possible causes of tiredness, further blood tests, a change in his medication, referral to an endocrinologist, time off work?
- What is his general health like – has diabetes been excluded?
- Does anyone in his family have hypothyroidism and what has their experience of the illness been?

Data gathering

Listed below is the additional information elicited from the patient with appropriate questioning.

- By tired, he means physical and mental lethargy – 'his get up and go has got up and gone'. He does not describe malaise or prodromal illness.
- He has been tired for 18 months, since prior to the diagnosis of hypothyroidism. Once the diagnosis was made and he started thyroxine, he hoped that the tiredness would lift.
- He is 'tired all the time'. He wakes up feeling as if he could go right back to sleep. In the evenings, he slumps in his chairs and nods off in front of the TV. He goes to bed at 9.30pm and wakes up at 5.30am and despite the eight hours of uninterrupted sleep, he is still tired.
- He takes his medication daily and says he is compliant.

Clinical Skills Assessment

- It was a 'tester' dose. There was difficulty in making the diagnosis – the first THS was normal, the 2nd TSH was 7.99. Because his usual doctor wasn't absolutely sure, he put him on thyroxine 75 µg five months ago and rechecked the TSH last month when it was 3.99.
- He does not have any other symptoms of hypothyroidism. His hair is thinning slightly, but he assumed that is normal for his age.
- He works as an infrastructure manager for a multi-national company.
- There are home and work stresses at present. His 16 year old teenage daughter is doing GCSEs at the moment. Unlike his wife, he worries whether she is revising enough, and there have been some arguments at home. He says 'it has been a bad month'. His job changed recently – instead of reviewing the budget for various building and maintenance jobs, he now has to visit sites scattered throughout the region. This involves approximately eight additional hours of driving each week, four on Monday and four on Wednesday. This also makes coming to the surgery on those days difficult, hence he has come to see you. The commuting, especially on the motorway, is challenging. He has not fallen asleep at the wheel but is worried about this. He does not think that he is stressed by the changes at work – 'this tiredness is not in my head'.
- He wants to know if he should increase his thyroxine dose.
- He is in good health usually. He is a non-smoker. He drinks four to six beers over the weekend. He tested negative for diabetes.
- Nobody else in the family has thyroid disease.

Targeted examination

- He does not have a goitre. See http://www.youtube.com/watch?v=JYb-io13fOA for a demonstration on how to examine the thyroid gland.
- He does not have oedema of the feet, hand or eye-lids.
- His weight is stable. Weight = 96 kg; height = 177 cm, BMI = 30.6.

Clinical management

- Discuss the possible causes of tiredness, checking all the time to see if the patient agrees with your suggestions. Look for nodding and non-verbal gestures of acceptance as you put forward each possibility.
- Discuss the significance of the negative examination findings.
- If he is not keen to explore psychological issues at present and if you assess that he is not depressed, then try to maintain rapport and address his ideas about increasing medication.
- His idea that his dose of thyroxine is too low may certainly be valid.
- Discuss possible options: increasing the dose of thyroxine and then review, perhaps with a blood test, in three months; or stay on the same dose but address issues at work and home that could be contributing to his tiredness.

- Address the patient's concerns and expectations. He is concerned about falling asleep at the wheel and expects that his tiredness will improve once he takes a higher dose. You advise him of what is an appropriate higher dose and issue the medication.
- Explain how to take the medication (are you issuing 100 µg, 50 µg or 25 µg tablets). Encourage compliance with the medication.
- Safety net: advise him of when you would next like to review him and under what circumstances he should return early for reassessment.

Interpersonal skills

Poor communication with the patient fails to explore how the patient has made sense of his symptoms, that is, his illness story is unheard (see Additional information below).

If the doctor interprets the patient's symptoms differently (for example, by insisting on psychological reasons for the tiredness), then their conflicting health beliefs may harm the doctor–patient relationship and prevent the development of an effective therapeutic alliance. On the other hand, acknowledging the validity of the patient's beliefs creates rapport and enables the development of an effectual therapeutic relationship.

Consequently, the poor communicator is unable to devise a management plan that is responsive to the patient's health beliefs and concerns. Instead, he adopts a rigid approach, investigates and medicates inappropriately and fails to forge a useful therapeutic alliance with the patient.

Additional information

Moncrieff G, Fletcher J. (2007) Tiredness. *BMJ*, **334**: 1221.
This 10-minute consultation article suggests that patients who present with tiredness consult for many reasons:
- it may be a symptom of physical disease, such as hypothyroidism, autoimmune disease, liver or kidney disease, or malignancy
- it may be a symptom of depression or a response to the stresses of life circumstances

It may be a tester symptom, where it is offered as an initial symptom to see whether the doctor is sympathetic and interested, before the main, perhaps sensitive, agenda is revealed. 'Patients may consider tiredness to be a more legitimate symptom to bring to a doctor than, say, unhappiness.'

How should doctor's deal with their patient's unhappiness? One approach is to employ active listening skills and allow the patient to tell their story.

Telling illness stories
From: http://www.aissg.org/articles/TELLING.HTM

'Illness stories are therapeutic for *tellers* who have a real opportunity to be heard and to hear themselves. As they tell and retell their story they can unravel the truth of their own experience of illness and begin to adjust to the person they have become. From this position they can begin to uncover the person they could become. Telling their story has given them the opportunity to step outside of themselves and witness who they are. This dis-identification allows new possibilities to emerge.'

Active listening skills
From: http://www.holisticlocal.co.uk/articles/view/293/The+Therapeutic+Relationship

'What are the skills required by the practitioner to instate a strong therapeutic relationship that can beget greater benefit for patients? The therapeutic skills [are]:

- unconditional acceptance
- empathy
- attending and listening
- open questioning
- reflection
- silence
- physical and behavioural techniques
- concreteness
- professionalism
- warmth and being genuine'

Test your knowledge

A 41 year old man presents with tiredness and weight gain. His thyroid stimulating hormone (TSH) and thyroxine are measured. Answer true (T) or false (F) for each of the following statements.
1. If TSH is raised and thyroxine is normal, he has sub-clinical hyperthyroidism
2. If TSH is raised and thyroxine is normal, the next screening test should be measuring his thyroglobulin antibodies
3. If TSH is raised, thyroxine is normal and he is positive for thyroid peroxidase antibodies, he should be treated with thyroxine
4. If TSH >10 mU/l, thyroxine is normal and he is negative for thyroid peroxidase antibodies, he should be treated with thyroxine
5. If TSH <10 mU/l, thyroxine is normal and he is negative for thyroid peroxidase antibodies, he should have a three month trial of thyroxine

Case 16 – Hyperthyroidism

Mrs CQ is a 39 year old woman who was last seen one month ago for her six-week post-partum check. She complained of tiredness and diffuse thinning of her hair. Her usual GP requested blood tests (see Appendix for details). She had blood taken one month ago and last week. She is returning to discuss the blood results.

Targeted history taking

- What are her current symptoms?
- What does she understand about her blood results?
- Does she have a family history of thyroid problems?
- Are her symptoms affecting her home or work life and, if so, how?
- Does she know of any treatments for hyperthroidism?
- What are her expectations of this consultation: general advice and education, referral to an endocrinologist, prescription of medication, further investigations?
- What is her general health like – is she on any medication such as amiodarone, which could cause thyroiditis, or is she asthmatic, which would be a contraindication to beta-blockers?
- Is she breastfeeding?

Data gathering

Listed below is the additional information elicited from the patient with appropriate questioning.
- Her main complaints are of hair thinning, tiredness, being short-tempered, having swollen ankles, and itchy legs – she scratches at night. She does not have any eye symptoms.
- After speaking to the phlebotomist when she presented for her 2nd blood test, she looked up hyperthyroidism on the internet. She thinks her symptoms fit in with the description of hyperthyroidism. What she doesn't know is how or why she developed it.
- She does not have a family history of hyperthyroidism.
- She works full time as a head teacher. Her baby is in nursery. He is bottle-fed. He sleeps through the night. Her husband is a computer programmer. He is bearing the brunt of her short temper. She is an organized and determined person so she is not letting the tiredness prevent her from working.
- She would like to start treatment as soon as possible so she can go back to feeling better again. When you discuss referral, she says she would like to be seen as soon as possible – should she buy BUPA insurance?

- She is usually in very good health and felt fine throughout her pregnancy. This is the first time she has been truly ill. She is not on any medication.
- She did not breastfeed.

Targeted examination

- Weigh the patient. *She now weighs 61 kg, and this is 15 kg below her pre-pregnancy weight.*
- Conduct a directed cardiovascular examination: *pulse 115/73; pulse 69 b.p.m. and regular. She does not have pedal oedema.*
- Symptomatic hyperthyroidism presenting within six months of childbirth is unlikely to be due to Graves' disease. Therefore it would be unusual for her to complain of eye symptoms (diplopia, discomfort or protrusion). Therefore, unless she complains of eye symptoms, a check for exopthalmos, proptosis, lid lag, ophthalmoplegia, visual acuity, and colour vision is not needed.

Clinical management

- Share the examination findings with the patient.
- Discuss the natural history and possible aetiologies of hyperthyroidism, including autoimmune and post-partum hyperthyroidism.
- Discuss management options: beta-blockers for symptom control and referral to endocrinology for further investigation with thyroid ultrasound and uptake scans. Carbimazole, to render euthyroid, is rarely used in post-partum hyperthyroidism.
- Address the patient's ideas: that her tiredness will improve by starting medication as soon as possible while awaiting referral.
- Address the patient's concerns regarding NHS treatment and her perceived need for private treatment.
- Address her expectations that treatment starts as soon as possible: organize referral and make a decision regarding beta-blockers. If you prescribe beta-blockers today, discuss the dose and potential side effects. Alternatively, provide Mrs CQ with an information sheet and arrange a follow-up appointment at which you can address appropriate and safe prescribing.
- Safety-net: outline follow-up and the conditions under which Mrs CQ should consult sooner or urgently.

Interpersonal skills

Good communication with the patient explores:
- her agenda and preferences – to be treated as soon as possible, either within the NHS or the private sector

- the impact of the illness on her life, particularly her relationship with her husband
- her preferences for treatment – the doctor works in partnership with the patient; he starts beta-blockers, at the patient's request, while awaiting the hospital appointment

A good communicator provides explanations about hyperthyroidism, including its investigation and management, which are understandable to the patient. When discussing the issue of private referral, good doctors do not allow their own views and values to inappropriately influence the patient's decision making. Hence, the patient's autonomy is respected.

Additional information

Are anti-thyroid drugs, such as carbimazole, used in the treatment of post-partum hyperthyroidism? Listed below are the summaries from two articles on the subject:
- Pearce (2006) says beta-blockers, and not anti-thyroid drugs, should be used in the treatment of post-partum hyperthyroidism
- Azizi (2006) says anti-thyroid drugs can be used

Pearce EN (2006) Diagnosis and management of thyrotoxicosis. *BMJ*, **332**: 1369–1373.

Painless postpartum lymphocytic thyroiditis occurs in up to 10% of women after giving birth, within six months after pregnancy. It is an inflammatory autoimmune disorder in which lymphocytic infiltration results in thyroid destruction and leads to transient mild thyrotoxicosis as thyroid hormone stores are released from the damaged thyroid. As the gland becomes depleted of thyroid hormone, progression to hypothyroidism occurs. Thyroid function returns to normal within 12–18 months in 80% of patients. Tests include the presence of thyroperoxidase antibodies, a low to undetectable thyroid radioactive iodine uptake. If treatment of the hyperthyroid phase is necessary, a beta-blocker is usually prescribed and not an anti-thyroid drug.

Symptoms of overt thyrotoxicosis include heat intolerance, palpitations, anxiety, fatigue, weight loss, muscle weakness, and, in women, irregular menses. Clinical findings may include tremor, tachycardia, lid lag, and warm moist skin.

In all forms of overt thyrotoxicosis:
- TSH is decreased
- free thyroxine (T4) or free thyroxine index or free tri-iodothyronine (T3), or both, are raised
- raised serum concentrations of thyroperoxidase (TPO) antibodies indicates an autoimmune thyroid disorder

A radioactive iodine uptake and scan should be performed when the cause of a patient's thyrotoxicosis cannot be definitively determined by history and physical examination. If radioactive iodine uptake is:
- normal (as in goitre) or elevated (as in Graves'), then treat with anti-thyroid drugs, radioactive iodine therapy, or thyroidectomy

- low, as in thyroiditis, then treat with beta-blockers to relieve symptoms and glucocorticoids to relieve anterior neck pain, if present

Azizi F (2006) Treatment of post-partum thyrotoxicosis. *J Endocrinol Invest*, **29**: 244–247.
- Thyrotoxicosis occurs more frequently during the post-partum period than at other times in women of childbearing age. Graves' disease and post-partum thyroiditis are two major causes of thyrotoxicosis in this period.
- The major task lies in differentiation of these two diseases in the post-partum period, since throtoxicosis caused by post-partum thyroiditis usually does not require treatment.
- Anti-thyroid drugs are the mainstay of the treatment of post-partum thyrotoxicosis. Recent investigations conclude that neither propylthiouracil nor methimazole cause any alterations in thyroid function and physical and mental development of infants breast-fed by lactating thyrotoxic mothers, and both can be safely administered in moderately high doses during lactation.

Carbimazole

Carbimazole decreases thyroid hormone synthesis and will control hyper-thyroidism within several weeks in 90% of patients. Minor side effects, such as fever, rash, urticaria, and arthralgias, occur in up to 5% of patients. Agranulocytosis occurs in approximately 0.5% of patients.

Appendix: Patient summary

Name	CQ
Date of birth (Age)	39
Social and Family History	Married, one child
Past medical history	Termination of pregnancy 2003
	Termination of pregnancy 1994
	Tonsillectomy 1993
Current medication	None
Blood tests	Test results from last week
TSH	0.01
T4	26.3 pmol/l (9–25)
T3	8.6 pmol/l (3.3–8.2)
Thyroid peroxidase antibody level	6 IU/ml (range 0–60)
LH	3.2 ((3–12)
FSH	6.3 (1–30)
Prolactin	70 (<600)
	Test results from one month ago
Haemoglobin	13.1g/dl (13.0–17.0)
TSH	0.35
Pulse	80 regular
BP	106/70
Height	168 cm
Weight	70 kg
BMI	24.8
TSH (17 months ago)	1.8

Test your knowledge

Regarding overt thyrotoxicosis, answer true (T) or false (F) for each of the following statements.

1. Symptoms include feeling cold, tiredness, weight gain and constipation
2. Clinical findings may include tremor, bradycardia, lid lag, and cold dry skin
3. Due to toxic nodular goitre, protrusion of the eyes and diplopia is clinically evident in 30% of patients
4. Thyroid stimulating hormone (TSH) is decreased and peripheral thyroid hormone is increased
5. In a patient with a low radioactive iodine uptake, treatment options include radioactive iodine therapy and thyroidectomy

Case 17 – Hypertension

Mrs SK is a 44 year old woman who has recently moved into the practice area. Her old notes have not yet arrived. She brings in her repeat prescription and asks for a re-issue. She is currently on bendroflumethiazide 2.5 mg, atenolol 100 mg and Cerazette 75 μg once daily. Her home BP readings over the last week are BP 132/98; 148/86; 138/94 and 150/78. *She comes across as a slightly anxious lady who is easily alarmed.*

Targeted history taking

- Why was she put on the medication?
- How long has she been on the medication?
- Are there any side effects or problems with taking the medication?
- How does she take her BP at home? Does she know the name of the device? Does she have it calibrated?
- Are the readings fairly typical for her?
- Is she aware of the alternative medication for hypertension and contraception?
- How does she feel about changing her tablets?
- What treatments, including lifestyle measures, has she tried already?
- Does she smoke? What is her general health like?
- Is she up-to-date with her annual blood tests and 3-yearly smears? Does she do breast self-examination?
- What are her expectations of this consultation: re-issue of current medication; further information about alternative treatments for BP and/or contraception; a change in medication today?
- Does she have a significant family history of cardiovascular disease?
- What job does she do? Who lives with her in her new home?

Data gathering

Listed below is the additional information elicited from the patient with appropriate questioning.
- She was diagnosed as hypertensive eight years ago.
- She has been stable on current anti-hypertensives for the last five years.
- She has not experienced any side effects on the medication. She has put on 4 kg in the last few years but says this could be due to 'getting old'.
- She bought a home-monitoring BP machine in Germany five years ago. It has a German name. It is a wrist monitor (she only tells you this if you ask directly). It has never been serviced or calibrated since purchase.
- The BP readings on the print-out she brings with her are pretty typical for her.
- She has not tried and does not know about other medication for BP.

- Mrs SK is quite worried by the questions you are asking her. *'Do you think my medicines are wrong doctor? or should I be on stronger pills?'* She was changed to progesterone oral contraception at age 35 years because she developed migraines on the combined pill.
- She expects you to make the decisions – *'what do you suggest I do doctor?'*.
- She exercises regularly and has a healthy diet.
- She is in good health, drinks a few half-pints of beer at weekends and has never smoked. She says she is a slightly anxious woman but she has been like this all her life; her mother was 'nervy'.
- She had a complete check-up, including her bloods a few weeks before she moved house. The surgery told her there was nothing to worry about. She is in-date with her smear. She self-examines her breasts for lumps regularly.
- She came in for her repeat prescription and wants you to make the decisions regarding her medication – *'you know best doctor'*.
- Her father had high blood pressure and had a stroke in his 50s. Both her brothers have hypertension.
- Mrs SK works part-time as a nursery nurse. She is studying towards her NVQs with a view to becoming a childminder on completion of the course. She lives with her husband and her 19 year old son, both smokers. They run a father/son plumbing business.

Targeted examination

- Measure her BP.
- Weight = 74 kg; height = 168 cm; BMI = 26.2.

Clinical management

- Briefly outline the aim of hypertensive management and the target BPs, which are <140/85 (JBS2) or <140/90 (NICE).
- Discuss the need to establish whether her BP is truly controlled. Her home readings indicate that her BP is possibly not reaching the target BP. However, she uses a wrist device that has not been calibrated in 5 years – how reliable are these results?
- Discuss her current drug regime and the two chief reasons for advising a change. First, beta-blockers may be less effective in reducing major cardiovascular events, particularly stroke than other drug combinations, hence in younger individuals ACE-Is or ACE-IIs are recommended by NICE as first line therapy. Secondly, co-prescribing a beta-blocker with a thiazide also carries an increased risk of developing diabetes.
- If her BP readings are within target, she has a choice of continuing with her current regime or changing to an ACE-I regime. NICE advises that beta-blockers may be continued if there is a particular reason for their use and if the BP is being controlled on them.

- If her BP readings are not within target, the dose should be stepped down and stopped gradually, and replaced with a more appropriate drug.
- Address the patient's ideas: BP can be monitored at home using automated devices; however, these must be appropriate devices that are serviced regularly.
- Address the patient's concerns that her tablets are 'wrong' or 'not strong enough'. Advise Mrs SK that most hypertensives will require at least two or three drugs to control their BP. The treatment of hypertension changes based on new and emerging evidence, so her current treatment is not 'wrong'. It needs updating for her to get maximal benefit.
- Address the patient's expectations: she expects you to make the decisions regarding her repeat prescription. If there is no particular reason for her to be on a beta-blocker/thiazide combination, and given her family history of stroke, it may be appropriate to change the antihypertensive regime. Discuss whether she is happy with your hypertensive management plan or whether she would like to read some patient literature first before making a decision.
- Consider the issue of contraception: it may be entirely appropriate to issue a repeat prescription of Cerazette, provide leaflets on alternative long-acting contraception and arrange a further discussion with the practice nurse, the Family Planning clinic, or you.
- Arrange follow-up based on the agreed management plan.

Interpersonal skills

Good communication with the patient:
- addresses her preference – you guide her in making decisions about complex medical management
- communicates risk to the patient without further alarming her
- provides explanations that enable her to understand what you are doing and the reasons for your actions

Therefore, despite the patient's willingness to leave all decision-making to the doctor, the doctor continues to consult with her at each stage to ascertain her preferences and agreement.

A poor communicator:
- adopts a rigid consulting style that fails to encourage the patient's self-sufficiency
- fails to empower the patient
- appears inappropriately paternalistic

Additional information

Stergiou G, *et al.* (2004) Self monitoring of blood pressure at home. *BMJ*, **329**: 870–871.

The advantages of self-monitoring are:
- the home readings are more reliable, that is, devoid of the white coat and placebo effects; multiple readings are averaged over time
- self-monitoring predicts cardiovascular outcome better than clinic measurements
- self-monitoring may improve control of BP by improving compliance as patients become more involved in their care
- self-monitoring might reduce healthcare costs by reducing the number of clinic visits

However, few of the devices available on the market are accurate. Wrist and finger devices are not recommended. Patients should be warned that devices for self-monitoring are often put on the market without having been independently validated. Two websites (www.bhs.soc.org and www.dableducational.org) provide information on validated devices for self monitoring.

Advice to patients undertaking self-monitoring:
- take the BP measurements over three to seven days, in the morning and evening; be seated; discard measurements taken on the first day
- do the readings for one week every three months
- do not monitor too often
- do not modify treatment without consulting a doctor or nurse
- if your average home BP reading is greater than or equal to 135/85 mmHg, you probably have high BP; < 130/80 mmHg indicates normal BP

Cappuccio FP, *et al.* (2004) Blood pressure control by home monitoring: meta-analysis of randomised trials. *BMJ,* **329**: 145.
- This paper presented a meta-analysis of 18 randomised controlled trials. Over a 2–36 month period, 1359 people with essential hypertension were allocated to home BP monitoring (study group) and 1355 allocated to monitoring within the healthcare system (control group).
- In the study group:
  ○ systolic BP was found to be lower (standardized mean difference 4.2 mmHg)
  ○ diastolic BP was lower by 2.4 mmHg
  ○ mean blood pressure was lower by 4.4 mmHg
- When publication bias was allowed for, the differences were attenuated: 2.2 mmHg for systolic BP and 1.9 mmHg for diastolic BP.
- The study concluded that the difference in BP control between the two methods is small but likely to be clinically important.

Relevant literature

NICE (2007) Hypertension – full guideline. See:
http://guidance.nice.org.uk/CG34/guidance/pdf/English.

Test your knowledge

A 51 year old Egyptian man presents with three blood pressure (BP) readings taken by the practice nurse. Answer true (T) or false (F) for each of the following statements.

1. Treat his BP if the readings are 160/102, 168/104 and 166/106
2. If readings are 148/92, 156/76 and 142/90, and his 10-year risk of cardiovascular disease (CVD) is 21%, treatment is needed
3. If hypertensive therapy is needed, the first choice should be a diuretic or calcium channel blocker
4. Suspect malignant hypertension if he has headache, palpitations, and pallor
5. Suspect malignant hypertension if his BP today is 174/108 mmHg

Case 18 – Grief

Mrs AC is a 54 year old woman who presents in emotional distress. She asks for 'something to help' with her grief. Her sister-in-law had a fatal MI in India three weeks ago.

Mrs AC usually consults annually for monitoring of her hypercholesterolaemia. She takes atorvastatin 10 mg at night. Her latest blood results, from 12 months ago, were: total cholesterol 5.1 mmol/l; HDL 1.4 mmol/l; triglyceride 2.01 mmol/l, and liver function tests were normal.

Targeted history taking

- What are Mrs AC's current symptoms?
- What does she think are causing these symptoms?
- Could there be other reasons for these symptoms?
- What treatments has she tried already?
- How are her symptoms affecting her home and work life?
- What are her expectations of this consultation: time off work, medication, advice, or signposting to mental health resources?
- What is her general health like – when is she intending to have her blood tests for cholesterol and liver function?

Data gathering

Listed below is the additional information elicited from the patient with appropriate questioning.
- Mrs AC feels tired and fatigued. She has headaches and interrupted sleep. She has difficulty concentrating on her work (she works in the local post office). She is weepy and 'shocked'.
- Adequate practical arrangements for her sister-in-law's funeral were made. She supported her husband during this process and was 'strong for him'. However, on returning home last week, she feels as if 'things have caught up' with her. She feels physically and mentally drained.
- Her sister-in-law's death also coincides with the anniversary of a miscarriage. She grieves both losses. She is well physically. She does not have a past history of anxiety or depression.
- She has tried hot milk with ginger at bedtime to help her sleep but this has not been helpful.
- She is very weepy and irritable. Little incidents, such as her co-worker forgetting to pass on a message, make her disproportionately angry. Later on, she feels guilty for her excessive emotional response. She does not want to burden her husband with her feelings; he lost his only sister and had to help with the funeral arrangements.

- She does not expect time off work; she believes it is important to maintain a routine. However, it takes a lot more concentration to do the work and she is tired. She would like to feel less tired and asks if taking St John's Wort or other tablets may help? She prefers alternative medicines.
- When specifically asked about the blood tests, she says that she is needle-phobic and has avoided this procedure, as she feels unable to cope with the venepuncture at present. She usually overcomes her dread of needles by sheer concentration and will-power.

Targeted examination

- A brief mental state examination may be all that is required.
- If appropriate, assess suicide risk.

Clinical management

- Discuss the natural history of a grief reaction. People may experience physical symptoms such as fatigue and headaches as well as psychological symptoms such as 'shock', i.e. feelings of unreality, detachment, disbelief or 'numbness'.
- As this is a normal grief reaction rather than a presentation of anxiety, depression, or abnormal grief (such as inhibited, delayed or prolonged grief), an explanation of the 'normality' of the above symptoms may be reassuring.
- Address the patient's ideas: she believes that she needs a tonic for the tiredness. Discuss ways in which tiredness can be improved, such as improving sleep, getting practical help with difficult chores, exercising, taking time out for self, and/or maintaining a routine that includes some enjoyable activities.
- Address the patient's concerns: she is concerned about burdening her husband by discussing her feelings with him. Explore whether this concern is well-founded and whether being more open with him could result in mutual support. Talking about the bereavement can often help to resolve the feelings. The amount of time and discussion needed for people to grieve varies according to the individual.
- Address the patient's expectations: she believes that St John's Wort may help with tiredness. St John's Wort could be useful. However, St John's Wort is known to interfere with many medications, including simvastatin. It *may* interact with atorvastatin – does she want to consider this option or other measures in the first instance? Negotiate a management plan. Consider prescribing sedatives (zopiclone or diazepam) for a few days.
- Discuss the needle phobia. Consider whether using a topical anaesthetic application or distraction techniques, such as breathing exercises, counting backwards from 300, or listening to music while having blood taken, may be useful.

- Briefly discuss the importance of cholesterol review and the need to reduce total cholesterol to <5 mmol/l, or preferable <4 mmol/l. Arrange follow-up with results of the blood tests to discuss lifestyle measures and perhaps an increase in the dose of atorvastatin.
- Safety net: outline when and why follow-up should be arranged for the grief reaction, needle phobia and cholesterol management.

Interpersonal skills

Good communication with the patient explores:
- her agenda (to improve her tiredness)
- health beliefs (St John's Wort and alternative medications are useful remedies)
- preferences (to delay venepuncture until she is better able to cope with the procedure)

A good communicator elicits social information that contextualizes the patient's problem, that is, obtains the information about not wanting to burden her husband with her emotional distress. By exploring the pros and cons of open discussion with her husband, the doctor and patient may be able to work in partnership to develop a shared management plan. Such discussion, in contrast to drug prescription alone, empowers the patient and encourages self-sufficiency.

Additional information

Parkes CM (1998) Coping with loss: Bereavement in adult life. *BMJ*; **316**: 856–859.
- A GP visit to the family home on the day after a death can give emotional support to the family. The bereaved may need reassurance that they are not going mad if they break down, that the symptoms of anxiety and tension are not signs of illness, and that it is OK for them to withdraw, for a while, from their accustomed tasks.
- As time passes people may also need permission to take a break from grieving – to return to work or do other things that enable them to escape, even briefly, from grief.
- The first anniversary is often a time of renewed grieving.

Charlton R, Dolman E. (1995) Bereavement: a protocol for primary care. *Br J Gen Pract*, **45**: 427–430.

Bereavement becomes a medical problem when the surviving intimates become ill. This paper proposes a bereavement protocol to minimize the effects of bereavement.

Relevant literature

For information on bereavement, see: http://www.rcpsych.ac.uk/mentalhealth
    information/mentalhealthproblems/bereavement/bereavement.aspx.
For information on complimentary therapies, see: http://www.rcpsych.ac.uk/mental
    healthinformation/therapies/complementarytherapy.aspx.
For information on St John's Wort and its interactions, see: http://www.info.doh.gov.uk/
    doh/EmBroadcast.nsf/f011981a95f31f4180256c07003d34a0/a4c8299ce082e
    6a980256dad004a0071?OpenDocument.
For information on needlephobia, see: http://www.needlephobia.co.uk/index.aspx.
For communication video-clips, see:
    http://www.tneel.uic.edu/tneel-ss/demo/connect/frame1.asp.

Test your knowledge

A 51 year old Caucasian woman presents with a blood pressure (BP) of 156/90 (average of three readings). Her fasting blood tests show:

cholesterol 7.2 mmol/l (3.2–6.5)   triglyceride 3.66 mmol/l (0.79–1.97)
HDL 1.0 mmol/l (1.2–1.7)   total cholesterol : HDL ratio 7.2

Answer true (T) or false (F) for each of the following statements.
1. If results vary when re-checking her fasting lipids, use the higher reading to decide whether treatment for hypercholesterolaemia is required
2. If blood was taken within 3 months of a major illness, re-check cholesterol levels outside the 3-month period
3. Levonorgestrel-containing contraception would not affect her cholesterol
4. If she smoked 20 cigarettes per day for 20 years and gave up smoking 4 years ago, her 10-year risk of cardiovascular disease (CVD) should be assessed as a smoker
5. If she has premature menopause, double her CVD risk
6. A triglyceride of 3.66 mmol/l requires referral to a lipid clinic for treatment with a fibrate

Case 19 – Obsessive compulsive disorder

Mrs TH is a 34 year old woman who presents in emotional distress. She says that her obsessive compulsive disorder (OCD) is back. She had been fine for 18 months, since the birth of her baby. During her pregnancy, she developed a fear of catching illnesses, such as toxoplasmosis. She washed the household surfaces and her hands several times each day. She saw a psychologist for talking therapies, having declined medication during pregnancy. She felt absolutely fine since the birth of her baby. Now, she is anxious about driving.

Targeted history taking

- What are her current symptoms?
- Elicit the thoughts that are making her anxious, that is, her obsessions.
- Elicit the way in which her anxiety manifests itself, such as her feelings and/or physical symptoms of anxiety such as headaches, palpitations and chest pain.
- Elicit the things she does to reduce the anxiety, that is, her compulsive behaviours.
- Has anything happened recently that could have provoked the anxiety, such as stress or life changes?
- How are her symptoms affecting her home and work life?
- Is there any associated co-morbidity such as depression?
- What treatments has she already tried?
- What are her expectations of this consultation: signposting to self-help information, referral to mental health services or initiation of medication?
- What is her general health like – how much is she smoking or drinking?

Data gathering

Listed below is the additional information elicited from the patient with appropriate questioning.
- She is afraid of driving. Her husband commutes and she has to drive the two older children to and from school each day.
- As school time approaches, she feels herself getting more anxious and fearful. By the time she leaves home, she is in a state of dread.
- She is worried about hitting cyclists and pedestrians. She worries whether her car is too close to them and whether she would know if she has injured them. She sees pictures of the injured people in her mind.
- Her palms are sweaty. She feels tense and fearful. She feels angry with herself for allowing these silly fears to take root. She feels exhausted from controlling the urge to go back along the route to check for injured people.

- She avoids driving whenever possible. She talks to her sister and her mum about her feelings. They are supportive. Her husband is understanding of her OCD and reassures her that she is not 'going mad'.
- Her husband went away on business three weeks ago. She had to look after her three boys on her own. She had to do more driving during this period. The symptoms started at this point. She has been driving for more than ten years and has never had any accidents or convictions.
- She is a housewife. The fear of driving now dominates a large part of her morning and afternoon. Once she returns home, she forces herself to not go back along the route to check for accident victims. She distracts herself by getting on with the housework and playing with the baby, but the images of accident victims keep popping into her mind. She feels exhausted and agitated. She is quite curt with the children on the drive to school because their noise may distract her. She feels guilty for treating them in this way.
- She sleeps from 9.30 pm to 6 am and wakes up tired. She does not wake during the night. Her appetite and weight are unchanged. She does not feel disinterested in things; however, she feels 'panicky' most of the time.
- She has tried re-reading her book, 'Overcoming Anxiety', which she found very useful during her pregnancy. It does not seem to help anymore. She has tried the relaxation and breathing techniques the psychologist previously advised. These helped to calm her but did not make the fear of driving disappear.
- She would like to feel better. She does not want a referral to community mental health because she associates seeing the psychologists with the way she felt during her pregnancy. She does not want to be reminded of this unhappy time. She would prefer that you treated her in your surgery.
- She is a non-smoker and she does not drink alcohol.

Targeted examination

- A brief mental state examination may be required.
- If she is washing her hands recurrently, briefly examine for dry or fissured skin.

Clinical management

- Discuss the natural history and possible aetiology of OCD.
- Reassure her that her husband is correct in saying that people with OCD are not 'mad'.
- Congratulate her on not getting into the ritual of checking for accident victims. Rituals may briefly reduce anxiety; however, they strengthen the belief that fixed patterns of behaviour can stop negative things from happening.
- Address the patient's ideas: she believes that seeing a psychologist will trigger the feelings she had during her pregnancy. It may be appropriate to gently

challenge the idea, perhaps by exploring how previous contact was useful. Ask Mrs TH if the she can think of anything to reduce her fear of contacting the mental health services, for example, would seeing them at an alternative venue be less stressful?

- Address Mrs TH's concerns: that she feels unwell with the recurrence of her OCD. OCD is treatable so encourage optimism and hope.
- Address her expectations: she would like treatment in primary care. Discuss possible options: referral to the practice counsellor for exposure and response prevention or cognitive therapy; or guided self-help using books such as *Overcoming Obsessive-Compulsive Disorder: a self-help book using cognitive-behavioural techniques* (by Veale and Willson); or treatment with SSRIs to reduce obsessions and compulsions. Negotiate a management plan. If you prescribe medication, take steps to encourage concordance.
- Safety-net: outline when and why you would next like to see Mrs TH. If you refer her, discuss when she is likely to hear from the team and what she should do if she has not heard from anyone within a specified period.

Interpersonal skills

Poor communication with the patient:
- fails to elicit a thorough history of her thoughts (obsessions), feelings (anxiety/dread) and behaviours (avoidance behaviour, constantly seeking reassurance)
- fails to explore how the patient's life is affected by the problem – how a large portion of the day is spent thinking about accident victims and how the emotional burden is fatiguing her
- fails to encourage self-sufficiency – referral to the mental health team or psychologist without exploration of her fears, and without offering self-help measures can be perceived as instructing the patient rather than adopting an approach that is responsive to the patient's preferences, feelings and expectations

Therefore, poor communicators show little understanding of their patients' illness and its psychosocial impact. Consequently, their management plan contains a number of instructions, most of which fail to empower the patient and nurture self-sufficiency.

Additional information

Heyman I, *et al.* **(2006)** Obsessive-compulsive disorder. *BMJ,* **333:** 424–429.
- Obsessions are intrusive thoughts (ideas, images, or impulses) that repeatedly enter a person's mind against his or her will, generating considerable anxiety.
- Compulsions are repetitive acts – attempts or rituals to reduce the anxiety caused by the obsessions, but the relief is only temporary.
- With time, 'automatic' rituals can increase, rather than reduce, the anxiety.

- Ritualising may maintain the problem – the patient fails to deal with their fears and their anxiety.
- The aim of exposure and response prevention, a psychological therapy, is to break this cycle by persuading patients to expose themselves to the feared situations and, at the same time, to refrain from performing any rituals.

Relevant literature

For a patient leaflet on OCD, see:
http://www.rcpsych.ac.uk/mentalhealthinformation/mentalhealthproblems/ obsessivecompulsivedisorder/obsessivecomplusivedisorder.aspx.
NICE (2005) Obsessive–compulsive disorder. See: http://www.nice.org.uk/CG031. Describes OCD management, including treatment in primary care.

Test your knowledge

Regarding obsessive compulsive disorder (OCD), answer true (T) or false (F) for each of the following statements.
1. If a selective serotonin re-uptake inhibitor (SSRI) is prescribed for the treatment of OCD, the response may take up to 12 weeks
2. If a selective serotonin re-uptake inhibitor (SSRI) is prescribed for the treatment of OCD, expect to continue it for at least 2 years
3. If a tricyclic antidepressant (TCA) is prescribed for the treatment of OCD, the best evidence is for imipramine

Regarding generalised anxiety, answer true (T) or false (F) for each of the following statements.
4. For the treatment of generalised anxiety, cognitive behaviour therapy (CBT) has the strongest evidence of benefit
5. It is appropriate to prescribe benzodiazepines for 2–4 weeks in a generalised anxiety crisis and in panic disorder

Case 20 – Tinea pedis

Mr RS is a 46 year old self-employed builder. He presents with athlete's foot, which he has had previously. He brings in a tube of terbinafine cream and asks for a script for more cream please. See Appendix for further details.

Targeted history taking

- What are his symptoms?
- When did he last have athlete's foot? Did the cream help to clear it up?
- What treatments has he tried already?
- Are the symptoms preventing him from doing any activities at home or at work?
- What does he think is the cause of the recurrence?
- You notice that his medical notes show a blood glucose result of 6.6 mmol/l in February 2004. Was this a fasting blood test? Was it followed up?
- You also notice that he has a family history of diabetes and cardiovascular disease. Could he give you more information on this?
- What are his expectations of this consultation: a script for terbinafine, further investigation, a discussion on possible reasons for recurrence?
- Discuss his general health: is he taking any medication, particularly immunosuppresives, or is he using any over-the-counter creams, or has he recently completed a course of antibiotics?

Data gathering

Listed below is the additional information elicited from the patient with appropriate questioning.

- He has very itchy, red toes. This started suddenly four weeks ago during the very hot weather.
- He had this in 2004. The doctor gave him some cream (*he points to the tube*) and it cleared up quickly.
- He tried washing his feet after work and drying thoroughly between the toes. He uses a new pair of socks with his work boots each day. He tries to walk about the house in sandals but now that his feet have become so red, his wife is concerned that he is passing the infection to everybody else and she wants him to wear socks all the time. He disagrees with this.
- The feet are itchy which can be very distracting at work. If he is busy, he can ignore it. If not, he finds that he is scratching the top of the boot with the heel of the other boot to alleviate the itch.
- He thinks the recurrence is due to wearing thick socks under work boots in the recent hot weather.

- He remembers that it was a fasting blood test in 2004. His doctor did the test when he had athlete's foot. He was told to come for a second test and to buy a bottle of Lucozade for the blood test but things at work got very busy and he was unable to attend.
- His mum has been diabetic since age 65. She takes tablets. His dad had a fatal MI aged 49. He used his mum's glucometer. The readings were 6 to 7, which his mum said were OK.
- He wants a script for the cream please.
- He is in good health and has not taken any tablets or over-the-counter medicines.

Targeted examination

- Ask the patient to show you his feet. *He produces a picture:*

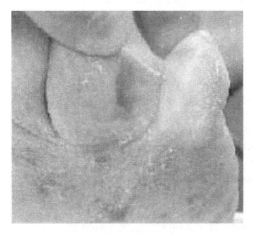

Reproduced from www.drfoot.co.uk with permission.

The toes are dry, erythematous and have fine scaling. There is no moistness or fissuring or evidence of secondary infection.

Clinical management

- Discuss the management of tinea pedis. Advise on foot hygiene and footwear (see: http://www.netdoctor.co.uk/diseases/facts/athletesfoot.htm).
- Discuss medication. He could buy imidazole antifungals such as clotrimazole (Canesten AF) or miconazole (Daktarin) from the pharmacy without a prescription. Provide a script if wanted. Improve concordance: discuss how to use the cream and advise use of the cream for a further two weeks after the symptoms have settled.

- Address the patient's ideas: Mr RS believes that terbinafine is obtained from the GP. Discuss seeking advice from the pharmacist and buying creams without a script. Mr RS also believes that blood glucometer readings of 6 to 7 are fine. Discuss his blood results and the importance of arranging a glucose tolerance test.
- Address the patient's concerns: Mr RS is concerned about the itchiness. Discuss the use of an antifungal containing hydrocortisone (such as Daktarin HC) for seven days.
- Link your health promotion to Mr RS's concerns about spreading the infection to family members. Discuss that spread between people can occur but most people have the immunity to deal with fungal infection. Socks do not protect against spread. In fact, not wearing socks at home is more beneficial to him. Discuss why some people, such as diabetics, are more likely to develop fungal infection.
- Address the patient's expectations: negotiate with the patient – provide a script for an antifungal and arrange the glucose tolerance test.
- Discuss whether Mr RS is happy with the arrangements and confirm his understanding of the glucose tolerance test.

Interpersonal skills

Good communication with the patient explores:
- his agenda – which is to get an effective cream; however, the medical agenda may be to get effective treatment for his athlete's foot, which includes arranging a glucose tolerance test. To do this, the doctor finds common ground with the patient and works in partnership with him. This may be achieved by asking what the surgery could do to help Mr RS to make an appointment. Should we send him a reminder, or shall we wait until his annual leave?
- preferences for treatment – Mr RS may want terbinafine cream, which the doctor may prescribe. However, by discussing over-the-counter alternatives and seeking advice from a pharmacist, the doctor has demonstrated that he has taken steps to enhance the patient's autonomy and alter his future health-seeking behaviour.

Additional information

Heneghan C, et al. (2006) Prevention of diabetes. *BMJ*, **333**: 764–765.

Two strategies currently exist for reducing the onset of diabetes – lifestyle interventions and drugs.

Lifestyle interventions
- Delivered over 2.8 years reduced the incidence of diabetes by 58%.

- However, these interventions are labour intensive – one study needed 16 one-to-one sessions delivered by case managers to achieve target weight reduction and exercise levels. Although lifestyle interventions produce successful results in research settings, they are difficult to replicate even in well-funded healthcare systems.

Drugs

Preventing diabetes with drugs, but are we medicalising a lifestyle issue?

- One study found a 31% reduction in the incidence of diabetes with **metformin** at 2.8 years.
- In people with obesity **orlistat** has been shown to reduce the risk of diabetes by 37% when compared with placebo.
- The **DREAM** trial, which cost £13 m, studied 5269 people over 30 years with impaired fasting glucose or impaired glucose tolerance, or both, and no previous cardiovascular disease. Subjects were randomized to receive either **rosiglitazone 8 mg daily** or placebo, or ramipril 15 mg daily or placebo. The primary outcome was a composite of incidence of diabetes or death over a three year median follow-up period. The trial was well executed. At the end of the study 306 (**11.6%**) of the patients taking rosiglitazone developed diabetes compared with 686 (**26%**) of those given placebo (hazard ratio 0.40, 95% confidence interval 0.35 to 0.46, $P < 0.0001$). Ramipril did not reduce the risk of diabetes. A key question that remains is whether rosiglitazone prevents the onset of type II diabetes or merely lowers blood sugar concentrations in patients with new onset diabetes.

Relevant literature

For patient information on athlete's foot, see:
    http://www.privatehealth.co.uk/diseases/skin-disorders/athletes-foot and
    http://www.netdoctor.co.uk/diseases/facts/athletesfoot.htm.
For medical patient information on athlete's foot, see:
    http://dermnetnz.org/fungal/tinea-pedis.html.

Appendix: Patient summary

Name	RS
Date of birth (Age)	46
Social and Family History	Married, four children
Medical history	
Active problems:	Snores (2.4.2007)
Significant past:	[V] Hypertension screening (2.2.2004)
Family history	FH: Diabetes mellitus,
	FH: hypercholosterolaemia,
	FH: cardiovascular disease,
	FH: hypertension, No FH: CVA/ stroke
Current medication	None
Values	
BP:	131/81 (three months ago)
O/E Height:	180 cm (11.5.2005)
O/E Weight:	82 kg (11.5.2005)
Body Mass Index:	BMI 25.3 (11.5.2005)
Blood glucose:	6.6 mmol/l (2.2.2004)

Test your knowledge

Answer true (T) or false (F) for each of the following statements.
Regarding retinal screening for diabetics:
1. direct ophthalmoscopy is acceptable
2. retinal screening using a digital camera is not possible in patients with cataracts
3. should occur at least once every 2 years

UKPDS has:
4. emphasised the importance (in diabetics) of achieving optimal blood pressure and blood glucose levels from the time of diagnosis
5. shown that in diabetics who are overweight (body mass index >25 kg/m^2) sulphonylureas may be particularly advantageous
6. observed the non-progressive nature of Type 2 diabetes, for example, people taking tablets seldom need to increase the dose, add other tablets or commence insulin treatment
7. shown that the additional cost of medication to improve blood pressure levels was not recouped by a reduced cost of hospital admissions

Case 21 – Migraine

Mr JE is a 22 year old man who presents asking for his migraine prophylaxis to be changed. He was prescribed amitriptyline 25 mg at night.

Targeted history taking

- Describe the migraine. What tablets does he use for treatment of the acute attacks?
- Where is the pain? Elicit intensity, aggravating and relieving factors.
- What is the frequency of the attacks without medication?
- What activities does the migraine limit?
- For how long has he been on amitriptyline? Does he have side-effects? Why does he want to change medication?
- Do the side effects interfere with his work and home life? How?
- Were other prophylactic treatment discussed with him?
- What are his expectations of this consultation: discussion about alternatives, an immediate change in medication, or referral to a neurologist?
- What is his general health like – does he have asthma?

Data gathering

Listed below is the additional information elicited from the patient with appropriate questioning.

- Mr JE has had migraine for two years. He gets a one-sided, intensely painful headache (*'like someone sticking a knife through my upper teeth into my eye socket'*), without warning (no aura). He needs to take his sumatriptan tablets immediately.
- Usually, he also needs to sleep and finds it difficult to continue working with the headache. His describes nausea, vomiting and photophobia. The migraine can occur at any time. If he hasn't eaten, is slightly dehydrated and working hard, he is more likely to have an attack.
- During the last semester at university, where he is studying aeronautical engineering, the attacks became frequent, almost weekly. It was difficult to attend lectures and to study. He almost lost his part-time job as a barman.
- He has been on amitriptyline for one month. It gives him a dry mouth and an increased appetite. He has put on 4 kg.
- He believes the amitriptyline has made him drowsy; studying and paying attention in class is difficult. His girlfriend complained that he was either studying or sleeping.
- Alternative prophylactic tablets were not discussed. His mum told him about feverfew but his research on the internet led him to believe that there is little evidence to support its use in migraine prophylaxis.

- He has an important examination in six weeks. He wants new tablets that prevent the migraine attacks but something that does not make him tired and drowsy.
- He has mild asthma, worse with a cold. He only uses his salbutamol inhaler when he has a cold or is in contact with cats.

Targeted examination

- Neurological examination between attacks is normal.

Clinical management

- Empathize with Mr JE: the migraines are severe, are adversely affecting his life, and are important to treat.
- Check that he uses his acute treatment appropriately.
- Discuss the side effects of amitriptyline and establish that these are definitely unacceptable to him.
- Establish the aims of treatment: to reduce the frequency of the attacks and the impact of the migraines on his life. However, the best that may be achieved with prophylaxis is a 50% reduction in frequency of the attacks.
- In view of his asthma, beta-blockers are contraindicated.
- Discuss second line migraine prophylaxis, such as sodium valproate 300–1000 mg twice daily or topiramate 25 mg once daily to 50 mg twice daily. *If you are not familiar with these drugs, use the BNF on your desk to check doses and contraindications.*
- Discuss discontinuing the amitriptyline and initiating the 2nd line drugs.
- Address the patient's ideas: that his symptoms are side effects of amitriptyline; and that there is no evidence for feverfew as a prophylactic treatment for migraine.
- Address the patient's concerns: that without migraine prophylaxis, the pending examination will provoke frequent attacks.
- Address his expectations: to discontinue amitriptyline and be prescribed evidence-based treatment.
- Safety-net: describe when and why he should next consult.

Interpersonal skills

Good communication with the patient:
- explores and empathizes with the adverse impact of the migraines, and amitriptyline, on the patient's life
- identifies key clinical clues, such as asthma being a contraindication to the prescription of beta-blockers
- responds to the patient's preferences for alternative medication, acknowledging the stress of impending exams

- discusses medication options and encourages concordance – works in partnership with the patient
- provides explanations that are relevant and understandable to the patient

Additional information

Fuller G, Kaye C. (2007) Headaches. *BMJ*, **334**: 254–256.
- Migraine can occur with or without an aura. A typical aura lasts from five to sixty minutes before the headache starts. It consists of transient visual, sensory, and speech disturbances. Visual symptoms are the most common manifestation of an aura and consist of flickering lights, spots or lines, or blind spots.
- Patients should continue taking prophylactic drugs that they find effective for at least four to six months. They should then withdraw these over two to three weeks to see whether the drugs are still necessary.
- First line drugs are beta-blockers and amitriptyline.
- Second line choices are sodium valproate and topiramate. Topiramate has recently been licensed for migraine prophylaxis; a dose of 100 mg a day is effective and well tolerated.
- Gabapentin is a third line prophylaxis.

Relevant literature

For diagnostic criteria and management guidelines, see:
    http://www.bash.org.uk/, in particular, consult:
    http://216.25.100.131/upload/NS_BASH/BASH_guidelines_2007.pdf.

Test your knowledge

A 21 year old, at her contraceptive pill check, gives a history of episodic headache. The last headache occurred 2 weeks ago. It lasted 6 hours, was unilateral, pulsating, and so intense she felt it was like hitting her head against a wall. Answer true (T) or false (F) for each of the following statements.
1. Three attacks of the above headache, with nausea, vomiting, photophobia or phonophobia meet the diagnostic criteria for migraine without aura
2. If she describes blurred vision or 'spots' preceding the development of the headache, this is diagnostic of migraine with aura
3. If she describes a jagged crescent in her vision preceding the development of the headache, this is diagnostic of migraine with aura
4. If she describes motor weakness in one arm preceding the development of the headache, this does not require specialist referral
5. Headaches lasting 1–2 hours, and described as unilateral pressure extending from the neck to the head, getting worse over the day, sound like tension-type headache rather than migraine

Case 22 – Non-accidental overdose

Mrs FM is a 38 year old woman who presents asking for a sick note for work. She says the hospital gave her a note for one week and advised her to see the doctor thereafter. She was admitted to hospital last week following an overdose and was discharged the next day. See Appendix for further details.

Targeted history taking

- Ask for further information regarding the circumstances of the overdose.
- Particularly, ask whether she was alone when she overdosed; did she time it such that she was unlikely to be found; whether she took precautions against being rescued; if she called anybody after taking the overdose; whether she wrote a suicide note or made any final plans?
- Was this an impulsive or premeditated act?
- How does she feel about the overdose now?
- Also enquire as to her feelings before the overdose – was she sad for most of the time?
- Does she feel hopeless about the future?
- Was this the first time she has tried to harm herself?
- Does she still think about harming herself?
- Were there any events that precipitated the act?
- What are her social circumstances: who lives with her at home and what job does she do?
- What advice did the hospital give? Has follow-up been arranged?
- What are her expectations of this consultation: a sick note, referral to the practice counsellor or psychiatry or alcohol services, discussion on recent overdose?
- Are there any on-going general health problems that need to be managed?

Data gathering

Listed below is the additional information elicited from the patient with appropriate questioning.

- Mrs FM took three overdoses last week. The admission to hospital occurred following the last overdose. The first overdose involved ten paracetamol; the second seven coproxamol; and the third involved a combination of twenty citalopram and fifteen ibuprofen. She took the third overdose after she dropped off her child at school.
- She took the tablets with vodka in the woods and sat there intending to die. Her husband, who does not routinely telephone her during the day, happened to call her on her mobile. When she told him she'd taken pills, he called for an ambulance and came to the woods to find her. She hadn't written a note or willed gifts to people.
- Although she wanted to die at the time, she thinks she acted impulsively. She used tablets that were in the house at the time.

- She is not sure how she feels about it. She is glad she did not die. Since the overdose, she has been able to talk more openly with her husband. They have discussed the stresses in her life over the past year: her dad being ill with end-stage heart failure; the stress that working with the elderly produces in her; and coping with a child who has behavioural difficulties.
- She has been sad for six months. She twice saw another doctor at the practice for help with her depression and alcohol problems. She was started on citalopram five weeks ago. When reviewed two weeks ago, things had seemed better. She is adamant that she does not wish to join AA having attended and disliked her first meeting.
- She is not hopeless about the future, just sad about the pain her father is in.
- She does not think about harming herself but she worries about how easy it felt for her to take the overdoses last week.
- Nothing precipitated last week's overdose. It was the accumulation of the on-going stresses.
- She lives at home with her husband and 6-year-old daughter. She works part-time in a care home for the elderly and is due back at work tomorrow.
- The hospital encouraged her to attend AA and she has an appointment with the specialist community addictions service in three weeks.
- She would like a sick note please and a script for citalopram.
- She does not have any on-going general health problems.

Targeted examination

- A mental state examination and assessment of suicide risk is required.

Clinical management

- It is important to form a good relationship with the patient. A trusting and comfortable relationship is required for disclosure of her history and feelings.
- Assess her suicide risk. The most widely used scales for assessing suicide risk are Pierce's Suicidal Intention Scale and Beck's Suicidal Intention Scale.
- Assess her support networks.
- Clarify what support the family is receiving with respect to her 6 year old daughter's behavioural problems. Are the daughter's problems related to her mother's alcohol dependency? Clarify whether there are any child protection issues here.
- Address the patient's ideas: that she lacks control over the current events in her life and the feelings she has. Consider asking her what needs to happen in her life for her to feel in control again. This may open up issues with which she can be helped.
- Address the patient's concerns: that she found it so easy to act on a fleeting impulse. Ask her what else she could do to prevent these impulses – she may identify that if she were not under the influence of alcohol she would be less impulsive. Ask her what else she could do if these impulses recurred; who could she phone? Does she have the telephone numbers readily available?

- Address the patient's expectations: for a sick note and a script for citalopram. It may be useful to ask the patient if time away from work increases her social isolation, or would the return to work expose her to further stress. With regard to medication, a script for a one-week supply is usually given.
- Arrange follow-up either in surgery or by telephone. Usually patients at low risk of suicide need review in a week; high-risk patients require referral to the mental health team.

Interpersonal skills

Good communication with the patient acknowledges her despair, perceived losses and daily difficulties. The doctor helps her to deal with her sense of hopelessness and lack of control by providing empathic support – he helps her to establish new and accessible goals. While exploring the impact of her actions on her life, the doctor focuses on working out daily problems rather than achieving psychological insight. Negotiation regarding the sick note, request for further medication and follow-up is undertaken in a sensitive and considerate manner. Non-judgemental clarification of all issues surrounding her daughter maintain the parent's trust and confidence while demonstrating an holistic, family-oriented approach, aimed at ensuring the entire family receive appropriate support.

Additional information

Foster T (2001) Dying for a drink: Global suicide prevention should focus more on alcohol use disorders. *BMJ*, **323**: 817–818.
- There is a strong link between alcohol use disorders and suicide. Many studies report a high prevalence of alcohol use disorders among people who successfully committed suicide – for example, 56% in New York, 43% in Northern Ireland, and 34% in Madras. The lifetime risk of suicide is 7% for alcohol dependence.
- Alcohol increases risk-taking behaviour. The biological explanation may be that alcohol affects serotonin neurons in the brain stem and reduces serotonin transporter function in the prefrontal cortex, both of which may decrease protection against suicidal impulses.
- Global suicide prevention strategies should include:
  - a focus on alcohol use disorders in terms of prevention
  - brief intervention by adequately trained and supported non-specialist staff, including in primary care
  - availability of multidisciplinary specialist alcohol services
  - aggressive treatment of co-morbid depression

Pfaff JP and Almeida OP (2005) Detecting suicidal ideation in older patients: identifying risk factors within the general practice setting. *Br J Gen Pract*, **55**: 269–273.
- Most GPs experience the death of a patient through suicide every 5 years.
- An average of six patients on a GP's list will deliberately self-harm each year.
- Patients who are experiencing suicidal ideation are three times more likely to have visited a GP in the last month compared with those without such thoughts.

Relevant literature

For guidance on detecting and treating suicidal patients in primary care, see:
http://www.gp-training.net/training/clinical/suicide.pdf.
NICE (2005) Youth suicide prevention. See:
http://www.nice.org.uk/page.aspx?o=503368. For information on preventing
suicide in teenagers, see table 6, page 45.

Appendix: Patient summary

Name	FM
Date of birth (Age)	38
Social and Family History	Married, one child
Past medical history	Alcohol problem
	Low mood

The medical record of her **last consultation** in surgery two weeks ago reads:

'Cut down drinking to weekends and two days per week. No problems at work or with family. Citalopram helped and feeling better. Still getting a few low days. Plan: continue citalopram for a further four months. Review in six to eight weeks.'

Current medication	Citalopram 20 mg once daily
Blood tests	Blood tests done two years ago
full blood count	normal
liver function tests	normal
BP	134/84

Summary of the A&E letter from last week:
- *'Overdose of paracetamol and salicylates.*
- *Alcohol involvement: suspected.*
- *Psychoactive drug involvement: no / information not available.*
- *Investigation: biochemistry, ECG, haematology.*
- *Treatment: parvolex and fluids.*
- *Repeat bloods normal.*
- *Assessed by psychiatry. Discharged – follow-up by GP.'*

Test your knowledge

Answer true (T) or false (F) for each of the following statements regarding deliberate self harm in teenagers.

1. The physical severity of the self-harm is a good indicator of suicidal intent
2. Telling other people beforehand about thoughts of suicide is a feature of high suicidal intent
3. Teaching problem-solving techniques is not helpful
4. If depression is present, cognitive behaviour therapy and fluoxetine are effective treatments
5. Problem-solving therapy starts with achieving psychological insight

Case 23 – Hernia

Mr TW is a 72 year old man who presents with a pain in his lower abdomen. He says 'I think I have a hernia, doc'. According to the computer record, he does not have any chronic diseases and does not take regular prescribed medication.

Targeted history taking

- What are his symptoms?
- When did the symptoms develop? Were there any precipitating events?
- Are there times when the symptoms are worse or better?
- Does he have any risk factors for the development of a hernia, such as heavy lifting, chronic coughing, constipation or obesity?
- Are his symptoms affecting any activities – work, hobbies, or social activities?
- What does he know about hernias and their treatment?
- What are his expectations of this consultation: advice, referral for surgery?
- Is he fit for surgery? Does he have any other problems with his health? What medication does he take?

Data gathering

Listed below is the additional information elicited from the patient with appropriate questioning.

- Mr TW feels a pain in his left groin, like a dull ache, 'a dragging feeling'. Sometimes he thinks he feels a lump in the mid-inguinal area but he is not sure.
- He felt a sudden pain in his left groin region three weeks ago. He thought he hurt a muscle while doing some building work in his garden.
- He has not noticed worsening or improvement of the inguinal discomfort with any particular activities. The discomfort sometimes radiates into his scrotum.
- He does not usually do manual labour. Three weeks ago, he helped build a garden wall. He does not have a chronic cough or suffer from constipation. Bowel movements are regular.
- He has not exerted himself recently because he is afraid he may make things worse. He stopped 'heavy' gardening.
- He knows that hernias are treated surgically, sometimes with a mesh.
- He expects you to confirm whether or not he has a hernia – he is not sure if he has felt a definite lump. If you think that he has a hernia, he would like a referral. He says his son is getting married in Papua New Guinea in six weeks. He and his wife had planned a four month trip to Papua New Guinea

and New Zealand. If he has the surgery done soon, will he be fit to fly? If not, can he safely wait for the surgery until his return? Should he wear a truss?
- He is in good health, walks two miles daily, and is not taking any regular medication.

Targeted examination

- Seek consent.
- Examine his abdomen for any masses.
- Examine his abdomen for an inguinal hernia, which is done more easily with the patient standing. If a lump is present, observe, palpate, percuss, and trans-illuminate.
- Assess the position, tenderness, shape, size, consistency and temperature of any lumps.
- Examine the opposite side.

In this case, assume that you are unable to detect a lump on clinical examination.

Clinical management

- Explain to Mr TW that the history is suggestive of a direct inguinal hernia. Doubt exists as to whether the hernia is present or not. Mr TW could 'wait and see' or he could be investigated further with herniography or ultrasound scanning.
- Address the patient's ideas: he suspects he has a hernia and hernias are treated surgically. Discuss the advantages and disadvantages of the different treatment options if he does indeed have an inguinal hernia: no treatment, surgical repair, or a truss. Conservative management is usually for elderly patient who are symptom free. However, hernias do not correct themselves and may deteriorate or complicate (strangulate or obstruct) with time. Surgery can be either open or laparoscopic. Provided the patient is fit and has adequate social care, surgery may be performed as a day case. Trusses may control symptoms but there is little evidence that they can prevent complications.
- Address the patient's concerns: he would like to visit his son without experiencing medical problems overseas. If he does have a hernia, chances are it is a small, direct inguinal hernia. Investigation and treatment can probably wait until he returns from his trip.
- Address the patient's expectations: he probably expects you to examine him to confirm whether or not he has a hernia, and to advise him about his options.
- If Mr TW asks for further information about local waiting times, trusses or complications, be prepared to answer his queries.
- Safety-net: outline what Mr TW should do if complications occur, or if the symptoms resolve completely.

Interpersonal skills

Good communication with the patient:
- estimates the likelihood of the diagnosis from the history
- balances the history with the negative examination findings
- explores the patient's health beliefs – that hernias usually require surgery
- negotiates further investigations, and the timings of possible referrals, taking into account the patient's plans and wishes
- provides sufficient information to the patient to enable the patient to make a decision

Therefore, the shared management plan is respectful of the patient's autonomy.

Additional information

BMJUpdates (2006) Inguinal hernia repair improves patients' general health compared with watchful waiting. *BMJ*, **333**.

The research question asked was 'should asymptomatic inguinal hernias be repaired?' The answer is 'possibly'. Surgery improves the general health of patients, without increasing the risk of long-term pain. However, the sample size was small and further research is required.

The original research came from **Fitzgibbons RJ** *et al.* (2006) Watchful Waiting vs Repair of Inguinal Hernia in Minimally Symptomatic Men. *JAMA*, **295**: 285–292.

Relevant literature

To refresh your technique on how to examine for hernias, see:
    http://medicine.ucsd.edu/clinicalmed/genital.htm.
For a discussion on hernia treatment options, see:
    http://hcna.radcliffe-oxford.com/hernia.htm.
For a discussion on investigations for hernia, see:
    http://www.rcsed.ac.uk/journal/vol44_6/4460026.htm.

Test your knowledge

Answer true (T) or false (F) for each of the following statements, regarding *paediatric* scrotal lumps.
1. If asymptomatic, bilateral and bluish in appearance, they are most likely inguinal hernias
2. Inguinal hernias are virtually all direct and often complete (that is, the sac comes all the way to the scrotum)
3. Inguinal hernias in uncomplicated cases are treated by a surgical herniotomy within 2 or 3 weeks of diagnosis
4. If the lump becomes tender, the infant starts to vomit and refuses to feed, treatment with antibiotics is indicated
5. If hydroceles persist beyond 2 or 3 weeks of diagnosis, they require an operation for the processus to be ligated

Case 24 – Osteoarthritis

Mr MO is a 78 year old man with longstanding osteoarthritis (OA) of both knees. He comes to see you for a repeat prescription. According to your records, he was issued 90 tablets of co-codamol 8/500 and 100 tablets of diclofenac E/C 50 mg three months ago; he had collected his monthly re-issue of his co-codamol over the last two months. See Appendix for further details.

Targeted history taking

- What medication is Mr MO taking?
- Does he know why he takes each drug? Does he still need them? Is the dose appropriate? Has he tried non-pharmacological treatments? *(Need)*
- When does he take his tablets?' Does he have any problems taking the tablets? Do the tablets work? What treatments has he tried in the past that didn't seem helpful? *(Open questions)*
- Are his symptoms adequately controlled? *(Tests and monitoring)*
- Have the guidelines, evidence base, or access to services for the management of his condition changed since his prescription was initiated? *(Evidence and guidelines)*
- Does he have any side effects? Is he taking alternative medications or over-the-counter preparations? Check for interactions. *(Adverse events)*
- Does the pain disturb sleep? Does his pain put him at risk in the activities he undertakes? Do the tablets reduce this risk? *(Risk reduction or prevention)*
- Can the treatment be simplified? *(Switches and simplification)*
- What are his expectations of this consultation: re-issuing of medication, changing the medication regime, a discussion on analgesia, or a referral to physiotherapy?
- What is his general health like – does he have asthma or indigestion?
- Are there any other issues he would like to discuss?

Data gathering

Listed below is the additional information elicited from the patient with appropriate questioning.
- Mr MO takes the white tablets and the little brown tablets. *'Its on my record doc.'* According to his records, he was issued 90 tablets of co-codamol 8/500 per month and 100 tablets of diclofenac E/C 50 mg three months ago.
- He takes the white tablets for pain. The brown tablets are anti-inflammatories. If he forgets to take them, his knees stiffen and hurt. He doesn't take them as prescribed – he only needs one co-codamol three times per day and the diclofenac when he has a bad day. He rubs topical *Deep Heat*

into his knees and, if they are stiff in the morning, he uses a heat pad. He does the exercises the physiotherapist gave him but not as regularly as he should.

- He takes his tablets after each meal and the diclofenac before bed. They are easy to swallow. He tried taking ibuprofen in the past but his daughter who is a healthcare assistant told him that diclofenac is stronger. He thinks they work better than ibuprofen.
- His tablets control his pain. He can't tackle the hills like he used to, and to travel distances, he cycles rather than walks. He doesn't want to take more tablets in case his body gets used to them.
- Mr MO attended physiotherapy and has been discharged from their care. He saw the consultant but he wasn't too keen on surgery. He has reduced his activities to suit the pain.
- He sometimes gets constipated. He takes lactulose. The doctor prescribed a large bottle of lactulose six months ago and he still has some left. Someone told him about willow bark and copper bracelets, but before he invests in them, he'd like your opinion please.
- The pain does not interrupt his sleep. If he has a very active day, he takes the diclofenac, which helps. Getting into and out of the bath is not a problem. He occasionally helps his son with odd-jobs but no longer kneels for long periods or works with ladders.
- He is very happy on his medication and would like you to re-issue the tablets. He is going to Scotland to stay with his daughter and asks for 200 of each tablet to be issued.
- He is in good health. His eyesight is much better after his cataract operation last year.

Targeted examination

- An examination may not be required unless the patient mentions specific side effects.
- Consider checking his BMI – obesity is a risk factor for OA of the knees.

Clinical management

- Discuss the benefits of taking regular paracetamol, which can be as effective as co-codamol 8/500 without causing constipation. Paracetamol is also safe and cheap.
- Discuss the degenerative nature of OA. There may be a small amount of inflammation in OA. The pain relief provided by the diclofenac may be due to its analgesic properties rather than its anti-inflammatory effect. Mr MO may be one of the 40% who do not respond to one NSAID, such as ibuprofen, but respond well to another, such as diclofenac (*BNF*).
- Long-term non-steroidals are no better than placebo for pain relief. However, a two-week course should be considered for the short-term treatment of 'flares' (Bjordal *et al.*, 2004).

- Consider topical NSAIDs, which are also effective for short-term pain relief.
- *Deep Heat* may act by counter-irritation where the knee pain is relieved by irritation to the skin. Capsaicin is an alternative.
- Discuss compliance with exercises and the importance of remaining active. Obesity puts extra strain on joints. Discuss non-weight-bearing exercise such as cycling and swimming.
- Discuss the non-pharmacological management of constipation.
- Address the patient's ideas: alternative medications for OA may be helpful. As regards alternative medicine:
  - there are been no or few trials, as in the case of willow bark or copper bracelets, so effectiveness is not tested
  - trials are difficult to design, as in acupuntucre
  - trials have been done, and the cod liver oil, glucosamine and chondroitin sulphate tested are shown not to be particularly beneficial; on the other hand, they are also not particularly harmful
- Address the patient's concerns: that his body will develop tolerance to the analgesia. OA is a chronic, progressive condition – most patients deteriorate but up to one-third can actually improve (Linsell *et al.*, 2005). It may not be a case of tablets becoming ineffective, rather the disease progressing such that other treatments, like surgery, become more beneficial.
- Address the patient's expectations: he would like a script for 200 diclofenac and co-codamol. Explain the NHS guidance that a prescriber writes a prescription that does not exceed a maximum quantity of 30 days supply for tablets. Negotiate the script with the patient.
- Take steps to encourage concordance.

Interpersonal skills

Good interaction and communication with the patient:
- explores his current understanding and use of the prescribed medication
- acknowledges his decisions and respects his autonomy
- empowers the patient to adopt self-treatment and coping strategies where possible
- explores his health beliefs and preferences (alternative medication) in a sensitive and informed manner
- negotiates and develops a shared plan with the patient, for example, provides two scripts, each for one month of medication

Additional information

Lewis T. (2004) Using the NO TEARS tool for medication review. *StudentBMJ*, **12**: 349–392.

The **NO TEARS** tool for medication review:
- **N**eed and indication
- **O**pen questions
- **T**ests and monitoring
- **E**vidence and guidelines
- **A**dverse events
- **R**isk reduction or prevention
- **S**implification and switches

Hunter DJ, Felson DT. (2006) Osteoarthritis. *BMJ*, **332**: 639–642.
- Laboratory findings are expected to be normal – it is a non-inflammatory arthritis.
- The clinical features of osteoarthritis are joint pain with activity, transient stiffness in the morning or after rest, reduced range of motion, joint crepitus or periarticular tenderness, and bony swelling.
- Glucosamine and chondroitin seem to have the same benefit as placebo, and there is controversy over whether they also have structure-modifying benefits.

Bjordal JM, *et al.* (2004) Non-steroidal anti-inflammatory drugs, including cyclo-oxygenase-2 inhibitors, in osteoarthritic knee pain: meta-analysis of randomised placebo controlled trials. *BMJ*, **329**: 1317.
- NSAIDs can reduce short term pain in osteoarthritis of the knee slightly better than placebo, but the current analysis does not support long term use of NSAIDs for this condition.
- As serious adverse effects are associated with oral NSAIDs, only limited use can be recommended.

Relevant literature

Linsell L, *et al.* (2005) Population survey comparing older adults with hip versus knee pain in Primary Care. *Br J Gen Pract*, **55**: 192–198.
For information on prescribing for the older patient, see:
http://www.npc.co.uk/MeReC_Bulletins/2000Volumes/pdfs/vol11n10.pdf.
For information on NO TEARS, see:
http://student.bmj.com/issues/04/10/education/362.php.

Appendix: Patient summary

Name	MO
Date of birth (Age)	78
Social and Family History	Married, four adult children
Past medical history	OA both knees for 12 years
Current medication	Co-codamol 8/500 four times daily/as required
	Diclofenac E/C 50 mg three times daily/as required
Blood tests	Blood tests done two years ago
full blood count	no abnormality detected
BP	108/74

Summary of orthopaedic consultant's letter (dated six months ago):
'Unfortunately this man's X-ray confirms moderate to severe OA of both knees. Currently he is mobile without walking aids and is only able to walk 20 minutes before resting. He remains active and is not experiencing any side-effects with medication. He is still driving. He remains sceptical about the longevity of the knee replacements and seems particularly worried about MRSA. I have not arranged routine follow-up but will be happy to see him when he is ready to consider surgery.'

Test your knowledge

Answer true (T) or false (F) for each of the following statements, with regard to the literature on the treatment of osteoarthritis.

1. A meta-analysis (1996) confirmed a significant beneficial effect of education on joint pain but not on disability
2. In patients with osteoarthritis of the knee, controlled studies have shown that regular telephone contact from a healthcare worker does not produce significant improvement in functional status
3. The two main approaches used by physiotherapists are muscle strengthening programmes specific for certain joints and general anaerobic conditioning
4. The use of acupuncture is supported by case series and uncontrolled studies
5. Trials that have compared random needling with acupuncture show measurable benefit for true acupuncture
6. Capsaicin, a naturally occurring compound, does not have significantly greater analgesic effects than placebo

Case 25 – Request for cosmetic surgery

Mr LW, a 21 year old man, consults you requesting referral for a nose reduction. He gives a history of fracturing his nose one year ago and having it straightened, but immediately re-injuring it. He says that since this second injury his nose has had a hump on it. He is very conscious of the hump and would like to have a straight nose again. See Appendix for further details.

Targeted history taking

- Explore his description of how his nose has changed shape.
- Assess whether he has any nasal passage compromise.
- For how long has he been conscious of the shape of his nose? Has anything happened or been said to cause this?
- Assess whether he is experiencing any psychological effects.
- Has he any past history of anxieties about his appearance?
- What is his job?
- Enquire about his physical health and whether he has any other symptoms.
- Enquire about his lifestyle and social life.
- Does he smoke or drink?
- What does he hope to gain from this consultation – your opinion or a referral?

Data gathering

Listed below is the additional information elicited from the patient with appropriate questioning.
- Since the second injury he reports that there is a bump on his nose.
- He can breathe easily through his nose.
- He has been conscious of the bump for about 6 months. He feels like everyone he talks to looks at it. He says that two of his work colleagues have commented on it – he says this confirms his feeling that it is very evident.
- He has talked about it to his mother. She says he 'still looks beautiful' to her! However, she has said that if it is really worrying him he should 'get it done'.
- He is very self-conscious about his appearance now. He used to enjoy going out clubbing, but now he will not go – 'who wants to talk to Mr Bentnose? What's the point?'. At this point you should explore whether anything else has happened to affect his self-confidence – why has he stopped socialising; is it entirely due to his nose?
- He has no past history of anxiety or self-image problems.
- He is an engineer. His appearance is not important to his job.
- He is in good health and enjoys football and going to the gym.
- He does not smoke. He used to drink heavily when he went out at weekends, but since stopping this, his alcohol consumption has reduced considerably.
- He would like to be referred to a plastic surgeon for a nose reduction.

Targeted examination

This falls into two parts:
1. Assessment of his nose:
   - examine the shape of his nose from front, side and from above, looking for asymmetry
   - examine his nasal passages for deviation of nasal septum or damage to the nasal septum
2. Assessment of his mental state
   - any evidence of depression, anxiety state, OCD, body dysmorphic disorder?

In this case – there is a very slight bump on one side of his nose, but you struggle to identify this. He is distressed, but not depressed.

Clinical management

- Discuss examination findings – minimal visible deformity, but this seems to be causing him disproportionate distress.
- Address patient's ideas: that everyone he meets immediately looks at his nose.
- Explore the benefits of surgery – would having an operation improve his self-confidence or are there other factors involved?
- Address patient's expectations: he expects a referral.
- Agree a management plan:
  - is a plastic surgery referral in his best interests?
  - do local guidelines for cosmetic surgery require a psychiatric assessment to confirm psychological distress?
  - is he eligible for NHS treatment?
  - would he benefit from counselling or exploration of why he has lost his confidence, whether he has an operation or not?

Interpersonal skills

Good communication with the patient enables:
- exploration of physical, psychological and social issues
- the patient to gain insight into reasons for his loss of confidence and whether an operation will benefit him
- reassurance of the patient following a focussed examination
- exploration of the patient's agenda: a plastic surgery referral
- exploration of the patient's health beliefs: an operation will result in a return of his self-confidence
- safety-net: what can be done if the operation does not have the desired effect

Good communication should incorporate:
- empathy and understanding
- support for the patient
- being non-judgemental

Additional information

This case requires sensitive exploration of the patient's anxieties and beliefs in a supportive and non-judgemental manner. The decision about whether to refer for surgery or whether there is an underlying psychological problem will be based on the doctor's assessment of the patient's mental health. Body dysmorphic disorder is believed to affect at least 1% of the UK population. It is more common in people with a history of depression and/or social phobia – and it usually starts in adolescence when people are most sensitive about their appearance. Minimal physical examination is required, and so the emphasis in this case is on interpersonal skills.

Phillips KA, Castle DJ. (2001) Body dysmorphic disorder in men. *BMJ*, **323**: 1015–1016.
- An American study reported that the percentage of men dissatisfied with their overall appearance (43%) has nearly tripled in the past 25 years and that nearly as many men as women are unhappy with how they look.
- The more severe form – body dysmorphic disorder (BDD) or dysmorphophobia – is relatively common but is poorly recognized. It affects men and women in equal numbers.
- People with BDD are excessively worried about an imagined or slight defect in appearance that result in clinically significant distress or impairment in functioning.
- Patients with BDD often present to non-psychiatric physicians, with reported rates of 12% in dermatology clinics and 7–15% in cosmetic surgery clinics.
- The most common preoccupations among male BDD patients involve their skin (e.g. acne or scarring), hair (thinning), nose (size or shape), or genitals.
- Male patients tend to exhibit time-consuming or repetitive behaviours such as mirror-checking, comparing themselves with others, and excessive grooming.
- Muscle dysmorphia is a form of BDD in which males think their bodies are puny when they tend to be excessively muscular. Social pressure for boys and men to be large and muscular is thought to be a contributory factor.
- The cause of BDD is unknown and probably multifactorial (genetic, neurobiological, evolutionary, and psychological).
- When it is recognized, treatment with CBT and serotonin re-uptake inhibitors has been shown to be effective.
- However, most men receive dermatological or surgical rather than psychiatric treatments. Outcomes of such treatments tend to be poor.
- Some patients become severely depressed and suicidal.
- People with BDD may not be able to hold down a job and may avoid socialising. They may find it difficult to have relationships.
- It is recommended that patients are educated about the disorder and psychiatric treatment options. Cosmetic procedures are probably best avoided while simply trying to talk patients out of their concern is usually futile.

Dufresne RG, Phillips KA, Vittorio CC, Wilkel CS. (2001) A screening questionnaire for body dysmorphic disorder in a cosmetic dermatologic surgery practice. *Dermatol Surg*, **27**: 457–462.
- The self-report questionnaire had a sensitivity of 100% and a specificity of 93%.

Relevant literature

Useful information for patients about plastic surgery including aesthetic surgery can be obtained from:
British Association of Plastic Surgeons (http://www.baps.co.uk).
The American Society of Plastic Surgeons website has some information for medical professionals as well as patients:
Plastic Surgery Information Service (http://www.plasticsurgery.org).

Appendix: Patient summary

Name	LW
Date of birth (Age)	21
Social and Family History	Single
Past medical history	Nothing of note
Recent reports	Last seen within practice 5 years ago with painful knee
	Letter from A&E 12 months ago: '*Punched. Fractured nasal bones. Referred ENT 7 days*'.
	Letter from ENT 10 months ago: '*Operative reduction fractured nasal bones 1 month ago. Bruising and swelling have now resolved. He is happy with the cosmetic result*'.
	Letter from A&E 10 months ago: '*Recent nose op. Hit on nose by football. Nose swollen. Fracture on XR. Refer ENT*'.
	Letter from ENT 9 months ago: '*Re-injured nose. There is minimal displacement. I do not feel further operative treatment is indicated at this time*'.
Current medication	None
Investigations	No information

Test your knowledge

Answer true (T) or false (F) for each of the following statements.
1. A simple nasal bone fracture is diagnosed clinically
2. Routine radiography of the nasal bones in a suspected simple nasal bone fracture is necessary
3. Trauma to the bridge of the nose, resulting in a nasoethmoid fracture, presents with persistent epistaxis or cerebrospinal fluid rhinorrhoea, or both
4. Plain radiographs can exclude nasoethmoid fractures
5. Delay radiology of a clinically suspected maxillofacial injury until an inebriated patient is more cooperative

Case 26 – Insomnia

DH is 25 year old temporary resident whose parents are registered with the practice. DH is on two-week leave from the Royal Air Force. He presents saying he would like some sleeping tablets please because he has had difficulty sleeping since his return from an overseas deployment two weeks ago.

Targeted history taking

- Clarify the nature of the sleep problem – is he experiencing difficulty in initiating or maintaining sleep, or is the sleep not refreshing? Is the problem affecting daytime mood or functioning?
- For how long has he had difficulty sleeping?
- What does he do or think about when unable to sleep?
- What does he think might be causing the problems with sleep: are there underlying medical, pharmacological or psychiatric issues?
- Medical causes: is his waking due to pain, cough, urinary frequency, sweats or itchiness?
- Pharmacological: could medication (e.g. corticosteroids), alcohol or coffee be affecting his sleep?
- Psychological: could anxiety, depression, post-traumatic stress disorder (PTSD), nightmares, or worry about not sleeping be affecting his sleep? Or does he have bad habits, such as sleeping during the day, or sleeping in an environment not conducive to relaxation? Has his routine changed?
- What has he already tried to improve his sleep?
- What are his expectations of this consultation: advice, a drug prescription, a second opinion (if he has already seen an RAF doctor), or psychological interventions?
- What is his general health like – has he had anxiety or addiction problems in the past?

Data gathering

Listed below is the additional information elicited from the patient with appropriate questioning.
- It takes DH an hour to fall off to sleep. Once asleep, he wakes up regularly throughout the early hours of the morning. It takes him up to an hour to get back to sleep. He feels mentally and physically tired throughout the day.
- He has had problems sleeping for two weeks, since his return from an overseas deployment. While overseas, he slept in shared accommodation with three other people. On returning home, he sleeps alone in a quiet and dark environment.

- He thinks about being back on deployment. He found the deployment, his first since joining up, difficult and he is not sure if being an aircraft engineer with the RAF is the career for him. He has only completed two of the nine years for which he has joined up.
- While overseas, there was an accident on the airfield. One of the helicopters landed awkwardly and slid towards the hangar in which he worked. He was not endangered. There was some slight damage to the aircraft but nobody was hurt. He does not experience nightmares or recurrent, intrusive thoughts about the incident.
- He does not have underlying medical or pharmacological issues that could be affecting his sleep.
- He tried drinking a 'bottle or two' of beer each night to help him sleep.
- He usually runs 3 miles daily but hasn't been doing much exercise on leave.
- He would like some sleeping tablets to help him sleep. However, if you prescribe these, he needs a note because the RAF sometimes do random drug testing and he could get into trouble if they find evidence of the sleeping tablets in his urine sample.
- He does not have a past history of anxiety or addiction problems.

Targeted examination

- Consider screening for anxiety and depression, perhaps using the hospital anxiety and depression (HAD) scale available on http://www.alanpriest. f2s.com/HAD2.htm, or the patient health questionnaire (PHQ 9), available on http://www.pfizer.com/pfizer/download/do/phq-9.pdf.
- If depressed, assess suicide risk.

Clinical management

- Discuss the diagnosis of insomnia and its probable causes. There is little to suggest PTSD. A good explanation can be reassuring.
- Address the stress: ask him what needs to happen for him make a decision about his career. To whom, in the RAF, could he speak about issues? From whom could he seek support while deciding? Encourage the patient to formulate an action plan.
- Discuss sleep hygiene measures, such as:
  ○ stimulus control, e.g. the use of the bedroom for sleep and sex only
  ○ temporal control, e.g. wake up at a specified time each morning and avoid daytime napping, no matter how tired
  ○ sleep restriction, e.g. curtail the amount of time spent in bed to the desired sleeping hours, such as 11pm to 6am
- Suggest lifestyle changes: reduce heavy night-time meals and alcohol. Increase daytime exercise.
- Discuss when drug treatments are indicated.

- If you decide to prescribe, discuss options: benzodiazepines, the newer hypnotic drugs (e.g. zopiclone), or sedative antidepressants. Negotiate the number of tablets prescribed, usually for less than one week.
- Address his expectation of a letter for the RAF drug-testing unit: explain that a copy of the medical record of this consultation will be sent to his RAF doctor. Should he test positive, the RAF doctor can check to see if the drug you prescribe is responsible for the positive urine test. Reassure him that this is unlikely to occur with the tablets you prescribe. A further note for the drug-testing unit may not be required.

Interpersonal skills

By dealing sensitively and responsibly with the patient's job stress, insomnia and concerns over drug testing within the context of his occupational contract with the RAF, the doctor demonstrates his ability to adopt a person-centred approach. The challenge here is negotiating decisions with patients who may have expectations the doctor is unwilling to meet. By exploring issues with the patient, clarifying what is and is not possible, and highlighting issues that will require the patient's further attention, the doctor empowers the patient.

Additional information

Insomnia
Buscemi N et al. (2006) Efficacy and safety of exogenous melatonin for secondary sleep disorders and sleep disorders accompanying sleep restriction: meta-analysis. *BMJ*, **332:** 385–393.
- A sleep disorder exists whenever a lower quality of sleep leads to impaired functioning or excessive sleepiness.
- Sleep disorders have a negative impact on quality of life, safety, productivity, and use of healthcare.
- Secondary sleep disorders are sleep problems that are associated with medical, neurological, or substance misuse disorders.
- Complementary and alternative medicine has been used increasingly to manage sleep disorders. One of the most popular treatments of this type is melatonin, a hormone that is secreted by the pineal gland and is linked to the circadian rhythm.
- There is no evidence that melatonin is effective in treating secondary sleep disorders such as jet lag or shiftwork. Melatonin seems safe with short-term use.

Glass J et al. (2005) Sedative hypnotics in older people with insomnia: meta-analysis of risks and benefits. *BMJ*, **331:** 1169.
- Benzodiazepines and the newer Z-drugs are effective for sleep disturbances in elderly people. However, there are risks associated with their use, such as ataxia, cognitive effects, and falls.

- In people over 60, the benefits associated with sedative use are marginal and are outweighed by the risks, particularly if patients are at high risk for falls or cognitive impairment.
- The number needed to treat for improved sleep quality was 13 and the number needed to harm for any adverse event was 6. This ratio indicates that an adverse event is more than twice as likely as enhanced quality of sleep.

Holbrook AM. (2000) The diagnosis and management of insomnia in clinical practice: a practical evidence based approach. *Canadian Medical Association Journal*, **162:** 216–220. See: http://www.pubmedcentral.nih.gov/picrender. fcgi?artid=1232275andblobtype=pdf.

NICE (2004) The newer hypnotic drugs. http://www.nice.org.uk/TA077.

Post-traumatic stress disorder
Bisson JI. (2007) Post-traumatic stress disorder. *BMJ*, **334:** 789–793.
Characteristic symptoms of post-traumatic stress disorder (adapted from DSM-IV):
- at least one of the re-experiencing phenomena
- at least three of the avoidance and numbing symptoms
- at least two of the increased arousal symptoms, such as difficulty sleeping, irritability or outbursts of anger, difficulty concentrating, hypervigilance, or an exaggerated startle response

For further information on PTSD, see: http://www.rcpsych.ac.uk/mentalhealth information/mentalhealthproblems/posttraumaticstressdisorder.aspx.

Test your knowledge

Answer true (T) or false (F) for each of the following statements, with regard to PTSD.
1. It arises from incomplete cognitive processing of the trauma
2. Intrusive nightmares and memory 'flashbacks' are symptoms and signs of hyperarousal
3. Anything reminiscent of the trauma is avoided
4. It is associated with decreased secretion of corticotrophin-releasing factor and hypocortisolaemia
5. There is evidence from randomised placebo-controlled trials of selective serotonin re-uptake inhibitors showing substantial benefit on core symptoms

Case 27 – Emergency contraception

Miss JD is a 27 year old woman who presents to your Monday morning surgery requesting emergency contraception (EC). See Appendix below for her summary details.

Targeted history taking

- Why does she believe EC is needed?
- What contraception does she usually take?
- How many pills has she not taken?
- When did the unprotected intercourse occur?
- How important is it for her not to become pregnant?
- Does she have any contraindications to progestogen-only EC or to the IUD? Has she had previous ectopic pregnancies or pelvic infection?
- Does she have valvular heart disease or any illness requiring prophylactic antibiotics?
- Is she at risk of sexually transmitted disease? Did the unprotected intercourse occur within a long-term relationship?
- What does she intend to do for long term contraception? If she does not want to start a family in the next year, has she considered long-acting contraception, such as the implant, injectables or intra-uterine devices?

Data gathering

Listed below is the additional information elicited from the patient with appropriate questioning.

- JD was away on a course last week and forgot to pack her progestogen-only contraception. She didn't take last week's tablets, from Monday to Thursday. She restarted once she got home on Friday night. On the Thursday night, she had intercourse with a colleague she met on the course. She thinks the condom slipped. She also had intercourse with her long-term male partner, without a condom, on Sunday morning.
- She has been on Cerazette, progestogen-only contraception, since 2005.
- She missed four pills last week.
- Unprotected intercourse probably occurred last Thursday night and definitely occurred on Sunday morning.
- JD is adamant that now is not the right time for her to become pregnant. She couldn't cope with a pregnancy.
- JD has not had any previous pregnancies or pelvic infection. She was treated for genital warts eight years ago.
- She does not have valvular heart disease. Her general health is good.

- She does not know the colleague she met at the course and could be at risk of an STD.
- She does not intend to have a family in the next year because she intends to concentrate on establishing her career. Her mum uses a Mirena IUS and is quite happy with it.

Targeted examination

- Is not needed. Arrange a follow-up appointment for cervical swabs, with or without an IUD insertion.

Clinical management

- Discuss with JD that she was very likely to have had unprotected sex last Thursday, that is, more than 72 hours ago. By restarting the Cerazette on Friday night, she was not protected for 48 hours, that is, until Sunday night. Hence, she also had unprotected sex on Sunday morning. She requires EC.
- Discuss her options: progestogen-only EC is licensed for use within 72 hours of the unprotected sex, with an efficacy rate at 72 hours of 58%. The copper IUD is indicated for presentation with 5 days (120 hours) and is 99% effective. As she has no contraindications to the copper IUD, one should be fitted as soon as possible, under antibiotic cover.
- Address the patient's (possible) ideas: she may only have known about progestogen-only EC (commonly called Levonelle, containing levonorgestrel 1.5 mg as a single dose). She may not have known that the copper IUD can be used effectively for up to 5 days.
- Address the patient's (possible) concerns: regarding the insertion of a copper IUD given a past history of genital warts; the possible need for antibiotics; whether swabs should be taken; or the efficacy of Levonelle if taken at 82 hours.
- Address the patient's (possible) expectations: for an out-of-licence prescription of progestogen-only EC (Levonelle); or for a Mirena IUS to be inserted – Mirena is not used for EC.
- Consider briefly discussing long-acting contraceptive alternatives and provide leaflets.
- Negotiate a treatment plan and make adequate follow-up arrangements.

Interpersonal skills

Good communication with the patient:
- elicits the patient's concerns regarding an unwanted pregnancy
- empathizes with her dilemma
- is respectful and non-judgemental
- explains the options clearly and acknowledges the patient's concerns
- respects her treatment preferences

- makes clear to the patient how the doctor's values or skills impact on arranging her treatment

Additional information

CKS Topic Review (2007) Contraception – emergency. See:
http://cks.library.nhs.uk/contraception_emergency/view_whole_topic_review

When a woman requests emergency contraception, **assess** the woman's:
- current risk for pregnancy
- need for future contraception
- risk for sexually transmitted infection
- risk for having had non-consensual sexual intercourse
- vulnerability

Discuss the different **methods of emergency contraception**, namely levonorgestrel or a copper IUD. The woman should make the final choice.
- Levonorgestrel is licensed for use up to 72 hours (3 days), and is recommended for use up to 120 hours (5 days), after unprotected sexual intercourse. Inform the woman that the effectiveness of levonorgestrel diminishes rapidly with delay in using it. Pharmacists will not provide levonorgestrel without a prescription if the time since unprotected sexual intercourse is more than 72 hours.
- An IUD containing at least 380 mm^2 of copper is the most effective method. It can be inserted up to 5 days after unprotected intercourse or, if the timing of ovulation can be estimated, up to 5 days after ovulation.

Follow up and aftercare
- Less than 6% of women vomit after taking levonorgestrel. If this happens within 2 hours of taking the drug, the woman should repeat the dose as soon as possible.
- Some women have light bleeding or spotting after taking levonorgestrel.
- No contraceptive method is perfect. If pregnancy is suspected (e.g. the next menstruation is abnormally late or light), the woman should have a pregnancy test.

Guidance from the Faculty of Family Planning
FFPRHC (2006) Emergency contraception. *Journal of Family Planning and Reproductive Health Care*, **32:** 121–128. See: http://www.ffprhc.org.uk/admin/uploads/449_EmergencyContraceptionCEUguidance.pdf.

Appendix: Patient summary

Name	JD
Date of birth (Age)	27
Social and Family History	Divorced, no children
Past medical history	Focal migraines on combined pills (2005)
Current medication	Cerazette, as directed.
Values	Tests done three months ago
BMI	27
BP	114/64
Smear	Normal

Test your knowledge

ET is a 30 year old woman with regular periods. Answer true (T) or false (F) for each of the following statements about her.

1. If starting the combined oral contraceptive (COC), extra precautions need to be taken for the first 7 days if started on the 6th day of her period
2. If starting on the 2nd day of her period, extra precautions need to be taken for the first 7 days
3. If she misses day 12 of her pill pack (Microgynon), and takes two pills on day 13, she needs emergency contraception if she had unprotected sexual intercourse (UPSI) on day 12
4. If she misses day 3 of her pill pack (Microgynon), and takes two pills on day 4, she needs emergency contraception if she had UPSI on day 3.
5. If she misses day 20 of her pill pack (Microgynon), and takes two pills on day 21, she needs to run pill packs together and not have a pill-free week, if she had UPSI on day 20

Case 28 – Bariatric surgery

Mrs RE is a 45 year old diabetic lady. She usually attends surgery one month after her annual hospital diabetic review for her repeat prescription (see Appendix for full details). When she consults today, she is quite upset with the diabetic consultant, Dr Wong.

Targeted history taking

- Why is Mrs RE consulting today?
- What specifically about Dr Wong has upset her – was it what he said or the manner in which he said it?
- What concerns her about the consultant's conduct? In other words, what would she like to see changed?
- What would she like to do about her feelings? Are her actions likely to benefit her or other patients? What specifically does she expect you to do?
- Would she like help in addressing her weight issues? What did she have in mind?
- What treatments has she tried? Were these beneficial?
- What are her expectations of this consultation: a medication review, resolution of the emotions generated by Dr Wong; or help with her weight?
- Besides diabetes, does she have any other health problems?

Data gathering

Listed below is the additional information elicited from the patient with appropriate questioning.

- Mrs RE is seeing you for her repeat prescription, but during the consultation it becomes evident that she is very angry at the perceived rudeness of the diabetic consultant.
- She usually sees Dr Anderson but on this occasion saw Dr Wong. She prefers *'nice Dr Anderson'*. Dr Wong's bluntness upset her – he does not understand how difficult it is to lose weight, especially with the avandmet tablets making her hungry. She is concerned that Dr Wong's rudeness may be upsetting other patients as well and *'someone should tell him he can't get away with behaviour like this'*. She expects you to advise her on the best course of action to take with respect to Dr Wong.
- She would love to lose weight. She would like to discuss bariatric surgery with you. She read that stomach stapling is quite effective.
- She has tried Weight Watchers, orlistat, sibutramine, exercise prescription programmes, and she has seen a dietician and a cognitive behaviour therapist. She loses weight but puts it back on. Twice, she has lost more than

30 kg, but within a year has returned to her pre-diet BMI. Diets end up making her feel depressed and food becomes her main focus.

- She expects you to advise her on resolving her anger with the diabetologist, to issue her repeat prescriptions, and give her information on bariatric surgery.
- She does not have other medical problems, and is generally fit for anaesthesia and surgery.

Targeted examination

- Weight, if appropriate.

Clinical management

- Acknowledge and respect Mrs RE's feelings.
- Consider signposting her to the Patient Advice and Liaison Service (PALS – http://www.pals.nhs.uk/), where trained staff will listen to her feedback and help her to resolve her concerns about the NHS.
- Encourage Mrs RE to provide her feedback to the hospital. Your intention, like hers, is to stimulate an awareness of the issues, and a reflection on events. If there are lessons to be learnt, then these will be identified and addressed.
- Demonstrate knowledge of the complaints procedure. Remember that you are not there to judge whether Mrs RE is right or wrong in her complaint. Your role is to clarify her options and assist her in the course she chooses. However, you may want to discuss whether in the long term, expending energy on pursuing a complaint is something she really wants to do. Would her energy be better spent on other things? Remind Mrs RE that her health is your primary concern.
- Discuss whether Mrs RE qualifies for surgery (using NICE criteria):
  - diabetic with BMI >38
  - she has exhausted all medical options, namely orlistat, sibutramine, CBT, dietary support and exercise prescription
  - she has no contraindications to bariatric surgery
  - she is aware of the risks of surgery
- Consider providing written information about specialized hospital obesity clinic and surgery. Give Mrs RE time to weigh the risks and benefits of surgery and to deliberate on her options. Make follow-up arrangements to confirm her decisions.

Interpersonal skills

Good communication with the patient:
- sets priorities – deals with anger towards the consultant and addresses obesity; the challenge here is establish that the diabetes is well controlled and to move on to the true presenting problems

- deals with the presenting problems making effective use of the doctor–patient therapeutic alliance – empathizes, but also reminds Mrs RE of her priorities and goals

In dealing with the complaint, repeat prescription, and obesity, the doctor has demonstrated an ability to explore multiple issues, both acute and chronic.

The doctor:
- adopts a person-centred approach and works in partnership with the patient – gives her the options, discusses with her the risks and benefits of each option, and allows her to reach her own decisions
- reconciles the health needs of the individual patient and the health needs of the community, balancing these with available resources – tactfully discusses bariatric surgery and its availability locally

Additional information

Kral JG. (2006) ABC of obesity: Management: Part III—Surgery. *BMJ*, **333**: 900–903.
- Bariatric surgery can prevent the progression of obesity towards diabetes, congestive heart failure, liver cirrhosis, and hypertension.
- Obesity surgery entails a trade-off between chronic diseases associated with obesity and the side effects and complications of surgery. Most obese adults who have chosen surgery and had complications (including death) have been satisfied with their choice because their lives as obese individuals were often not worth living.
- Indications for surgery are:
  - a body mass index (BMI) of ≥40 or 35–40 with obesity-related co-morbidity
  - patients should have seriously tried to lose weight by other means
  - candidates do not have behavioural conditions (such as borderline personality disorder) that are likely to interfere with postoperative care
  - age criteria are usually a minimum of 20–25 years and a maximum of 60–65

NICE (2006) Obesity: the prevention, identification, assessment and management of overweight and obesity in adults and children. See: http://www.nice.org.uk/guidance/CG43.

Test your knowledge

Mrs FW speaks to the receptionist advising her that she (Mrs FW) wishes to make a complaint about the practice nurse. Answer true (T) or false (F) for each of the following statements.

1. The receptionist should give Mrs FW written information about the practice's complaints procedures
2. The receptionist should refer Mrs FW to the practice nurse to discuss the issue informally
3. The written complaint should normally be acknowledged within five working days
4. An explanation should normally be provided within 14 working days
5. The practice should keep a record of the complaint, its investigation and outcome
6. A record should also be kept in the patient's medical records
7. The complaints administrator should disassociate herself from the practice nurse while investigating the complaint
8. Mrs FW and the practice nurse should be reassured that only those who need to know will learn of the complaint

Case 29 – Multiple sclerosis

Mrs YC is a 43 year old lady with multiple sclerosis (MS), which was diagnosed three years ago in Oxford. She moved to your practice area six months ago and saw the local neurologist recently (see Appendix for full details). Mrs YC presents today with urinary difficulties.

Targeted history taking

- What exactly is the problem with urination: frequency, urgency, dysuria, nocturia, incontinence?
- For how long has she had the problem?
- Are there aggravating and relieving factors?
- Are there bowel problems, particularly faecal incontinence?
- Is sensation in the genitalia and perineum altered?
- Does the problem affect her home or work life? How?
- What does she think is causing the problem?
- What treatments has she tried already?
- Has she seen the MS nurses or physiotherapist recently and are they aware of the problem?
- What are her expectations of this consultation: further investigation, medication, a discussion regarding her options?
- What is her general health like: are her usual MS symptoms well controlled?

Data gathering

Listed below is the additional information elicited from the patient with appropriate questioning.

- Mrs YC has a problem with urgency and frequency. She is unable to feel her bladder filling until the very last moment. Then, she feels she has to go immediately or will wet herself. She is losing confidence.
- She has had the problem for four months but it seems to be getting worse. She read about pads and mattress protectors on the MS Trust website and has obtained some from the MS nurse.
- Coffee aggravates the problem and, to reduce night-time waking, she no longer drinks fluids after 8pm.
- She has good control over bowel function. There have not been any episodes of faecal incontinence.
- Sensation in the genital and perineal area is unaltered.
- She usually copes with going to the toilet every two hours and by using pads. In familiar environments, she knows where the toilets are, so usually the urge incontinence is manageable. However, this weekend she is attending an out of town wedding – she would like not to be embarrassed by incontinence or be worried about smelling of urine.

- She thinks the problems are due to her MS – she looked on the internet for information.
- She expects you to treat a urine infection if one is present and would like medication to keep her dry during the wedding.
- Her usual MS symptoms are well controlled.

Targeted examination

- Perform a dipstix examination of the urine. The patient has thoughtfully brought a urine sample, if you ask. *For this case, assume urinary dipstix is negative for blood, leucocytes and nitrites.*
- A neurological examination of the perineum may not be indicated.

Clinical management

- Discuss urge incontinence as a common problem in MS – 87% of MS patients have bladder problems; 70% say it has a moderate to severe adverse effect on their lives (MS Trust, 2007).
- Reassure the patient that urinary symptoms can be treated; there are several options.
- Outline that a post-void residual bladder volume measurement using ultrasound scanning is needed – make arrangements for this, perhaps by referring to the MS nurses.
- Address the patient's ideas: MS or a UTI may be causing her urinary symptoms.
- Address the patient's concerns: that her urgency and frequency will result in an embarrassing situation at the wedding.
- Address the patient's expectations: for medication to be prescribed today because the wedding she wishes to attend occurs this weekend.
- Discuss medication options: anti-cholinergics such as oxybutynin or tolterodine, or desmopressin. If you prescribe, take steps to encourage concordance by explaining how the drug works and how to take the drug. If you are unable to remember the details, check the *BNF* on your desk.
- Consider physiotherapy options for long-term benefit: pelvic floor exercises +/– electrical stimulation of the pelvic floor.
- Make arrangements for follow-up: perhaps to review medication, or to arrange referral to physiotherapy, or to review with bladder diary.

Interpersonal skills

Good communication with the patient:
- explores her symptoms – are these the symptoms and signs of MS or a UTI
- explores her health beliefs and is considerate of the information she obtained from the internet

Multiple sclerosis

- establishes her preferences for treatment – negotiates medication and referrals
- explores her understanding of the diagnosis and treatment plan offered – a good 'handover' occurs (Neighbour, 2005)
- negotiates follow-up – 'safety nets'

Therefore, once the patient's ideas, concerns and expectations have been elicited, and the clinical priorities negotiated, the management plan is developed in true partnership with the patient.

Additional information

Murray TJ. (2006) Clinical review: Diagnosis and treatment of multiple sclerosis. *BMJ*, **332:** 525–527.
Disease-modifying drugs moderately reduce the number and severity of attacks, the number of new lesions on magnetic resonance imaging, and progression. In relapsing-remitting multiple sclerosis, early therapy has better outcomes. Late therapy when there are no relapses has doubtful benefit.

Marcus R. (2007) Should you tell patients about beneficial treatments that they cannot have? Yes. *BMJ*, **334:** 826.
- Depriving a patient of such knowledge deprives him of choice. If patients are empowered by knowledge, they can lobby government or appeal to a local or wider community for financial support. They may also wish to spend their own money on treatment.
- Many doctors are salaried employees of the state and hence have a supposed dual loyalty – to their patients and to their employer. Do doctors owe a primary duty to the state or the patient?
- Marcus argues that the doctor, as the patient's advocate, betrays his patient's trust if he does not inform him about beneficial treatments he cannot have.

Physiotherapy for urinary problems in MS
http://www.mstrust.org.uk/publications/wayahead/08012004_03.jsp

Treatments options for urinary problems in MS
http://www.msrc.co.uk/index.cfm?fuseaction=showandpageid=751
http://www.mstrust.org.uk/publications/factsheets/bladder.jsp

Relevant literature

Neighbour R. (2005) *The Inner Consultation*. Radcliffe Medical Press, Oxford.

Appendix: New patient summary

Name	YC
Date of birth (Age)	43
Social and Family History	Married, two children
Past medical history	Multiple sclerosis. Demyelination seen on MRI in 2004
	Relapsing and remitting course since original presentation with diplopia
Current medication	None
Blood tests	Blood tests done eight months ago
Lupus anticoagulant screen	not detected
Prothrombin time	11.2 sec (10–14)
Thrombin time	9.4 sec (11–14)
INR	0.9
TSH	5.46
BP	108/74

Summary of neurologist's letter from last month:

'Unfortunately this lady's MRI scan has shown multi periventricular subcortical white matter lesions with a lesion in the right cervical hemi cord C2–C5 and lower dorsal hemi cord T9 T10 consistent with demyelination. Currently she is mobile with some right arm and leg weakness and she finds that stamina is a problem and that she is only able to walk 20 minutes before the right leg starts to drag. She is still driving when she is up to it. I have arranged to see her once more in four months' time and I will refer her to the MS nurses and send her some literature concerning MS.'

Test your knowledge

Answer true (T) or false (F) for each of the following statements about Mr FG who developed MS at the age of 36.

1. Being male is associated with a better prognosis
2. Presenting at the start of the illness with optic neuritis is associated with a better prognosis
3. If Mr FG presents at the start of an acute disabling relapse, methylprednisilone (500 mg orally daily) for 3–5 days can hasten recovery
4. If Mr FG presents at the start of an acute disabling relapse, methylprednisilone (500 mg orally daily) for 3–5 days can shorten the long-term course of the illness
5. Baclofen, an anti-inflammatory, should be reduced over several weeks because abrupt withdrawal may provoke seizures
6. Musculoskeletal pain may be treated with gabapentin, amitriptyline or carbamazepine

Case 30 – Balance problems

Mrs YC is a 43 year old lady with multiple sclerosis (MS), which was diagnosed in Oxford three years ago. She presents today complaining of 'my balance is shot', aching more and recent home stresses. Her computer record does not indicate any sickness absence since she joined your practice six months ago. See Appendix for further details.

Targeted history taking

- How have her symptoms changed and over what period?
- What does she think has caused the change?
- What job does she do?
- Who lives with her?
- How have her symptoms affected her home and work life?
- Is her sleep disturbed? What activities are limited?
- Enquire about what she means by 'my balance is shot', taking care to exclude transverse myelitis – weakness and sensory loss in both legs with loss of control of bowels and bladder.
- What are the home stresses and how are these affecting her?
- What treatments has she tried already?
- What are her expectations of this consultation: time off work, further investigation, a change in medication?
- What is her general health like – does she have other on-going medical problems?

Data gathering

Listed below is the additional information elicited from the patient with appropriate questioning.

- Mrs YC says her balance gets worse sometimes. She starts to walk like a 'drunken sailor'. Then after a few days, it improves spontaneously. The balance worsened four days ago, for no particular reason. The backs of her legs ache, probably because she has been sitting more over the last four days.
- She thinks the change in weather may have caused a change in symptoms. Also, she is worried about her 19 year old daughter who has returned to live at home until she finds a new job. Mrs YC works thirty hours per week at a local supermarket. The company is good to her and provides her with clerical or till work if her mobility is affected.
- She lives with her husband, her 15 year old son and now her 19 year old daughter.
- Due to her balance difficulties, she is not confident in moving hot pots around the stove or showering if someone else is not at home, in case she

falls. Currently, juggling home life to meet work commitments is difficult. She feels clumsy and unsure at work, and is worried about losing her balance and having accidents in front of customers.

- Her sleep is disturbed mainly because she is worried about her daughter. The poor sleep and tiredness add to her balance difficulties and she is afraid of falling. She does not feel depressed, just worried.
- Further questioning on 'my balance is shot' elicits a history of walking like a 'drunken sailor', as if the floor below her is rolling. She does not have vertigo or loss of power or altered sensation in the legs. The desomopressin helps with urinary frequency and she has good bowel control.
- The company for which her daughter worked closed suddenly after declaring bankruptcy and the staff were laid off without the last month's pay. Jobs in this area are difficult to find and she would like to see her daughter be self-sufficient and independent.
- She rested over the weekend. She spent time reading and napping when the family went out. She felt she had more energy and less anxiety after the rest.
- She would like some time off work just until her balance improves and she gets her confidence back. She is due to see the physiotherapist next week.
- She does not have other on-going problems requiring attention at present.

Targeted examination

- In view of her balance difficulties, it may be useful to examine for nystagmus, diploplia, Rhomberg's sign, and to conduct a heel–shin test.
- Observe her gait, heel-to-toe walking and finger-to-nose testing – is there intentional tremor?
- Based on her history (lower limb weakness and sensory problems are not reported), a brief neurological examination of her lower limbs may not be required.
- Please note that a full neurological examination is not required. The examination should be focussed so that any significant pathology responsible for 'a drunken gait' is unlikely to be missed.
- *In this case, assume that the examination findings are unremarkable.*

Clinical management

- Discuss the examination findings.
- Discuss the natural history of relapses and remissions in MS.
- Reassure the patient that, in view of her spontaneous recovery from balance problems in the past, further investigation such as imaging is not required. Negotiate the use of time as a diagnostic tool.
- Address the patient's ideas: she believes that her relapse may be due to 'stress' or a change in the weather.
- Address the patient's concerns about falling and her loss of confidence.

- Encourage her to continue with her daily activities and exercises in a paced manner to maintain strength and endurance.
- Address the patient's concerns about falling at work and needing time off. Negotiate time off and discuss strategies to maintain confidence. A question such as 'when your balance plays up, what else could you do to improve your confidence? Could using your stick help?' opens the discussion.
- Discuss whether she intends to discuss strategies for improving balance and mobility with the physiotherapist next week.

Interpersonal skills

Good communication with the patient:
- explores the possible physical, psychological and social issues affecting her presentation today
- reassures the patient following a focussed examination
- negotiates the use of time as a diagnostic tool
- addresses the social factors (daughter moving back into the family home) in the management plan

Therefore, a shared management plan incorporates strategies for dealing with 'stress at home', by exploring possible lifestyle changes, such as:
- taking time off work or making time for herself
- consciously considering how she would like to interact with her daughter
- possibly seeking support from her husband
- perhaps considering a change in her working hours

Additional information

Murray TJ. (2006) Clinical review: Diagnosis and treatment of multiple sclerosis . *BMJ*, **332:** 525–527.

Classification of MS
- 85% of patients have relapsing-remitting MS: the first attack is categorised as clinically isolated syndrome.
- thereafter, there are episodic relapses and remissions, partial or complete.
- 15% of patients present with slowly progressive pattern called primary progressive multiple sclerosis.

Treatment
- Bladder frequency and urgency often responds to oxybutynin.
- Pain and spasms from spastic limbs usually respond to baclofen.
- Tricyclic antidepressants are useful for treating emotional lability with pathological laughing or crying.
- Amantadine reduces fatigue in half the patients.
- Pain, sexual dysfunction, weakness, dysesthesia, tremor, ataxia, and cognitive change are more difficult to treat.
- 50% of patients will become depressed and may require treatment.

Appendix: Patient summary

Name	YC
Date of birth (Age)	43
Social and Family History	Married, two children
Past medical history	Multiple sclerosis. Demyelination seen on MRI in 2004
	Relapsing and remitting course since original presentation in 2003 with diplopia
Current medication	Desmopressin 200 µg at night
Blood tests	Blood tests done nine months ago
Lupus anticoagulant screen	not detected
Prothrombin time	11.2 sec (10–14)
Thrombin time	9.4 sec (11–14)
INR	0.9
TSH	5.46
BP	108/74

Physiotherapy report from last practice (dated seven months ago):
- Lower limb examination
  - right hip flexion 3/5
  - non-specific lower limb paraesthesia
  - rest of neurology – no abnormality detected

Notes from last consultation one month ago:
New patient, moved into practice area six months ago. Refer today to local neurologist, MS nurses, and physiotherapist. Reports recent eye check at optician was fine. Active problems:
- nocturia (takes desmopressin 200 µg at night, to good effect)
- reduced power in the right hip and after 20 minutes of walking, drags her right leg – uses a cane

Test your knowledge

Answer true (T) or false (F) for each of the following statements.
1. A sudden onset of decreased vision and soreness when moving the eye suggest central vein occlusion
2. In a 70 year old, presentation with a sudden, severe loss of central vision suggests optic neuritis
3. In a 70 year old, presentation with a sudden, painless and complete loss of vision in one eye suggests central artery occlusion
4. In a 70 year old, a history of a film that grows on the eye causing double or blurred images suggests a cataract
5. Dry macular degeneration typically results in a less severe, more gradual loss of vision than wet macular degeneration.

Case 31 – Tonsillitis

Mrs PC is a 37 year old woman who consults infrequently. She presents complaining of having a headache, feeling unwell, feverish and tired. See Appendix for summary details.

Targeted history taking

- What are her current symptoms?
- For how long has she had these symptoms?
- Does she have cough, sore throat, urinary symptoms, or diarrhoea and vomiting?
- In what way are the symptoms affecting her home and work life?
- Does the fever disturb sleep?
- What treatments has she tried already?
- Does she have any illnesses or does she take any medication that may be lowering her immunity?
- What does she think is causing her illness?
- Does she have a past history of recurrent infection, or complicated illness? Does she have any particular concerns?
- What are her expectations of this consultation: an examination and reassurance, further investigation, medication, a sick note?
- What is her general health like – is she taking contraception?

Data gathering

Listed below is the additional information elicited from the patient with appropriate questioning.

- She gives a four day history of feeling unwell, having hot and cold temperature spells and feeling very tired. When she feels cold, she shivers and cannot get warm. She has a generalized dull headache. She is so tired, she fell asleep at 8 pm last night and slept right through to the morning. This is very unlike her.
- It started four days ago, at the same time as her daughter's illness. Her 3 year old girl is at nursery and seems to have caught something that is going around nursery.
- She does not have cough, urinary symptoms, or diarrhoea and vomiting. She has a sore throat and thinks her neck glands are swollen. It hurts to swallow but it is not too painful.
- Her husband and au pair are helping at home. She works as a senior administrator and her commute takes 45 minutes. She felt too ill and tired to drive to work today.
- Sleep is unaffected. She has not had feverish dreams or delirium.

- She has tried taking regular paracetamol for the fever, which has helped. She took paracetamol an hour before this consultation.
- She is very rarely ill. She does not have any illnesses, nor does she take any medication that may be lowering her immunity.
- She thinks she has the same viral illness as her daughter and just needs some time at home to recover. However, her sister-in-law had bacterial endocarditis last year which presented as a feverish illness, which she ignored until she became very ill. Now her sister-in-law has a damaged heart valve.
- Mrs PC does not have a history of recurrent sore throats. She just wants to get 'checked out' and for you to confirm she has a self-limiting viral illness.
- She expects to be examined and reassured. She does not want antibiotics; she prefers homeopathic medicines.
- She takes Cileste for contraception and is on day 18 of her pill.

Targeted examination

- Examine the tonsils. *The patient hands you a picture of enlarged, follicular tonsils:*

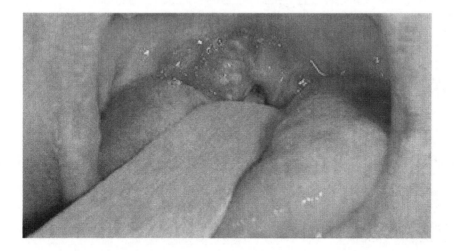

- Assess if cervical lymphadenopathy is present. *Not present.*
- Measure her temperature. *The patient hands you a card with her temperature recorded as 37.8°C.*
- If she looks very ill and possibly septic, measure her pulse and respiratory rate.

Clinical management

- Discuss the difficulty in diagnosing viral versus bacterial tonsillitis. The follicular appearance, the history of fever and malaise point to a bacterial infection.
- Explain that swabs are not routinely indicated in patients whose immunity is not compromised.
- Discuss the Centor criteria, a validated system for grading the severity of sore throats. As Mrs PC has pus, the absence of a cough, tender cervical lymph adenopathy and a history of fever, she has a severe infection according to the Centor criteria. Hence, antibiotics could be prescribed, either today or by issuing a delayed script.
- Address the patient's ideas: she believes she has a self-limiting viral infection. In the absence of near-patient testing, you are unable to confirm or disprove this belief.
- Address the patient's concerns: ignoring an illness at its early stages can result in potentially serious complications. Antibiotics for streptococcal sore throat can reduce the incidence of acute rheumatic fever and glomerulonephritis, both of which are rare in the UK.
- Address the patient's expectations: she prefers homeopathic remedies and would prefer not to take antibiotics. Discuss the use of a delayed script. Safety-net – discuss the symptoms of the best-case and worst-case scenarios and outline what she should do in their eventuality.
- If you do prescribe, consider antipyretic analgesics and/or antibiotics – penicillin V 500 mg (SIGN guidelines) four times daily for ten (10) days, or erythromycin or azithromycin for five (5) days.
- Discuss contraceptive pre-cautions when antibiotics are used. Since Mrs PC is on day 18 of the combined pill, she should run pill packs together, omit the pill-free interval, and use condoms for the duration of the antibiotics, plus an additional seven days.

Interpersonal skills

The candidate demonstrates poor interpersonal skills if he/she:
- does not work through the diagnostic sieve to elicit why the patient is 'feeling unwell and feverish'
- does not inquire sufficiently about the patient's perspective and health understanding – her niggling concern about serious complications from seemingly self-limiting illness
- uses a rigid approach to consulting that is insufficiently responsive to the patient's contribution – launches into a discussion about antibiotics without appreciating the patient's preference for homeopathic medicines
- fails to empower the patient – fails to safety-net

On the other hand, good communication:

- responds to the person's concerns with understanding – discusses the rare complications of bacterial tonsillitis in a sensitive and understandable manner
- backs his or her own judgement appropriately – discusses the Centor criteria and appropriate use of throat swabs
- acts in an open and non-judgemental manner – respects the patient's decision not to have antibiotics but allows for re-consultation or provides a delayed script should symptoms worsen

Additional information

Pichichero ME. (1998) Group A beta-hemolytic streptococcal infections. *Paediatric Review*, **19:** 291–302.

Only about 20–30% of paediatric patients present with classic streptococcal tonsillopharyngitis, which is characterized by:
- an acute onset
- concurrent headache
- stomach ache
- dysphagia

and examination is characterized by:
- intense tonsillopharyngeal erythema
- yellow exudate
- tender/enlarged anterior cervical glands

Treatment
- Penicillin is recommended by the American Academy of Paediatrics and American Heart Association as first-line therapy for GABHS infections; erythromycin is recommended for those allergic to penicillin.
- Treatment duration with penicillin should be 10 days to optimize cure in GABHS infections.
- A five day regimen is advised for azithromycin (a macrolide).
- Prevention of rheumatic fever is the primary objective for antibiotic therapy of GABHS infections.

Relevant literature

MeReC (2003) Antibiotic prescribing and resistance. *MReC Briefing*, **21:** 1–8. See: http://www.npc.co.uk/MeReC_Briefings/2002/briefing_no_21.pdf. Provides details of the Centor criteria.

Appendix: New patient summary

Name	PC
Date of birth (Age)	37
Social and Family History	Married, three children
Past medical history	1993 – traumatic fractured right ankle
Current medication	Cileste one tablet as directed
Clinical values	last seen 3 months ago
BP	124/78
Height	172 cm
Weight	74 kg
BMI	25

Test your knowledge

Answer true (T) or false (F) for each of the following statements.
1. Because of the increased risks associated with other analgesics, paracetamol is the analgesic of choice in sore throat
2. If the sore throat persists, a throat swab to identify group A beta-haemolytic streptococcus (GABHS) is helpful
3. Antibiotic therapy has been shown not to alleviate symptoms in viral sore throats
4. Return to usual activities after tonsillectomy takes on average 2 weeks
5. In children under 16 years, emergency re-admissions within 4 weeks of discharge after tonsillectomy occur in 1 in 20 cases

Case 32 – Menstrual problems

Ms JB is a 27 year old woman who has recently joined your practice. She presents with menstrual problems.

Targeted history taking

- Is she using contraception?
- What menstrual problems is she experiencing and for how long have these symptoms occurred?
- Establish the details of her menstrual cycle – length, number of days of bleeding, regularity, inter-menstrual or post-coital bleeding?
- What investigations has she had in the past and what have these shown?
- What treatments has she tried already? Did they help?
- Has she had problems with fertility?
- In what way do her symptoms impact on her home and work life?
- What are her expectations of this consultation: an exploration of the problem, further investigation, a prescription for medication?
- What is her general health like – are her smears up-to-date?

Data gathering

Listed below is the additional information elicited from the patient with appropriate questioning:

- Ms JB is not using contraception. She stopped taking Marvelon one year ago when her relationship ended.
- Over the last eight months, her periods have become infrequent, her skin has become greasy and she has started to get acne. Most distressing, is the increasing facial hirsutism. Her arms have always been hairy but now her face is getting a fine down along the sides, just below her ears.
- The time between the last two periods was 42 days and this is typical of the last 3 cycles. She bled for 4 days, of which 2 days were heavy. She does not experience inter-menstrual or post-coital bleeding.
- She had a scan when she was 18 years old, which showed ovarian cysts but she is unable to remember the details. The scan was done in Germany; her parents were based there with the Army. She is not sure if she had blood tests.
- Since the age of 18, she has been on contraception, except for when she had her baby 4 years ago. She has tried several different types of pills and has experienced problems with them.
- She did not have difficulty falling pregnant. Fertility is not an issue at present.
- The hair on the arms and face socially embarrasses her. Since her relationship ended, she has not had the confidence to meet new people. She works from home as a freelance graphic designer.
- She expects you to address the problems of her hirsutism, acne and oligomenorrhoea. She does not have much confidence in oral contraceptives. She vaguely remembers having break-through bleeding and premenstrual tension on Marvelon, Yasmin and Dianette.

- She does not have other medical problems and her smears are up-to-date.

Targeted examination

- An examination of her face, back and/or forearms may be needed.
- When you ask to examine her back, *the patient produces an image*:

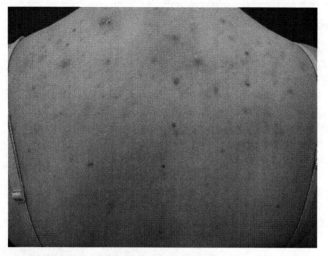

- When you ask her to push her hair back to look at her face, *she shows an image*:

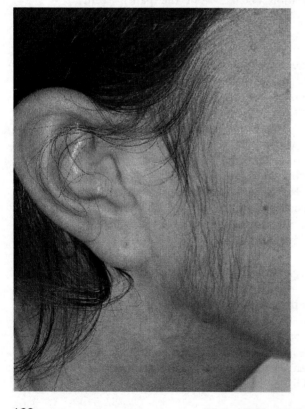

Both images reproduced with permission from the New Zealand Dermatological Society.

- Calculate BMI – *26*
- Measure BP – *118/72*

Clinical management

- Discuss the possibility of polycystic ovarian syndrome (PCOS) and your reasons for suspecting this.
- Outline the tests you would like to perform (LH, FSH, prolactin, testosterone, oestriol, fasting glucose and cholesterol. Renal and kidney function could also be tested if therapy with metformin is a possibility). Consider repeating the ultrasound scan. Discuss with Ms JB how these tests would change your management and elicit her views on further investigation.
- Address the patient's ideas: that combined pills are likely to cause PMT and break-through bleeding again. Discuss whether the pill side effects were completely unacceptable or whether it is reasonable to try Dianette or Yasmin again.
- Address the patient's concerns: regarding her hirsutism and reassure that a number of treatment options are available.
- Address the patient's expectations: the best option for treating all three of her problems (acne, hirsutism and oligomenorrhoea) may be the combined pill (Dianette or Yasmin). Other treatment options for hirsutism include spironolactone, eflornithine or cosmetic (laser) treatment. However, while the latter treatments may address the hirsutism, they do not address her menstrual problems.
- Discuss whether she would like a leaflet on PCOS and time in which to decide which option she'd prefer. If she agrees to further investigation, organize these.
- Make follow-up arrangements.

PS. You may not have time in which to discuss, in detail, the patient's ideas, concerns and expectations. You may have to make follow-up arrangements to review Ms JB, perhaps with the results of her blood tests. In which case, you need to advise her that you will address these issues at the later appointment.

Interpersonal skills

Good communication with the patient explores:
- her agenda – understands that the patient wants something done for her acne, hirsutism and oligomenorrhoea, and reassures her that these issues will be addressed
- your agenda – you make explicit to Ms JB why you want to investigate her symptoms further
- negotiates a management plan – prioritizes the order in which investigations and treatment need to be carried out, for example, hormone assays should be taken before initiating the combined pill.

Some candidates may have difficulty in completing this consultation in ten minutes. Good interpersonal skills are required to make the patient feel understood and to propose a staggered management plan to which the patient agrees.

Additional information

Franks S. (1995) Polycystic ovary syndrome. *N Engl J Med*, **333**: 853–861.

Diagnosis is usually made on the basis of a combination of:
- clinical features – oligomenorrhea, hirsutism, acne, androgen-dependent alopecia, with or without obesity
- ultrasonographic features – bilateral ovarian enlargement (>9 cm in maximal diameter), 10 or more follicles 2–10 mm in diameter per ovary, and increased density and area of stroma
- biochemical criteria – elevated serum concentrations of androgens, particularly testosterone and androstenedione and hypersecretion of luteinizing hormone, but with normal or low serum concentrations of follicle-stimulating hormone

The **differential diagnosis**: pituitary or adrenal diseases, for example, hyperprolactinemia, acromegaly, and congenital adrenal hyperplasia.

The **management** encompasses:
- the treatment of hirsutism and anovulation
- the long-term consequences of the syndrome, including the metabolic sequelae

In effect, this means that the majority of patients with the PCOS should be considered for treatment.

Test your knowledge

Answer true (T) or false (F) for each of the following statements, with regard to polycystic ovarian syndrome (PCOS).
1. Screen women with PCOS, at high risk for diabetes, for glucose intolerance (with an oral glucose tolerance test) every 3 years
2. Women with PCOS at high risk of diabetes include:
   (a) women with a body mass index greater than 20 kg/m^2
   (b) South Asian women with a body mass index greater than 25 kg/m^2
   (c) women who have a waist circumference greater than 62 cm
   (d) women over 40 years of age
3. Women with PCOS troubled by facial hirsutism are treated with eflornithine cream (Vaniqa)
4. Evidence suggests an increased risk of ovarian cancer when clomifene is used for 6 to 12 cycles
5. Clinical features of PCOS include truncal obesity, oligo- or amenorrhea, and hirsutism
6. Women with PCOS in middle age have a 50% risk of developing type 2 diabetes
7. Women with PCOS have risk factors for cardiovascular disease (CVD), namely obesity, hypertension, hypoandrogenism and hypoinsulinaemia

8. In women diagnosed as having PCOS before pregnancy, metformin taken throughout pregnancy is not shown to reduce their chances of developing gestational diabetes
9. In amenorrheic women with PCOS, induce a withdrawal bleed every 3–4 months to reduce the risk of endometrial hyperplasia and carcinoma

Case 33 – Irregular heart beats

Mr NM, aged 41, presents saying he has noticed that his heart has been beating irregularly over the last 48 hours. See Appendix for summary details.

Targeted history taking

- What exactly does he mean by an irregular heart beat?
- For how long did the irregularity last? Elicit intensity, aggravating and relieving factors. What, if any, was the effect of exercise on the symptoms?
- Were there associated symptoms?
- Does he have risk factors for cardiac disease? Family history, smoking, high cholesterol, diabetes, or a sedentary lifestyle?
- What job does he do? What is his home life like?
- Is he going through a stressful time at the moment?
- What does he think is the problem and its cause?
- What are his expectations of this consultation: an examination, further investigation, a cardiology referral?
- What is his general health like – how much caffeine does he drink and how much exercise is he getting?

Data gathering

Listed below is the additional information elicited from the patient with appropriate questioning.

- He describes being aware of the forceful beating of his heart. It seems to miss a beat, have a forceful beat and then speed up for a minute or two. When he took his pulse during an episode, it was 80 and felt regular.
- The 'odd heart beat' where he was aware of the beating of his heart lasted from a few seconds to two minutes. This would be followed by a normal period, of at least one hour. It started two days ago and kept recurring, every few hours. He was aware of his heart beat, intermittently throughout his night shift and when he was trying to rest at home. He is unable to identify any aggravating or relieving factors. He has not exercised during this period.
- There was no associated chest pain, shortness of breath or light-headedness. He is systemically well and has not lost weight or had health problems recently.
- He is worried because he has a family history of cardiac disease. His dad died of an arrhythmia at age 64 and his older sister had an MI last year at age 51. He now smokes 10 cigarettes per day. His girlfriend made him cut down this year. He previously smoked 20 per day for 20 years. He has also cut down alcohol to 4 beers a night over the weekend. He last had his cholesterol

measured 10 years ago and didn't have any problems. His urine test for an insurance medical recently didn't pick up diabetes. He tries to play golf once a week.

- He works in an engineering firm, but his job is mainly desk-based and administrative now. He went through a stressful divorce last year, but 'a new regime' has taken over this year. He now feels settled and happy in his new relationship.
- While on night shift, he looked on the internet and read about heart-block. He is a bit worried that he may have an arrhythmia.
- He expects an ECG, which he read about on the internet.
- He drinks approximately six cups of strong tea each day. Except for weekly golf, he does not get much exercise.

Targeted examination

- Examine the pulse – are there missed, weak or abnormally strong beats?
- Examine the JVP – atrial contraction against closed A–V valves produces cannon waves.

Clinical management

- Reassure the patient that ectopics, either atrial or ventricular, are frequently found in normal people.
- Discuss the natural history and aetiology of ectopics. The outlook is usually excellent and treatment is usually unnecessary.
- However, the patient's idea that his family history is significant is entirely valid. Ventricular ectopics are sometimes a manifestation of sub-clinical heart disease and should therefore prompt general cardiac investigation (ECG, measurement of fasting glucose, cholesterol and/or TSH).
- Address the patient's concerns about having a significant arrhythmia such as heart block and perhaps provide more appropriate patient information.
- Address the patient's expectations: arrange an ECG and blood tests.
- Provide brief lifestyle advice – stop smoking, more exercise and a healthier diet. Advise on reducing caffeine intake.
- Make follow-up arrangements.
- Be prepared to answer questions about 'how much exercise', or 'what exactly is a healthy diet' or 'is it ok to start exercising straight away?'

Interpersonal skills

Good communication with the patient:
- elicits his concerns regarding an underlying cardiac problem
- avoids lecturing the patient about his lifestyle
- explores his expectations and negotiates appropriate investigation

- provides an explanation about ectopic heart beats in a way which is understandable to him
- gives targeted lifestyle advice and sets realistic goals in partnership with the patient

Poor communication with the patient:
- does not elicit the reason for the patient's heightened anxiety, that is, his family history and his internet research
- instructs the patient rather than mutually agreeing goals
- uses inappropriately technical language
- is patronizing or paternalistic in his reassurance

Appendix: Patient summary

Name	NM
Date of birth (Age)	41
Social and Family History	Divorced
Past medical history	Travel advice July 2005
	Upper GI endoscopy May 2000
Current medication	None
Values	Tests done five months ago (insurance medical)
Urine dipstix	no glucose, protein or blood detected
BP	114/81
Height	172 cm
Weight	71 kg
BMI	25

Test your knowledge

Answer true (T) or false (F) for each of the following statements.
1. Atrial flutter is suspected in a 75 year old man presenting with palpitations and an irregular pulse of 150 bpm
2. The ECG findings of atrial flutter are saw-tooth flutter waves with 3:1 or 4:1 conduction
3. Third-degree block presents with tachycardia
4. Atrio-ventricular block is a cardiac presentation in Lyme's disease
5. Where potassium is increased in Addison's disease, the ECG shows saw-tooth flutter waves
6. Wolff–Parkinson–White is suspected in a young man presenting with palpitations and light-headedness whose ECG shows narrow, bizarre complex tachycardias

Case 34 – Psoriasis

42 year old Mrs SN presents asking for your opinion on a 'Miracle Creame' for Anna's psoriasis. Anna is her 12 year old daughter. Mrs SN hands you an internet print-out – see Appendix below.

Targeted history taking

- What type of psoriasis does Anna have and what is her current treatment regime?
- What did they expect of the psoriasis and/or its treatment? Are these expectations being met?
- Is Anna, or her mother, experiencing any problems or side effects with the current treatments?
- What does Anna think of the 'Miracle Creame'? Is she likely to use the treatment regime as directed?
- What expectations do Anna and/or her mother have of the cream? What would be a good result?
- What could the possible harms be of using this cream? How expensive is it?
- What does Mrs SN think about the other evidence-based treatments, available on the NHS, for Anna?
- How is the psoriasis affecting Anna? What is the impact of psoriasis on school and home life?
- What are Mrs SN's expectations of this consultation: your opinion on the product, your advice regarding the treatment of psoriasis, a change in Anna's prescriptions, or a referral to dermatology?
- Is Anna generally well?

Data gathering

Listed below is the additional information elicited from the patient with appropriate questioning.
- Anna developed guttate psoriasis suddenly four months ago following a throat infection, which was treated with antibiotics. Thereafter, she was prescribed several different emollient creams for the psoriasis. At the moment, Anna bathes in baby oil softened water using a moisturising soap. She towels dry and applies an emollient. A few minutes later, she applies eumovate steroid cream. She applies the emollients at least twice daily.
- Anna and her mother thought the guttate psoriasis would be self-limiting and are surprised that it persisted this long. They expected the creams to make the plaques vanish. The plaques are still present on her arms and chest and are itchy and unsightly.

- The current regime of emollients and steroid are tolerated, but time consuming. Mrs SN worries about the long-term effect of steroids on the skin: 'it thins the skin'.
- Mrs SN has not spoken to Anna about the 'Miracle Creame' because she wanted to get your opinion first. The internet article says all other creams should be discontinued, presumably because they contain non-natural, synthetic ingredients. Does this include Anna's prescribed emollient? Mrs SN thinks Anna will use the 'Miracle Creame', especially if it simplifies and shortens the daily routine. She is not sure how Anna would feel about the smell of bananas though.
- Mrs SN expects to use the cream on Anna for two or three months. Hopefully, this cream will push the guttate psoriasis into complete remission. A poor result would be the lack of a cure and the development of chronic psoriasis.
- MRS SN thinks that because the 'Miracle Creame' is made from natural ingredients, it should not cause any harm, unlike steroids. It costs £25 per tube, per month.
- Mrs SN is not aware of other treatments such as phototherapy, which are available on the NHS.
- Anna is getting self-conscious about her appearance. She now refuses to swim; chlorine also stings. Anna does not want to wear summer clothes, despite the heat because people might see the plaques. Also, the whole routine takes so long. Anna has been late for school on a few occasions.
- Mrs SN wants to know what is the best course of action for Anna. She doesn't mind paying for the 'Miracle Creame' if you think it will help Anna.
- Anna is otherwise fit and well.

Targeted examination

- None needed as it is the patient's mother who presents for advice.

Clinical management

- Address the mother's ideas: that guttate psoriasis is self-limiting. Discuss the natural history of guttate psoriasis – it often runs a self-limited course, lasting from a few weeks to a few months, but in approximately two-thirds of cases, it develops into chronic plaque-type psoriasis. Be sensitive and empathetic. Be hopeful – it may be too early to assume that it has become a chronic disease.
- Address the mother's concerns: that steroid creams thin and damage the skin. Discuss the role of steroid in the treatment of a T cell autoimmune-mediated condition.
- Address the mother's expectations: of inducing remission. Anna needs to be re-examined – is the guttate psoriasis taking a bit longer than expected to

clear, or has it developed into chronic type psoriasis? If it has developed into chronic psoriasis, discuss the availability of treatment options such as vitamin D analogues, phototherapy or a coal-tar preparation, such as Exorex, which contains extracts from bananas. All these treatments are available on the NHS.

- Discuss the likelihood of the 'Miracle Creame' inducing remission, being used regularly, and its possible harms. Give your opinion of the internet regime, its possible benefits and harms. Once the information is provided, allow Mrs SN to evaluate the risks and benefits of the treatment. Negotiate and develop a shared plan.
- Incorporate Anna's and her mother's values and preferences for treatment. If Mrs SN wants to use 'Miracle Creame', then negotiate a trial of treatment. How would Mrs SN decide whether the cream is beneficial? Arrange follow-up against agreed success criteria.
- Discuss the availability of support from other team members, such as the practice nurse or health visitor who has an interest in dermatology.
- If required, provide written information in support of the discussion.

Interpersonal skills

Good communication with the patient:
- explores and acknowledges the reasons for the mother's attendance – her wish to do more for her daughter; concerns about Anna's recent self-conscious behaviour; and her fear that long-term use of steroid cream may be harmful to Anna's skin
- appreciates that Mrs SN may have an underlying fear that her daughter's guttate psoriasis may be evolving into a chronic plaque-type disease
- explores her expectations of treatment – by discussing the natural history of the disease and explaining how treatments work, Mrs SN is empowered
- achieves a shared understanding, and negotiates an appropriate and acceptable management plan

Therefore, finalising on a decision for which both parties take responsibility, maintains the doctor–patient relationship.

Poor communication:
- fails to appreciate that bringing in an article on a 'Miracle Cure' may be Mrs SN's attempt at signalling concerns with Anna's current treatment
- dismisses the 'Miracle Cure' out of hand without taking time to consider with Mrs SN its possible acceptability, benefits and drawbacks
- is patronizing and fails to foster a therapeutic doctor–patient relationship

Additional information

NICE (2001) Referral guidelines for psoriasis. See: http://www.nice.org.uk/pdf/Referraladvice.pdf.

✪✪✪✪   the patient has generalised pustular or erythrodermic psoriasis

✪✪✪   the patient's psoriasis is acutely unstable

✪✪✪   the patient has widespread guttate psoriasis (so that he/she can benefit from early phototherapy)

✪✪   the condition is causing severe social or psychological problems

✪✪   the rash is sufficiently extensive to make self-management impractical

✪✪   the rash is in a sensitive area (such as face, hands, feet, genitalia) and the symptoms particularly troublesome

✪✪   the rash is leading to time off work or school which is interfering with employment or education

✪✪   the patient requires assessment for the management of associated arthropathy

✪   the rash fails to respond to management in general practice. Failure is probably best based on the subjective assessment of the patient. Sometimes failure occurs when patients are unable to apply the treatment themselves

✪✪✪✪   is seen immediately

✪✪✪   is seen urgently

✪✪   is seen soon

✪   has a routine appointment

Relevant literature

Catherine H, Smith CH, Barker JNWN. (2006) Psoriasis and its management. *BMJ*, **333**: 380–384.

Appendix

Al-Preve Miracle Cure

After bathing/showering with a glycerine soap, just peel a banana, and rub the inner soft skin (the one next to the banana) on your patch of psoriasis. The peel is the scrub. Rub it in thoroughly. Later, once your skin has absorbed the oils from the peel, we suggest you use a common gentle skin cream to help keep the psoriasis patch soft. Our best-selling cream is 'Al-Preve', which does not contain the dyes and perfumes that make the psoriasis sting. It is a simple cream with vitamins and is made from entirely natural ingredients. If you discontinue all other products and use 'Al-Preve' at least once a day, the nasty, white flaky skin will soften up and eventually you will see a miraculous thing – pink healthy skin emerging.

Test your knowledge

Answer true (T) or false (F) for each of the following statements.

1. Methotrexate is indicated for treatment of localised plaque psoriasis such as on the elbows or knees
2. For scalp psoriasis a tar-based shampoo should be tried first
3. When there is significant scaling, use tar-based cream first or other treatments will fail
4. Emergency referral is indicated in cases of generalised erythrodermic or generalised pustular psoriasis
5. If the patient developed psoriasis soon after starting on NSAIDs and paracetamol, the provocative agent is likely to be the paracetamol

Case 35 – Onychomycosis

Mrs DM is a 58-year-old woman who presents for treatment of her fungal toenail infection. At the end of your consultation, she says, 'By the way doctor,..'

Targeted history taking

- How many nails are affected?
- For how long has she had the problem? Why is she presenting today?
- What symptoms does the infection produce?
- What does she think has caused or aggravated the problem?
- What treatments has she tried already?
- What are her expectations of this consultation: a prescription, advice regarding over-the-counter medication, or further investigation?
- What is her general health like – does she have other dermatological conditions such as psoriasis, predisposing factors such as immunosuppression, or is she taking any medication, such as HRT, which could interact with anti-fungals?

Data gathering

Listed below is the additional information elicited from the patient with appropriate questioning.

- Most of the nails on both feet are affected. The large toenails are thickened and discoloured.
- She has had the problem for three years. Except for the cosmetic appearance, it has not caused many symptoms. However, her son is getting married in Greece in two months and she would like to wear open-toe sandals to the wedding.
- She gets an occasional itchiness around the big toes and has to stop herself from scratching her toes. She would like to treat the unsightly appearance of the nails.
- She cannot think of any reasons for developing the infection. She has good hygiene, wears comfortable shoes, and is in good health.
- She tried some mycota powder, which her husband was prescribed for his athlete's foot, but this has not helped.
- She would like some 'strong tablets' to get rid of the infection in time for the wedding in two months.
- Her general health is good. She stopped taking HRT for menopausal flushing two years ago.

Targeted examination

- Expose her toenails – *she produces a photograph of her toenails*:

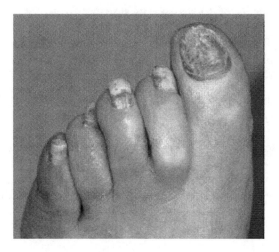

- Examine the surrounding skin for fungal infection.
- Examine her fingernails.

Clinical management

- Discuss the natural history and epidemiology of fungal nail infections. Up to 10% of the population can suffer from fungal nail infections. In 80% of cases, the toenails are affected. Age, diabetes and occlusive footwear are risk factors.
- Address the patient's ideas: that it is definitely a fungal infection. 50% of cases of nail dystrophy are fungal in origin but such cases cannot always be identified accurately on clinical examination. If treatment is given and the appearance of the nails does not improve as the nail grows out (this process takes up to 12 months), then it is not known if this is treatment failure or an incorrect diagnosis. To confirm the diagnosis, nail clippings and subungual debris should be sent to the laboratory in a prefolded envelope designed for this purpose.
- Address the patient's concerns: that the appearance of the nails precludes the wearing of open-toe sandals. Discuss ways in which the appearance may be improved, such as using a nail varnish.
- Address the patient's expectations: that a script for an anti-fungal be provided today and for the appearance of the nails to improve within two months. Topical treatments need to be used for 6–12 months. Treatment with systemic terbinafine can take up to 4 months to eradicate the organism. However, this does not always result in a normal appearance of the affected

nails, as it takes 6–12 months for the nails to grow out. Also, the nail may have been dystrophic to begin with, predisposing to fungal infection.
- Discuss the risks and benefits of not awaiting microscopy results before initiating treatment.
- Discuss the risks and benefits of topical versus systemic treatment for a cosmetic problem.
- Negotiate whether scrapings are done (advise patient on the technique of collecting a suitable sample) and whether a script is provided.
- If needed, arrange follow-up.

When you complete this consultation, the patient says, *'By the way doctor, my husband still gets up at night to pee despite his prostate operation. Has the operation not worked?'*
- You may want to advise Mrs DM in general terms about the causes of nocturia.
- You could outline that there are treatments, such as restricting fluid intake 3–4 hours before bedtime, taking a small dose of diuretic at 4 pm or using desmopressin. However, her husband would require assessment first and should therefore be encouraged to attend.

Interpersonal skills

Good communication with the patient explores:
- her agenda – to improve the appearance of her toenails, using tablets, within two months
- health beliefs – that anti-fungals would solve the problem
- preferences – for immediate initiation of tablet treatment

The doctor deals with the nail infection and addresses the patient's concerns regarding her husband's nocturia. The challenge here is to be sensitive to the patient's queries and to provide information without breaking confidence or destroying hope.

In dealing with both issues, the doctor has demonstrated an ability to behave as a 'family doctor', utilizing a person-centred approach in dealing with problems in the context of a patient's circumstances.

Additional information

Prodigy Guidance (2006) Fungal and candidial nail infections. See: http://cks. library.nhs.uk/fungal_candidal_nail_infection/view_whole_guidance.

- Mycological investigation is necessary before starting treatment, except if after discussing the treatment options, the person decides that they would not opt for treatment if fungal infection were found.
- Nail clippings and subungual debris are required. Nail clippings of the diseased part of the nail may be best taken with chiropody nail clippers.

- All samples should be put on to black card so that the material is easily visible.
- People should not have been on antifungal treatment within the previous 2 weeks and specimens should be kept at room temperature.
- If using oral terbinafine, prescribe 250 mg once a day. Supply 28 tablets, which in 2006 cost approximately £35. For fingernail infections, terbinafine needs to be taken for at least 6 weeks and possibly for up to 3 months. For toenail infections, terbinafine need to be taken for at least 3 months and possibly for up to 6 months.

Roberts DT, Taylor WD, Boyle J. (2003) Guidelines for treatment of onychomycosis. *Br J Dermatol*, **148**: 402–410. See: http://www.bad.org.uk/healthcare/guidelines/Onychomycosis.pdf

Test your knowledge

Answer true (T) or false (F) for each of the following statements.
1. With regard to microscopy samples, subungual debris taken from the most proximal part of the infection is likely to yield the best results
2. With regard to onychomycosis, the most common cause of treatment failure in the UK is incorrect diagnosis
3. With regard to onychomycosis in the elderly, especially those with diabetes or peripheral vascular disease, fungal nail infection can predispose to cellulitis
4. Fungal elements are protected in keratin; hence disinfecting the floors of communal bathing places is difficult
5. If the nail remains dystrophic following eradication of fungus, an alternative oral antifungal should be commenced

Case 36 – Transient ischaemic attack

Mr BY is a 72 year old man with hypertension. He presents today with '*My missus sent me in because I had a problem with my eye yesterday*'. See Appendix for further details.

Targeted history taking

- Describe the eye problem.
- What was he doing when the symptoms started?
- For how long did the episode last?
- Did it resolve completely?
- Did he have any other symptoms, such as weakness, numbness or tingling, speech disturbance or balance problems?
- Did anyone else witness what had happened? What did they say about how he appeared to them?
- Has this happened before?
- Has he had previous strokes, TIAs, coronary heart disease, migraines or epilepsy?
- Is he taking his hypertension medication?
- Is he still smoking?
- Does he have a family history of strokes, TIAs, or coronary heart disease?
- Has he experienced any other illness recently?
- What are his expectations of this consultation: a diagnosis or explanation of what happened, further investigation, a change in medication, or referral to hospital?
- Quite a lot has been discussed today. What is he going to say to his wife?

Data gathering

Listed below is the additional information elicited from the patient with appropriate questioning.

- Mr BY noticed blurring in his right eye. The eye didn't feel irritated. He kept rubbing but his vision became greyer and more indistinct. He could see perfectly with his other eye. Eventually he couldn't see out of the right eye at all; it was black. Just when he was about to call the out-of-hours services, the vision in the eye reappeared, like the fog disappearing. His eye is fine today, but his wife insisted that he get checked out.
- He was watching the evening news on television.
- It lasted until the weather report, so probably fifteen minutes in all.
- The symptoms resolved completely.
- He has not experienced any other symptoms. His arms and legs were fine – no weakness, numbness or tingling. His speech and balance were undisturbed.

- His wife saw what happened but said he looked normal. She thought he was 'having a joke'.
- He has not experienced anything like this before.
- He has not had previous strokes, TIAs, coronary heart disease, migraines or epilepsy. He occasionally gets lower back pain, but that is from years of manual labour.
- He cut down and now smokes six cigarettes per day, mainly after meals or with tea. He tried NRT but it didn't work for him.
- His father died young, he thinks from 'thrombosis'. His mum died of bowel cancer. His older sister is overweight and diabetic. His younger sister has hypertension.
- He has been in good health recently.
- He expects reassurance that what happened is just one of those things, but appears quite shaken by the experience. His wife does not drive and relies on him to do the driving.
- He intends to tell his wife that his examination today was fine, but the doctor wanted to run some more tests.

Targeted examination

- Perform a targeted neurological examination.
- How fluent is his speech? Is he alert and co-operative? *Yes.*
- Examine his carotid and peripheral pulses for abnormalities of rate or rhythm. *No abnormalities found on examination.*
- Listen for a carotid bruit. *No bruit heard.*
- Check BP in both arms. *BP in the right arm is 142/92 and in the left arm is 138/90.*
- Perform fundoscopy in a darkened room. Say to the patient that ideally you would prefer to dilate the pupils using a solution of 1% cyclopentolate. See http://medicine.ucsd.edu/clinicalmed/eyes.htm.
- *The patient hands you a card with a picture of your examination findings.*

Clinical management

- Discuss the examination findings.
- Explain your clinical suspicion of a TIA, particularly amaurosis fugax (retinal ischaemia).
- Score Mr BY according to the Oxfordshire Community Stroke Project ABCD score (see under Additional information below). Given that he is >60 years of age (score = 1); has a BP of 142/92 (score = 1); no unilateral weakness or speech disturbance without weakness (score = 0); and the duration of the episode was 15 minutes (score = 1), he scores a total of 3.
- Since the ABCD score <4, and he recovered within 30 minutes, he should be referred urgently to the TIA/neurovascular clinic to be seen within one week.

- Explain to Mr BY that further tests (carotid dopplers) will be done. If he has a stenosis > 70%, then he could have an operation within two weeks, to prevent further TIAs and strokes.
- Make an appointment with the practice nurse; an ECG should be done immediately. Blood tests can be arranged for later in the week.
- While awaiting cholesterol results, consider starting a statin – it may stabilize the atheroma.
- Mr BY is already on aspirin, but you may want to check compliance, increase the dose to 300 mg once daily, or change to clopidogrel 75 mg once daily.
- Advise smoking cessation and promote healthy lifestyle measures.
- Advise Mr BY that anyone who has had a single TIA should not drive for one month and that he must inform his insurance company. If he has more than one TIA, he must inform the DVLA and he probably won't be allowed to drive for 3 months.
- Invite Mr BY to make a follow-up appointment, perhaps with his wife, to discuss any information that he has not been able to digest in consultation today.

Interpersonal skills

Good communication with the patient:
- involves taking a good history, to quickly establish the nature of the problem
- explains the findings of the focussed examination to the patient
- constructs an evidence-based management plan with the patient
- negotiates which tests are arranged in primary care
- addresses the patient's anxiety regarding driving
- recognizes that the patient has been given a large amount of information and therefore offers a follow-up appointment for further discussion

Additional information

The following table is adapted from the **Oxford Community Stroke Project** (OCSP), see: http://www.stroke.org.uk/document.rm?id=384 (accessed 24 July 07).

Scoring system for risk of stroke after TIA (ABCD)		
Age	Age >60	1
Blood pressure	BP>140 systolic and/or >90 diastolic	1
Clinical features	Unilateral weakness	2
	Speech disturbance without weakness	1
	Other	0
Duration of symptoms	>60 min	2
	10–59 min	1
	<10 min	0

Fairhead JF, Rothwell PM. (2006) Underinvestigation and undertreatment of carotid disease in elderly patients with transient ischaemic attack and stroke: comparative population based study. *BMJ*, **333**: 525–527.

This study showed that:

- even though the incidence of symptomatic carotid stenosis increases steeply with age, and
- there is good benefit from endarterectomy in elderly patients, and
- there is a willingness in older patients to have surgery,
- GPs underinvestigate patients aged ≥80 with transient ischaemic attack or ischaemic stroke.

Are GPs ageist?

For comprehensive guidance on the investigation and management of TIA, see: http://www.crestni.org.uk/tia-guidelines.pdf, particularly pages 29 and 30.

For an eye atlas or information on eyes, see: http://www.mic.ki.se/Diseases/C11.html.

Appendix: Patient summary

Name	BY
Date of birth (Age)	72
Social and Family History	Married, with two children who live nearby.
Past medical history	Hypertension since 1998. Intermittent lower back pain.
Current medication	Bendroflumethiazide 2.5 mg once daily × 28 Atenolol 50 mg once daily × 28 Aspirin 75 mg once daily × 28 Ibuprofen 400 mg thrice daily or as required × 100 Paracetamol 1 g four times daily or as required × 100
Private prescription	Sildenafil 100 mg as directed × 4
Blood tests	Blood tests done three months ago.
BP	148/90
Urea and electrolytes	within normal range
Liver function tests	within normal range
Serum cholesterol	6.5
Cholesterol/HDL ratio	6.0
Fasting triglycerides	1.8
Fasting glucose	5.4
Current smoker	10 cigarettes per day

Test your knowledge

Answer true (T) or false (F) for each of the following statements.

1. The proposed new definition of TIA is a 'brief episode of neurological dysfunction caused by a focal disturbance of brain or retinal ischemia, with clinical symptoms typically lasting less than 1 hour, and without evidence of infarction'

2. TIA patients, unless normotensive, should have their BPs reduced by 10/5 mmHg

3. ACE-Is and ARBs, but not thiazide diuretics and beta-blockers, are beneficial in reducing cardiovascular events and stroke incidence in patients with diabetes

4. Patients with TIA who are heavy drinkers should reduce their consumption of alcohol to no more than 2 drinks per day for men and 1 drink per day for non-pregnant women

5. For patients with recent TIA and ipsilateral carotid artery stenosis, there is no indication for carotid endarterectomy if the degree of stenosis is <75%

Case 37 – Newly diagnosed diabetes mellitus

Mrs SB is a 49 year old lady who presents today to discuss her recent blood results. See Appendix for full details.

Targeted history taking

- What does she already know about the blood tests?
- Does she know why the blood tests were done?
- Does she have any symptoms of diabetes?
- What does she know about treatment? What help or advice is she likely to need?
- What is her job?
- Who lives with her?
- Are her symptoms or treatment likely to affect her home and work life?
- What are her expectations of this consultation: an explanation of test results, further investigation, referral to diabetic clinic / dietician / eye screening services, or the initiation of medication?
- What is her general health like – does she have other on-going medical problems that require attention?
- Is she a smoker? Does she have a family history of diabetes or vascular disease?
- Does she drive?

Data gathering

Listed below is the additional information elicited from the patient with appropriate questioning.

- The phlebotomist said the first glucose result was slightly raised when she had her blood taken last week. She thinks that the recent blood tests confirmed diabetes.
- She knows that she has to have annual blood tests for her high cholesterol. She knows that her gestational diabetes and impaired fasting glucose put her at risk of eventually developing overt diabetes.
- As regards symptoms, she is tired, but she does not know if this is due to interrupted sleep from menopausal flushing. She recently had thrush, but does not give a history of recurrent infections or polyuria or nocturia.
- She knows that she should lose weight but has tried several diets, including Weight Watchers over the years. She has been overweight since her late 20s. She says doctors always tell her to lose weight. *She becomes tearful at this point.*

- She is a housewife.
- She lives with her husband.
- She and her husband have an active social life. They eat with friends or meet for drinks at least weekly. Her friends know her as someone who enjoys her food and drink. She does not want to be one of these fussy women at dinners that count calories and ask people to prepare special food for her.
- She expects you to advise her of the treatment for her diabetes.
- Her BP was a bit high when she saw the doctor three weeks ago. She takes a tablet for her high cholesterol. She does not report side effects.
- She is a non-smoker. She was adopted and is unaware of her family history.
- She does drive.

Targeted examination

- It may be useful to repeat her BP measurement.

Clinical management

- Discuss the blood results: there are three issues that need addressing, her new diagnosis of diabetes, her BP and her cholesterol management. Negotiate the agenda for today's consultation.
- Explore and discuss what the patient already understands about diabetes and how it is treated. Discuss tiredness as a possible symptom of diabetes.
- Discuss dietary measures and lifestyle changes: give dietary advice, offer referral to a dietician, and encourage regular physical activity. Inform her that glycaemic control in the newly diagnosed diabetic should ideally be reviewed at two to three monthly intervals.
- Inform the patient that she will require further examination and tests (such as checking her peripheral pulses, sensation in her peripheries, and microalbuminuria testing). Hence, an appointment with the practice nurse is needed.
- Respond to her cue regarding weight issues. Give specific advice about weight loss. Consider medication to help with weight loss, such as sibutramine or orlistat.
- Ideally, her BP should be <130/80 and she should be initiated on an ACE-I. Consider, with the patient, when you would start anti-hypertensive medication.
- Consider, with the patient, how the cholesterol could be reduced further – perhaps by better compliance (if that is an issue), or better dietary control, or increasing her exercise levels, or by increasing her medication (for example, by adding ezetimibe).
- Advise the patient to contact the DVLA to inform them of her diagnosis.
- Arrange follow-up. Specify when you would like to see Mrs SB again and what you would be assessing at follow-up.

Interpersonal skills

Poor communication with the patient:
- fails to explore the impact of her obesity on her life, hence missing the opportunity to be responsive to the issue with which she has the greatest difficulty
- fails to provide explanations that are relevant to the patient, who in the consultation revealed an understanding of gestational diabetes and impaired fasting glucose. By being overly simplistic, the doctor wastes time and may appear patronizing. By reading too much into the patient's use of medical terminology, the doctor may provide too little understandable information. The responsive doctor checks to see if the patient has understood him at each stage of the consultation.
- fails to encourage the patient to seek information and help from various members of the primary care team. The patient is not empowered.

Good communication with the patient:
- encourages the patient to present her agenda
- informs the patient of the medical agenda – there are three issues regarding her recent tests which need addressing
- negotiates how the limited time available for this consultation is utilized, thereby constructing a plan which will deal with all the important issues, but prioritizes appropriately and in response to what the patient also wants

Therefore, a shared management plan incorporates strategies for dealing with the patient's difficulties in losing weight, by exploring possible lifestyle changes, such as
- smaller portion sizes rather than needing different food
- the omission of snacking
- increasing activity levels
- considering drug treatments for obesity

Additional information

Smith SM (2003) Newly diagnosed type 2 diabetes mellitus. *BMJ*, **326**: 1371.
Diagnosis – is based on:
- random venous plasma glucose > 11.0 mmol/l, or
- fasting venous plasma glucose > 7.0 mmol/l, or
- by oral glucose tolerance testing.

Two raised readings – a diagnosis of diabetes has serious implications and should be confirmed by repeat testing on a subsequent day.
At the initial appointment:
- exclude secondary causes, such as pancreatic disease, hormone-induced diabetes, and drugs that may precipitate diabetes, such as steroids or thiazide diuretics. Take a history of smoking, diet, and exercise habits.

- do an initial physical examination: measure BP, measure weight and height to calculate body mass index and check for any existing complications
- arrange for initial investigations: haemoglobin A_{1c}, full blood count, renal profile, fasting lipid profile, and microalbuminuria testing
- initiate a change in diet. Focus on the need for a healthy balanced diet, with restriction of refined sugars. Most patients should have a three month trial of dietary treatment before starting on oral hypoglycaemic agents.
- provide written information and instructions. Initial education may involve just a simple explanation of the nature of diabetes and clear advice on action to be taken if the condition deteriorates before the next review.
- should patients be referred immediately? This is generally indicated if the patient is clearly unwell, has ketonuria, or if the blood glucose concentration is > 20 mmol/l. Recent weight loss is an indication of severity of disease.
- ensure that the patient has a follow up appointment to see you

Other tasks:
- cardiovascular risk profiling is essential, but including it in the initial consultation is likely to overwhelm most patients
- organizational tasks include recording of findings and inclusion of the patient on the practice register and recall system; referral for assessment of eye complications; and referral to dietician, chiropodist or podiatrist, and community diabetes educator, if available

Relevant literature

NICE (2002) Type 2 diabetes. See:
http://www.nice.org.uk/page.aspx?o=guidelineg.

Test your knowledge

Answer true (T) or false (F) for each of the following statements, with regard to diabetes mellitus in the UK.
1. One in five people over the age of 85 have diabetes
2. Type 2 diabetes is one-and-a-half times more prevalent in the most affluent one-fifth of the population
3. Diabetes accounts for more than one in six people starting renal replacement therapy
4. In one-third of cases of hyperosmolar non-ketotic syndrome (HONK), it is the first manifestation of type 2 diabetes
5. Diabetic ketoacidosis (DKA) is precipitated by insulin over-use, severe illness (e.g. myocardial infarction) or infection (e.g. pneumonia)

Appendix: Patient summary

Name	SB
Date of birth (Age)	49
Social and Family History	Married, one child
Past medical history	Menopausal symptoms for eight months
	Hypercholesterolaemia since 2005
	Impaired fasting glycaemia since 2002
	Oesophageal reflux since 2001
	Gestational diabetes in 1991
Current medication	Atorvastatin 40 mg at night
	Enzira suspension i.m. injection last November
Blood tests	Tests were done two weeks ago.
Plasma fasting glucose *	7.2 mmol/l (3.65–6.5)
HbA1c*	6.2% (4.3–6.1)
	Blood tests were done three weeks ago.
Plasma fasting glucose*	7.1 mmol/l
Total cholesterol	5.6 mmol/l
Total cholesterol:HDL ratio	5.1
HDL	1.1 mmol/l
LDL	3.5 mmol/l
TSH	1.58
Liver function tests	normal
Renal function tests	normal
BP	138/90
O/E weight	87 kg
Body mass index	38.7

Notes from last consultation three weeks ago

- Candidial vulvuvaginitis.
- Vulval itch, soreness, redness, with white discharge, unresponsive to pessary. Known to have impaired fasting glycaemia. On atorvastatin – needs repeat of bloods. See practice nurse for fasting glucose, cholesterol, LFTs, UandEs and TSH (tiredness – ?menopausal, ?hypothyroid).
- Prescribed fluconazole 50 mg × 3 – repeat in one week if needed.

Case 38 – Cognitive impairment

Ms AE is a 56 year old woman who presents asking for advice regarding her elderly mother who refuses to consent to blood tests. Ms AE seems rather angry when you invite her into your consulting room.

Targeted history taking

- Why is she angry?
- What seems to be the matter with her mother?
- Why were the blood tests requested? Who requested them?
- Why is Ms AE asking for your advice?
- What is the impact of her mother's illness on Ms AE? How does Ms AE feel about her mother's illness?
- What ideas does she have regarding the investigation and treatment of her mother?
- What are her main concerns regarding her mother?
- What are her expectations of this consultation: discussing whether blood tests are definitely needed, making alternative arrangements for tests, the provision of support during a difficult period, or signposting to appropriate services?

Data gathering

Listed below is the additional information elicited from the patient with appropriate questioning.

- Ms AE is angry because the surgery has not returned her calls regarding her mother. She realizes that you are the locum doctor. She understands that Dr Brown is on sabbatical, but every time she called in the last two weeks, she spoke to a different receptionist who promised that someone would call. Nobody did. She is worried about her mother and wants some advice today. You had appointments free so she booked in to see you. She wants this problem with her mother sorted out today.
- Dr Brown thinks that her mother has dementia and has requested some blood tests. Her mother has refused to have these tests done at the surgery. Her mother is an 84 year old Italian lady who has lived with Ms AE since she moved to England 30 years ago. Her mother thinks she (Ms AE) is trying to put her in a home so she refuses to leave the house.
- Dr Brown requested the blood tests because he wanted to see if there was anything that was causing her mother's dementia. Ms AE hopes that her mother's strange behaviour is due to a treatable illness, such as thyroid disease.

- Ms AE is seeing you because you had appointments and she is tired of chasing around after Dr Brown's replacement.
- Ms AE is struggling to cope with her mother's illness. Eight years ago when her Italian aunt, who had lived with her, became demented, the stress of caring for elderly relatives contributed to the breakdown of her marriage. Her aunt was eventually put in a home where, three months later, she fell, breaking her hip. Ms AE is now retired. Her mother is increasingly fearful of being left on her own. She is suspicious of strangers and is rude to Ms AE's visitors. Ms AE feels trapped by her mother. She also feels too guilty to put her mother in a home.
- Ms AE wants the blood tests to be done to rule out reversible causes of dementia. Her mother does not want to come to surgery and when the district nurse came to take blood, she refused. She then accused Ms AE and the district nurses of trying to kill her. She wants to help her mother but her mother refuses to consent to treatment.
- Her main concern is that her mother and her cannot continue as they are. If her mother refuses treatment, and continues behaving in her current, suspicious manner, then Ms AE is trapped at home with her. If her mother were more manageable, Ms AE feels she could cope with looking after her at home.
- Ms AE wants her mother to have the blood tests and for you to organize the procedure. She feels that she cannot make decisions regarding the care of her mother without knowing the results of these tests.

Targeted examination

- Not required.

Clinical management

- Establish the reason for the patient's anger. Be understanding and listen to what she says. Consider asking if she wishes for further action to be taken – does she want to speak to the practice manager, would she like you to raise the issue with the practice manager, or does she want to make a formal complaint?
- Establish the reasons for wanting the blood tests, and empathize with the difficulties she is experiencing in getting these organized.
- Consider verbalizing aloud the available options. Discuss the pros and cons of each option. Encourage Ms AE's contribution to each offer. For example, Ms AE may reject the offer of the district nurse visiting again, or referral to the psychogeriatrician, but she may take up the offer of a home visit and an attempt by you to take the blood.
- Discuss the consent procedure. Consider aloud what you would do if her mother refuses to allow you to take the blood.

- Discuss how you would assess whether her mother is competent to refuse treatment – would her mother be able to comprehend, believe and weigh up the information to come to a decision about providing blood for testing. Based on the history Ms AE has provided, it seems that her mother may believe that you, like the district nurse, are trying to kill her. If this is the case, then her mother's decision-making is not valid.
- If her mother's decision-making is not valid, that is, her mother is not competent, then the decision to take blood depends on you and Ms AE. Ask Ms AE what constitutes a reasonable attempt at blood taking?
- Address the patient's ideas: that blood testing is needed.
- Address the patient's concerns: that the surgery, in Dr Brown's absence, is not being helpful in resolving the dilemma she has with her mother's illness.
- Address the patient's expectations: that an agreeable and shared management plan is made today.
- Arrange follow-up: discuss when the blood will be taken and outline what decisions Ms AE should be prepared to make at this encounter.

Interpersonal skills

Good communication with the patient:
- acknowledges and apologizes for the difficulties Ms AE has had in speaking to a doctor about her mother's illness
- is sensitive to Ms AE's dilemma and respects the difficult choices available to her
- provides her with reasonable options, that is, takes the consultation forward

The candidate displays poor interpersonal skills if he is insensitive, unwilling to help, and directive, that is, if he tells Ms AE what she should do without listening or trying to meet her half-way.

Additional information

NICE (2006) Dementia: Supporting people with dementia and their carers in health and social care. See: http://guidance.nice.org.uk/cg42.

Presentation
People with dementia can experience some or all of the following: memory loss, language impairment, disorientation, changes in personality, difficulties with activities of daily living; self-neglect; psychiatric symptoms (for example, apathy, depression or psychosis); and out-of-character behaviour (for example, aggression, or sleep disturbance).

Blood tests
The following blood tests should be performed at presentation, usually within primary care:

- routine haematology
- biochemistry tests (including electrolytes, calcium, glucose, and renal and liver function)
- thyroid function tests
- serum vitamin B_{12} and folate levels

Helping carers
Healthcare professionals are advised to make time available to:
- discuss the diagnosis and its implications with the patient, and with their consent, with family members, and
- to provide patients and relatives with ongoing support

Capacity
If patients do not have the capacity to make decisions, health and social care professionals should follow the Department of Health guidelines:
- Reference guide to consent for examination or treatment (2001)
- Seeking consent: working with older people (2001)
- Seeking consent: working with people with learning disabilities (2001)

all available from http://www.dh.gov.uk.

From April 2007, health and social care professionals need to follow a code of practice accompanying the Mental Capacity Act 2005 (summary available from http://www.dca.gov.uk/menincap/bill-summary.htm). The Act has five key principles:
- adults must be assumed to have capacity to make decisions for themselves unless proved otherwise
- individuals must be given all available support before it is concluded that they cannot make decisions for themselves
- individuals must retain the right to make what might be seen as eccentric or unwise decisions
- anything done for or on behalf of individuals without capacity must be in their best interests
- anything done for or on behalf of individuals without capacity must be the least restrictive alternative in terms of their rights and basic freedoms

Referral
Patients with mild cognitive impairment should be referred to memory assessment services, which are provided either within memory assessment clinics or community mental health teams. More than 50% of people with mild cognitive impairment later develop dementia.

For information on the management of patients with dementia, see SIGN guidance (Feb 2006): http://www.sign.ac.uk/pdf/sign86.pdf.

Test your knowledge

Answer true (T) or false (F) for each of the following statements.

1. Reversible causes of dementia, such as those due to hypothyroidism or vitamin B12 deficiency, are relatively common (5–10%)
2. With regard to dementia, the ability of clinical examination to predict a structural lesion is 90%
3. Bright light therapy is recommended for the treatment of cognitive impairment
4. Severity of Alzheimer's disease should not be a contra-indication to the use of donepezil
5. A Cochrane systematic review suggests that *Gingko biloba* is more potent in establishing cognitive improvement than cholinesterase inhibitors
6. Patients may have to take *Gingko* for 52 weeks before there is an improvement in cognition
7. Anti-inflammatories are recommended for treatment of cognitive decline in patients with Alzheimer's disease

Case 39 – Gout

Mr CJ is a 22 year old man who has come to discuss his blood results. He says he saw a doctor last week with a painful left foot. The doctor was not sure if Mr CJ had gout so he requested some blood tests. See Appendix for details of results.

Targeted history taking

- How is Mr CJ feeling now?
- Which part of the foot was affected and is the foot still painful?
- What activities did the pain limit?
- What is his job and was he able to work?
- What treatment did he find useful?
- Does he know why the bloods were taken and what they were intended to investigate?
- Explore possible reasons for the raised ALT:
  - how much does Mr CJ drink?
  - is he taking any drugs, including herbal remedies?
  - does he have hepatitis or risk factors for hepatitis, such as recent travel or unprotected sex or tattoos?
  - does he have diabetes, obesity, hyperlipidaemia (all of which are suggestive of fatty liver disease)?
  - does he have coeliac disease?
  - has he been feeling systemically unwell with fever and/or weight loss?
- What advice was he given about last year's blood results? Has he followed the advice?
- What are his expectations of this consultation: advice, further investigation, or referral to hospital?
- What is his general health like: does he have other on-going medical problems?

Data gathering

Listed below is the additional information elicited from the patient with appropriate questioning.

- Mr CJ feels that the pain is much better, having improved from 8/10 to 1–2/10 once the anti-inflammatories kicked in.
- The left toe was painful at the MTP joint *(which he points to)*. What surprised the doctor last week was the lack of redness and swelling of the joint. The doctor told him that gout usually causes the skin to become red and shiny. While Mr CJ's joint was very tender to touch, it looked normal and he can now weight-bear without difficulty.
- The pain had limited walking and any pressure put through the foot was agonizing.

- Mr CJ works at the bank. A colleague gave him a ride to work and he was able to continue with his mainly sedentary job. His DIY at home was put on hold.
- He found elevating the foot and using an ice-pack after work helped. The diclofenac also gave good relief, unlike the ibuprofen which he tried before he saw the doctor.
- The doctor he saw last week wanted to check his bloods to see if his uric acid was raised. Also, the tests he had last year after the first episode of foot pain, which was also thought to be gout, had shown some problems. He hadn't re-attended surgery last year for those tests to be repeated, so the doctor repeated them to see if the liver problem has persisted.
- Mr CJ says he has cut down his drinking from 5 to 8 beers three times per week to 5 beers per night on Fridays and Saturdays. The drinking increases during rugby season. He is not taking any drugs, has not travelled recently and has not had unprotected sex. He had a tattoo at a reputable parlour four years ago. He has not experienced polyuria, polydipsia or nocturia. He feels well in himself and has no digestive complaints.
- Last year he was advised to cut down his drinking, which he did. He now walks to work, weather permitting. He tries to eat fewer pre-prepared meals but cooking is not something he enjoys.
- He expects to be told that he has gout and that he should eat less meat. Should he have an X-ray of the foot?
- His general health is fine.

Targeted examination

- Weigh the patient and calculate his BMI – is he obese?
- Does he have central obesity? If so, consider measuring his waist circumference.
- Examine the abdomen for hepatomegaly.
- *In this case, assume that he is centrally obese and the examination of the liver is unremarkable.*

Clinical management

- Discuss the blood results and examination findings: he has a raised ALT, serum urate, triglycerides and BMI, all of which possibly suggest fatty liver with or without metabolic syndrome.
- Discuss what should be done about the raised ALT: he needs to stop drinking alcohol completely and recheck his LFTs in four to six weeks. If the ALT remains high, then further blood tests (viral serology, ferritin, prothrombin time) and an ultrasound scan may be needed.
- Reassure the patient that, in the early stages, the liver recovers well if a healthier lifestyle is adopted.
- Negotiate goals for the patient to work towards and ask him what help he may need in reaching these goals. Consider food diaries and review with the practice nurse for healthy eating advice.

Clinical Skills Assessment

- Address the patient's ideas: that eating too much meat causes gout. A low protein diet is less important than a healthy, balanced diet. Discuss the importance of a low calorie diet rich in dietary fibre, with unsaturated fats, carbohydrates with a low glycaemic index and plenty of fresh fruit, that is, a 'Mediterranean diet'.
- Address the patient's concerns about being told to eat less pre-prepared food and being advised to cook from scratch. Cutting out snacks, eating more fruit, drinking < 21 units of alcohol per week, and exercising for 150 minutes per week would be an excellent start.
- Address the patient's expectations that an X-ray be done: an X-ray may be useful if the diagnosis of gout is in doubt. Two blood tests have already confirmed a marginally raised serum urate, and sepsis or rheumatoid arthritis is not suspected.
- Confirm his understanding of gout, its treatment with anti-inflammatories, its link with metabolic syndrome, and the treatment of these conditions by lifestyle modification.
- Arrange follow-up tests and review in four to six weeks.

Interpersonal skills

Good communication with the patient:
- explores what the patient already knows and understands about his health
- highlights issues the patients prioritizes, such as 'lack of interest in cooking' and 'too much meat'. Therefore, the doctor provides focussed information and advice, using motivational interviewing skills.
- negotiates which diagnostic tests are needed and justifies why some investigations (such as the X-ray) are not currently indicated
- links the clinical presentation of gout with the abnormal blood tests
- explains the global picture of increased cardiovascular risk to the patient in simple terms

Poor communication with the patient:
- does not enquire sufficiently about his health understanding (gout, meat, alcohol)
- instructs the patient rather than seeking common ground (lectures the patient on alcohol units and calories without establishing what is realistic for him)
- uses inappropriate or technical language (in explaining the abnormal blood test results)
- appears patronizing or inappropriately paternalistic (when discussing the management plan)

Additional information

Hayden MR and Tyagi SC. (2004) Uric acid: A new look at an old risk marker for cardiovascular disease, metabolic syndrome, and type 2 diabetes mellitus: The urate redox shuttle, *Nutr Metab (Lond)*, **1**: 10. Published online October 2004.

- In 1923, Kylin described the importance of hyperuricaemia and the clustering phenomenon of three clinical syndromes: hypertension, hyperglycaemia, and hyperuricaemia.
- In 1988, Reaven described the important central role of insulin resistance in the metabolic syndrome. The four major players in the metabolic syndrome are hyperinsulinaemia, hypertension, hyperlipidaemia, and hyperglycaemia, each of which is an independent risk factor for CHD.
- In a like manner, hyperuricaemia, hyperhomocysteinaemia, and highly sensitive C-reactive protein (hsCRP) each play an important role in expanding the original metabolic syndrome in the atherosclerotic process.
- Elevations of uric acid > 4 mg/dl should be considered a 'red flag' in those patients at risk for cardiovascular disease – a global risk reduction programme should be employed to reduce the complications of cardiovascular disease.

Khunti K, Davies M. (2005) Metabolic syndrome. *BMJ*, **331**: 1153–1154.

What is metabolic syndrome?

Metabolic syndrome is characterized by hyperinsulinaemia, low glucose tolerance, dyslipidaemia, hypertension, and obesity, conditions that increase the risk of developing heart disease and diabetes.

What does it look like?

The clinical identification of metabolic syndrome is based on measures of:
- abdominal obesity
- atherogenic dyslipidaemia
- hypertension
- glucose intolerance

Clinical criteria

People meeting three of the following criteria qualify as having the metabolic syndrome:
- raised blood pressure (> 130/85 mmHg)
- a low serum concentration of HDL cholesterol (< 1.04 mmol/l in men and < 1.29 mmol/l in women)
- a high serum triglyceride concentration (> 1.69 mmol/l)
- a high fasting plasma glucose concentration (> 6.1 mmol/l)
- abdominal obesity (waist circumference > 102 cm in men and > 88 cm in women). A new definition has central obesity as an essential criterion, with a range of cut-offs for waist circumference for people from different ethnic groups.

Lifestyle changes

Advice from the University of Southampton School of Medicine, see: http://www.metabolicsyndrome.org.uk/Treatment/default.htm.

- The risk of developing the metabolic syndrome increases with weight gain. Therefore, weight loss is one of the cornerstones of management. The general aim is to decrease calorie intake while increasing energy expenditure.
- Cycling or jogging three times a week over 20–26 weeks has been found to reduce cholesterol by 14% and triglycerides by 34% while doubling HDL.

- There is some evidence that specific dietary changes can have benefits in addition to weight loss alone.
  - Eat more dietary fibre and consume less dietary fat.
  - Replace dietary saturated fats with equal amounts of unsaturated fats to lower LDL cholesterol and triglycerides.
  - Eat foods with a low glycaemic index – by slowing digestion and absorption, they have much less of a dyslipidaemic effect.

Relevant literature

For advice on what to do with asymptomatic patients with abnormal liver function tests, see: http://www.clinicalanswers.nhs.uk/index.cfm?question=1118.

For the investigation algorithm of abnormal LFTs, see:
http://www.northsomerset.nhs.uk/Publications/newsletters/Practice_Briefing/Issue%2010/ManagementOfPersistentMinorElevationsOfAlt3urIInAd-V_011.pdf.

Appendix: Patient summary

Name	CJ
Date of birth (Age)	22
Social and Family History	Single, no children
Past medical history	Tonsillitis 2001
	Minor head injury 1997
Current medication	Diclofenac 50 mg thrice daily
Blood tests	Blood tests done last week
CRP	8 (<8)
Alkaline phosphatase	181 IU/l (95–280)
Total bilirubin	6 μmol/l (3–17)
ALT *	66 IU/l (10–45)
Plasma creatinine	112 μmol/l (70–150)
Plasma urate *	534 μmol/l (210–480)
Plasma albumin	48 g/l (35–50)
	Blood tests from one year ago
Alkaline phosphatase	177 IU/l (95–280)
Total bilirubin	12 μmol/l (3–17)
ALT/SGPT *	92 IU/l (10–45)
Plasma creatinine	100 μmol/l (70–150)
Plasma urate *	522 μmol/l (210–480)
Plasma albumin	47 g/l (35–50)
Fasting glucose	4.9 (3.0–5.5)
Serum cholesterol	5.5 (3.65–6.5)
HDL	1.24 (0.8–1.8)
Fasting triglyceride *	2.6 (0.55–1.9)
O/E height	176 cm
O/E weight	94 kg
BMI *	30.3
BP	128/78

Test your knowledge

Answer true (T) or false (F) for each of the following statements, with regard to the management of acute gout.

1. Affected joints should be rested
2. Anti-inflammatory drug therapy should be commenced immediately and continued for 4 weeks
3. Colchicine, an effective alternative, should be used in doses of 500 µg once daily
4. Patients already established on allopurinol should discontinue their allopurinol
5. In patients with heart failure, diuretic therapy should not be discontinued
6. In patients taking diuretics for hypertension, an alternative antihypertensive agent should be considered

Case 40 – Renal colic

Mr DC is a 25 year old man who was seen by the Out-of-Hours service three weeks ago with an episode of presumed renal colic. He saw your partner in a 5 minute emergency appointment the next day when his pain had gone completely and all she was able to do was to examine him briefly, check his urine and arrange some tests. She asked him to return the next week for the results and to take a full history. She is now on leave and he has come to see you. See Appendix for further details.

Targeted history taking

- Enquire how he has been since last seen – any recurrences?
- Any family history of kidney stones?
- Any past history suggesting structural abnormalities or problems with his renal system? Any history of UTIs?
- Dietary history, in particular, fluid intake, animal proteins, salt and calcium.
- Occupational history – ambient temperature and opportunities to drink fluid and to micturate.
- Any other health problems suggesting inflammatory bowel disease, chronic diarrhoea or malabsorption? Any gout?
- Any drugs that may affect stone disease? – including ephedrine, calcium and vitamin D tablets.
- Enquire about his physical health and whether he has any other symptoms.
- Does he smoke or drink alcohol?
- Why did he not return as requested?
- What does he hope to gain from this consultation– an explanation of the test results, further investigation, or a prescription for medication (analgesia)?

Data gathering

- He has had no further episodes of severe pain although he had some mild discomfort one morning two weeks ago.
- Family history – negative.
- No history of GU problems.
- Works as a chef in the hot kitchen of a local hotel. Late nights – very busy – no time to go to toilet so does not drink much when working. Gets home late, has a couple of packets of crisps or pretzels, drinks a pint of milk and then goes to bed. Has cereal and milky coffee for breakfast.
- He is usually very well, but has an erratic lifestyle due to his working hours.
- He takes one multivitamin a day because he frequently misses meals but eats one very healthy meal late afternoon.
- He is otherwise well.

- He does not smoke and drinks occasionally.
- He had not returned because he has trouble making appointments that do not clash with his working hours. He is reluctant to take time off work when he feels very well.
- He expects you to tell him that he is well and that he will not be troubled by a renal stone again.

Targeted examination

- *In this case an examination is not indicated.*

Clinical management

- Reassure him that all investigations are normal.
- Discuss natural history of condition:
  - most calculi pass spontaneously within 4 weeks, but this needs to be monitored
  - high risk of future episode (recurrence rate at least 50%)
  - complications
- Discuss prevention – increase fluid intake, lower salt intake and normal calcium intake (recommendation for diet low in animal protein and salt is supported by epidemiological studies and a normal calcium intake is recommended).
- Discuss whether to proceed with further investigations – unenhanced helical CT, consider stone analysis.
- Management of future attacks – analgesia, admission criteria.
- The importance of making follow-up appointments.

Interpersonal skills

Good communication with the patient:
- by taking a comprehensive and structured history and by interpreting investigation results, you have gathered and used relevant information to identify predisposing factors
- explores the patient's health beliefs – risk of recurrence
- by considering his occupation and dietary habits you enable Mr DC to make informed lifestyle changes to reduce the chances of recurrent attacks
- a person-centred approach enables a shared approach to a management plan and encourages compliance with further investigations and essential monitoring
- is it appropriate to admonish him for not attending when requested?

Additional information

The incidence of renal stone disease is rising. While an acute episode would be difficult to stage in an examination, a follow-up case requires candidates to demonstrate knowledge of the management of an acute attack, as well as structured history-taking and interpretation of results. This case shows the importance of taking an occupational history as all the prevention strategies relate to this.

Miller NL, Lingeman JE. (2007) Management of kidney stones. *BMJ*, **334**: 468–472.

Natural history
- Kidney stones affect 5–15% of the population.
- Recurrence rates are around 50%.

Initial evaluation
Important factors to identify in the history.

Systemic disease:
- primary hypoparathyroidism
- renal tubular acidosis
- cystinuria
- gout
- diabetes mellitus
- inflammatory bowel disease
- renal insufficiency
- sarcoidosis
- medullary sponge kidney

Anatomical features:
- horseshoe or solitary kidney
- obstruction
- previous surgery to kidneys or ureters

Kidney disease:
- infections
- positive family history
- previous stones

Drugs affecting stone disease:
- carbonic anhydrase inhibitors (topirimate)
- ephedrine
- guaifenesin
- calcium + vitamin D
- triamterene
- indinavir or sulfadiazine

In the acute phase
- Microscopic haematuria is a positive predictor of stone disease, but may be absent.
- Exclusion of infection is important (nitrites or leucocytes on dipstick).
- Unenhanced helical CT is the best radiological test.
- Most ureteric calculi <5 mm will pass through within 4 weeks; if they do not pass within 4 weeks intervention is indicated to prevent complications such as ureteral strictures and impaired renal function.
- NSAIDs are effective in relieving pain.

Urgent intervention is indicated if:
- infection with obstruction
- intractable pain, vomiting or both
- impending acute renal failure
- obstruction in a solitary or transplanted kidney
- bilateral obstruction

For follow-up
- Plain abdo X-rays or CT can be used to monitor disease activity.
- Patients with risk factors should have a metabolic work-up.

Management
- General advice:
  - increase fluid intake to produce a urine output of at least 2 litres a day
  - decrease animal protein intake
  - restrict salt and oxalate intake
  - dietary restriction of calcium intake is not recommended
- Shock wave lithotripsy can treat 80–85% of simple stones.
- Complex and staghorn calculi are best treated by percutaneous nephrolithotomy.
- Ureteroscopy is useful when other treatments fail or when other factors such as pregnancy, coagulopathy or morbid obesity prevent lithotripsy.

Relevant literature
For educational information for patients and information on research, see:
International Kidney Stone Institute (http://www.iksi.org).

For information on diagnosis and treatment of kidney stones, see:
American Urological Association (http://www.urology.health.org).

For information on kidney stones, see:
Patient UK (http://www.patient.co.uk).

For information for patients and clinicians on kidney stones, see:
Royal Infirmary of Edinburgh Renal Unit
(http://renux.dmed.ed.ac.uk/EdREN/EdRENINFObits/KidStonesLong.html).

For information for patients, see:
National Kidney Foundation (http://www.kidney.org/atozTopic.cfm?topic=13).

A US website with information for patients, see:
The National Institute of Diabetes and Digestive and Kidney Disease
(http://www.kidney.niddk.nih.gov).

Appendix: Patient summary

Name	DC
Date of birth (Age)	25
Social and Family History	Single
Past medical history	Nil
Recent reports	Printout from PCT Out-of-Hours service dated 3 weeks ago:

"05.15 hrs. Acute onset loin to groin colicky pain, right side 2 hours ago. Afebrile. Rolling round in pain. Tender renal angle. Blood ++ on dipstick. Diagnosis renal colic. Given 100 mg pethidine + stemetil i.m. Pain settled well. Prescription left for oral pethidine x20 tabs. Advised see own GP for further investigation. See SOS if recurs."

Your partner in a 5 minute emergency appointment the next day recorded:

"Renal colic last night. Pain settled after i.m. pethidine from PCT OOH. First ever episode. Urine blood+. Abdo NAD. BP 105/70. Enc fluids. Has collected script for pethidine so use this if recurs. For urine and blood tests see in one week with results."

Current Medication	None
Investigations	
Urine MC&S	RBC nil, WBC nil, No growth.
FBC, U&Es	NAD

Calcium, phosphate, magnesium, uric acid – normal
24-hour urine pH, calcium, oxalate, sodium, uric acid – normal
Plain abdo X-ray reported: '*No radio-opaque calculi seen in kidneys, which do not appear to be enlarged, or along the line of the ureters or within the bladder. Unenhanced helical CT is the best radiographic technique for diagnosing urolithiasis – please contact the department if you wish to arrange this.*'

Test your knowledge

Answer true (T) or false (F) for each of the following statements, with regard to the immediate management of renal colic.

1. If diclofenac (75mg i.m.) does not relieve the pain within 30 minutes, a 2nd dose can be given
2. If diclofenac gives inadequate pain relief, diamorphine (5–10 mg) by intramuscular, but not subcutaneous, injection should be given
3. Telephone the person after 1 hour and admit to hospital if there is no response to analgesia.
4. Patients who are not admitted on presentation should be referred urgently for diagnostic investigations (such as intravenous urogram) to be carried out within 7 days
5. The absence of haematuria excludes the diagnosis of renal colic
6. Advising people to filter their urine to capture the stone is no longer recommended

Case 41 – Neck of femur fracture

Mrs BB is a 76 year old lady who usually sees one of your partners. She has recently had a fractured neck of femur treated operatively followed by an admission for rehabilitation in a local nursing home. She comes to see you following her discharge from the nursing home to tell you that during her admission all her medication was stopped. See Appendix for details of her medication list and past history.

Targeted history taking

There are two parts to this:
1. Relating to her fractured neck of femur:
   - review how she broke her hips – has she got osteoporosis, is she having falls or giddy turns?
   - review progress following her fractured neck of femur, in particular, mobility, safety in her home, activities of daily living, and any on-going treatment such as physiotherapy/OT
   - home circumstances – type of accommodation (sheltered, home, own home), social support (health visitor, district nurse, home help), aids at home
2. Relating to her past history and medication:
   - you will need to review the patient's past history and medication list and reasons for taking each item.
   - review her present condition relating to each of her identified problems – have they changed since her medication was stopped?
   - any other symptoms
   - does she smoke or drink alcohol?
   - explore her views on having her medication stopped
   - explore her views on taking medication – is she keen to minimize medication?
   - what does she hope to gain from this consultation– an explanation regarding initiation or stoppage of medication, or reintroduction of all her medication?

Data gathering

Listed below is the additional information elicited from the patient with appropriate questioning.
   - She tripped over a rug in her bedroom and fell, fracturing her neck of femur 3 months ago.
   - She has been discharged by the orthopaedic team as she is mobile on one stick.
   - The physiotherapist is not planning to see her any more and she has been told it might be a good idea to continue to use one stick.
   - Her son and daughter have agreed to take her into town to shop once a week. They have told her she should not drive her manual car any more.

- She lives in a one bedroom first floor flat in a converted manor house in the countryside, 4 miles outside town.
- She has not taken any of her usual medication since she was admitted to hospital 3 months ago.
- She feels well:
  - CVS – no exertional chest pain or dyspnoea, ankle slightly puffy only, but can wear normal shoes
  - RS – no cough, wheeze, dyspnoea
  - GI – eating well, no heartburn, indigestion, abdominal pain, bowels normal
  - GU – no dysuria, frequency, incontinence
  - NS – no neurological symptoms, sleeping well
  - LS – knees and back hurt, but has found that losing a lot of weight and being made to be more mobile has improved these
  - Skin – still dry and itches at night in bed, varicose eczema has virtually gone since losing weight and increasing mobility
  - Endocrine – losing weight, no cold intolerance, hair not dry or coarse, no lassitude
- She is a non-smoker and has a glass of sherry before dinner every day and an occasional malt whisky after dinner.
- She is very much of the opinion that if you need tablets you should take them, and that each of her medications was started for a definite reason and so she should continue to take them.
- She is very unhappy that the hospital stopped everything.
- She expects you to restart all her medication without question.

Targeted examination

This is a relatively common scenario in general practice but could be difficult to complete in 10 minutes unless a systematic approach is taken to obtain facts and perform a targeted examination, leaving time to discuss your findings and formulate an agreed action plan.
- The extent of the examination required will depend on what symptoms she has and whether they have changed since stopping her medication. Given the time constraints, you might consider negotiating reviewing some rather than all of her problems in this consultation. In this case, you will have to identify which are the most important conditions to review – this will need to be a joint decision balancing clinical seriousness and how troublesome they are to Mrs BB.
- *In this case you note:*
  - *general condition – she has no signs of hypothyroidism apart from dry skin*
  - *CVS – you aim to exclude heart failure – chest examination, heart sounds and BP are all normal; she has very slightly puffy ankles with mild varicose eczema, but nothing to suggest the skin is at risk*
  - *you have observed she is walking with no apparent pain or great difficulty with one stick*

Clinical management

- Discuss your clinical findings – absence of symptoms and few physical signs.
- Discuss the need for regular review of conditions treated with repeat prescriptions to ensure that the need for medication is extant, especially when there is multiple pathology.
- Discuss the natural history of her conditions.
- Discuss whether any blood tests should be taken, e.g. TFTs.
- Reinforce her view that medication should only been taken when necessary.
- Explore her views relating to the hospital stopping her medication – is she criticising them, or your practice for prescribing so many medications?
- Negotiate which, if any, of her list of medications she needs to continue to use.
- Reassure her that you are not depriving her of necessary treatments.
- Congratulate her on her recovery from her fracture.
- Discuss her altered mobility and ask if her children will be able to bring her to the surgery regularly.

Interpersonal skills

Good communication skills enable you to:
- establish a rapport with a patient who you do not normally see
- explore possible physical, psychological and social issues
- reassure patient following a focussed examination
- ascertain whether stopping all her medication has been detrimental
- enable her to understand the need or not for any medication
- negotiate reducing the list of repeat medication
- ensure she is safe in her home and has mobility provided by her children
- support both your partner's and the hospital's actions in a non-judgemental manner
- use time as a diagnostic tool – she has not deteriorated since stopping her medication, so was it necessary in the first place?

Additional information

Lewis T. (2004) Using the NO TEARS tool for medication review. *BMJ*, **329**: 434.
- >33% of patients aged over 75 years in the UK take more than 4 drugs.
- 5–17% of all hospital admissions are related to adverse drug reactions.
- The **NO TEARS** tool:
  - ○ **N**eed and indication
  - ○ **O**pen questions
  - ○ **T**ests and monitoring
  - ○ **E**vidence and guidelines
  - ○ **A**dverse events
  - ○ **R**isk reduction or prevention
  - ○ **S**implification and switches

Appendix: Patient summary

Name	BB
Date of birth (Age)	76
Social and Family History	Lives in a flat in an exclusive conversion of a listed house 4 miles out of town.
	Daughter and son live nearby with their respective families.
Past medical history	pre-1982 IBS
	Hayfever
	Hypothyroidism
	1987 OA knees
	1988 atrophic vaginitis
	1991 stress incontinence
	1994 ankle oedema
	1995 dry eyes
	1996 OA back, hands and hips
	1997 analgesic induced constipation
	1998 leg cramps; haemorrhoids
	1999 poor sleep; hypertension
	2002 dizzy spells
	2003 dry skin; mild intermittent indigestion
	2005 varicose eczema
Recent reports	Patient of one of your partners who is on leave.
	GP notes show she was taken to A&E 3 months ago following a fall and was admitted with ?fractured neck of femur. No discharge letter has been received from the local hospital.
Current medication	Mebeverine 1 t.d.s. prn
	Loratadine 10 mg daily
	Beclomethasone nasal spray 2 puffs b.d.
	Thyroxine 25 µg once daily
	Ibuprofen 400 mg t.d.s. prn
	Lactulose prn
	Senna prn
	Co-codamol 30/500 2 q.d.s. as required
	Bendrofluazide 2.5 mg mane
	Aspirin 75 mg mane
	Prochlorperazine 1 t.d.s. prn
	Oilatum bath oil
	Aqueous cream
	Gaviscon prn
	Ibuprofen gel
	Simple linctus
	Anusol ointment
Investigations	Routine bloods tests 4 months ago in the practice:
Hb	12.1
MCV	84.2
U&Es	normal
Cholesterol	4.9
Triglycerides	1.0
Fasting glucose	4.9
TSH	normal

Test your knowledge

Answer true (T) or false (F) for each of the following statements, with regard to postmenopausal women with osteoporosis and fragility fracture.

1. Drug therapy is indicated in women aged 75 years and older, without the need for prior dual energy X-ray absorptiometry (DEXA) scanning
2. Ibandronate and etidronate reduce the incidence of both vertebral and non-vertebral fractures
3. Ibandronate taken monthly may be considered as an alternative to the other daily and weekly bisphosphonate preparations
4. An active, but not past, history of venous thrombosis precludes the use of raloxifene and strontium ranelate
5. When investigating osteoporosis, if the ESR is raised, then serum and urine electrophoresis are indicated to exclude renal osteodystrophy
6. If repeat DEXA scanning is thought to be appropriate, in general this should not be carried out unless the person has been taking treatment for at least 2 years

Case 42 – Drug use

JO, a 19 year old single man, presents to you asking for help for his drug problem. See Appendix for details.

Targeted history taking

You need to collect a lot of information:
- Drug history:
  - what is he taking, how much, when, and how?
  - how much is he spending a day to support his habit?
  - if injecting does he use clean needles? Has he ever shared needles?
  - when did he start using drugs?
  - obtain a full drug history
  - smoking and alcohol
  - any prescribed drugs from other sources?
  - any previous attempts to stop? If so when, how and why did they fail?
- Forensic history – police/criminal history
- Medical history:
  - screening questions for GI and liver problems
  - general health
  - is he eating normally?
- Mental health problems:
  - in past?
  - currently – specifically depression
- Social – check what support is available: parents, friends, girlfriend?
- Past history
- Assess motivation to stop
- Clarify his expectations of this consultation – an exploration of his options for treatment and/or support, medication, referral, or signposting to drug-related services?

Data gathering

Listed below is the additional information elicited from the patient with appropriate questioning.
- He has been smoking cannabis for 4–5 years and started taking heroin 8 months ago. He injected with friends a couple of times 6 months ago using fresh needles and syringes, but was frightened by the experience and has not injected again. He is spending about £80 a day at present.
- He drinks 5–6 units a day – usually vodka. He smokes 15/day.

- He tried to cold turkey a month ago while his parents were on holiday, but he could not cope on his own.
- No forensic, relevant past medical history or any mental health issues.
- His girlfriend of 2 years' standing left him 2 months ago because she could not stand him taking drugs. He tried to cold turkey as a response to this.
- All his circle of friends takes drugs.
- He lives with his parents. He thinks they are unaware of his problem and says they disapprove strongly of drugs.
- He says he really wants to stop – family pressure, lost one girlfriend and does not feel he will attract and keep 'nice' girls with his current habit, cannot support his habit financially any more without resorting to criminal activity and he is also worried about his long term health although he says he does not really know the risks.
- He has heard that GPs can prescribe methadone and thinks this would be the best option for him.

Targeted examination

A brief physical examination incorporating:
- general assessment – nutritional status
- oral health
- inspect common injection sites to confirm his story
- *In this case he looks well and has no abnormal physical findings. He tells you that he does not inject and inspection of common injection sites confirms this.*

Clinical management

- Risk reduction:
  - support his decision not to inject
  - check vaccination status
  - discuss screening for hepatitis C and HIV
- Confirm drug taking:
  - drug screening
  - urine or saliva?
- Notification to regional database
- You could discuss management options:
  - specialist hospital assessment and stabilization
  - shared care protocol – substitution therapy
  - detoxification
- Follow up :
  - to discuss results
  - to agree management plan
- Referral: negotiate making a referral to a specialist after follow-up appointment
- Support for JO and his parents: drug support agencies, both local and national

Interpersonal skills

Good communication skills are required in order to:
- gather information in a non-judgemental way
- explore possible physical, psychological and social issues
- support him in giving up his drug habit
- enable you to engage with him and encourage compliance with whatever programme you agree
- be supportive and motivational

Additional information

Drug abuse is common and many GPs offer shared-care substitute treatments. This case tests data gathering and management of a common problem and maintaining a positive approach. Development of a supportive trusting relationship will encourage compliance in future and contribute to the potential success of any treatment.

Pilling S, Strang J, Gerada C. (2007) Psychosocial interventions and opioid detoxification for drug misuse: summary of NICE guidance. *BMJ*, **335**: 203–205.
- Drug misuse is an increasing problem.
- It impacts negatively on individuals, their families and society in general.
- GPs care for at least one-third of opioid misusers in treatment.
- Two new NICE guidelines identify the most effective, safe detoxification regimens for primary and secondary care, the most cost-effective psychosocial interventions and effective ways to engage patients.
- The community-based detoxification regimen is derived from consensus rather than being evidence-based.
- Community-based detoxification should not be offered to patients who:
  - have failed previous community-based detoxification
  - have other health problems requiring medical/nursing care
  - require complex polydrug detoxification
  - have considerable social problems that may adversely affect community-based detoxification
- Offer buprenorphine or methadone first-line.
- Lofexidine should be considered especially when there is mild or uncertain dependence, but adjunct medication is usually required to manage withdrawal symptoms.
- Benzodiazepines, minor analgesics or antidiarrhoeals should not be used routinely.
- Opportunistic brief interventions focussing on motivation should be offered.
- Information about self-help groups should be offered routinely (e.g. Narcotics Anonymous).
- Contingency management includes use of incentives such as vouchers or privileges and drug testing. There is evidence from overseas trials that

behaviour can be influenced positively by incentives rather than threats or punishments, which have little influence on this patient population.

The NICE guidelines can be found at:

Drug misuse: psychosocial interventions. (2007) see: www.nice.org.uk/CG051.
Drug misuse: opioid detoxification. (2007) see: www.nice.org.uk/CG052.

Appendix: Patient summary

Name	JO
Date of birth (Age)	22
Social and Family History	Single. Unemployed.
Past medical history	Fractured wrist 6 months ago
	Amoebiasis after holiday in India 14 months ago
	Indigestion 18 months ago – given 10 mg omeprazole once daily for one month
Recent Reports	14 months ago – Hep A & B and Typhoid vaccs.
	Last seen 4 months ago: *'Discharged by Trauma Clinic. Wrist now feels ok. Final sick note. Not happy being signed off as fit to work.'*
Current Medication	None
Investigations	None

Test your knowledge

Answer true (T) or false (F) for each of the following statements, with regard to hepatitis C.

1. 60% of people will fight the infection and naturally clear it from their bodies within 2–6 months
2. 20% will progress to cirrhosis over a period of 20–30 years
3. Since September 1991, all blood donated in the UK is checked for the hepatitis C virus
4. Methotrexate and ribavirin can clear the virus in approximately half those treated
5. If hepatitis C is cleared with treatment, patients are immune to future infections of hepatitis C

An introduction to case-based discussion (CbD)

What is CbD?

'Case-based discussion (CbD) is a *structured interview* designed to explore *professional judgement* exercised in clinical cases which have been selected by the GP trainee and presented for evaluation' (RCGP, 2007).

What is a structured interview?

CbD is a formal discussion that is conducted in accordance with national (RCGP) guidance. The guidance specifies the length of the interview, the competencies to be assessed, the case-mix required, the number and timing of discussions throughout the training period and the marking schedule. This provides a measure of standardisation of assessment throughout the UK.

The CbD is not an oral or viva exam. Consequently, it does not carry a pass/fail assessment, nor should it feel intimidating. On the other hand, it is one of the many mini-assessments required to provide evidence for workplace-based assessment (WPBA), one of the three components of the global assessment (nMRCGP) which licenses the trainee for practice as an independent GP. Therefore, it is a component of continuous assessment.

The CbD structured interview requires two major skills from trainers:

- **questioning skills** – devising questions targeted at specific areas of performance. For example, if the area of 'practising holistically' is being assessed, then trainers are required to devise appropriate and searching questions to assess how the trainee has thought through the steps of 'practising holistically'.
- **feedback skills** – to offer trainees specific feedback, arising from the CbD, to assist them with their development and progression towards independent general practice.

CbD requires two major skills from trainees:

- **demonstrating the steps of decision-making**. The trainee must overtly show this skill. To use an analogy, in a driving test, the learner driver demonstrates to the examiner his driving skills – his ability to recognize problems on the road and to take appropriate action. He is not passed because he gets from A to B. Similarly, the CbD tests the skills of decision-making and the trainee must be overt in his demonstration of decision-making skills. He has to show each step of the process. The CbD is not assessing the final action the trainee took with the patient, but the steps in decision-making which he discusses during the interview.
- **accepting feedback**. It is hoped that the action a trainee takes in his last three

months of GP training is different to his actions in his first three months. The reason for the difference is experiential learning – the learning about being a GP that the trainee acquires by doing and reflecting on the job. Therefore, the initial CbDs, when judged against what an independent and safe GP would do, are very likely to identify several learning needs. The trainee's responsibility is to consciously identify, with the trainer, what these learning needs are and to develop an action plan for meeting these needs. Hence, the trainee needs to accept feedback.

What is professional judgement?

According to the RCGP (2007), 'Professional judgement may be considered as the ability to make holistic, balanced and justifiable decisions in situations of complexity and uncertainty. It may include the ability to make rational decisions in the absence of complete information or evidence, and to take action or even do nothing in such situations. It requires a selection of attributes: recognising uncertainty/complexity, application or use of medical knowledge, application or use of ethical and legal frameworks, ability to prioritise options, consider implications and justify decisions.'

The oral exam of the old MRCGP, an exit or summative assessment exam, also tested the trainee's decision-making skills and their underpinning professional values and behaviour. When oral examiners were asked how they would recognize good decision-making steps, independently of the final outcome of decisions, Simpson (2004) wrote that oral examiners were looking for eight stages of decision making:

1. recognize the dilemma
2. identify possible options and solutions
3. recognize the implications of these options
4. prioritize and weigh each option
5. choose an option
6. justify choice
7. check that the option works and does not need further modification or reassessment
8. reflect on what has been learnt from the experience.

Likewise, CbD tests decision-making, albeit in continuous assessment format. Trainees get good assessments if they:

- recognize the dilemma. Many of the problems require GPs to balance conflicting issues – for example, demand versus resources available, doing good as opposed to harm, the needs of the individual versus the needs of society.
- present a greater number of options together with the implications of each. Trainees should be able to discuss the advantages and disadvantages of each option – this demonstrates a deep understanding of the issue and shows the ability to anticipate the potential consequences of the decision.
- are prepared to justify why they dismissed some options as well as why they chose others.

- are able to make a decision or reconsider the decisions they made. When asked to reconsider, trainees are expected to reassess a plan of action and justify their choice. There is no textbook answer or college line to be regurgitated – trainers are looking for sound, ethical and evidence-based decision making.
- are able to construct an evaluation plan for their decision – in six month's time, how will they know that they made the correct decision? Therefore, by identifying their learning needs at the end of the discussion, they demonstrate an awareness and an approach to continuing professional development.

When does CbD occur?

CbD occurs throughout GP training.

- For Structured Training Year one (ST1) and ST2, a minimum of three cases should be discussed prior to each interim review. There will be two reviews each year, and therefore a minimum of six cases each year, bringing up a total of twelve cases by the end of ST2.
- For year ST3, prior to the 30 month review, at least 6 cases should have been discussed. Prior to the final review, 6 more cases should have been discussed, bringing the total to twelve cases in the ST3 year.

Where does CbD occur?

CbD occurs in both hospital and GP settings. Each CbD is a mini-assessment within WPBA. The nMRCGP is an integrated assessment programme that includes three components:

- Applied Knowledge Test (AKT)
- Clinical Skills Assessment (CSA)
- Workplace-Based Assessment (WPBA)

Each of these three components is independent and will test different skills, thereby providing mini-assessments of the trainee over the entire training period. Together these three components will cover the curriculum for specialty training for general practice, to inform a global assessment.

Why does CbD occur?

CbD occurs to test how GP trainees make decisions in everyday practice. Everyday practice is real-life, with over-running surgeries, staff that interrupt clinics, and patients who don't always speak fluent English. These are not the carefully constructed scenarios of exam situations. CbD tests professional judgement within the contextual stresses in which GPs make decisions.

Miller (1990) proposed that one could assess skill at four levels of increasing sophistication:

1. Knowledge – for example, the trainee *knows* the indications and contra-indications for safe Combined Pill prescribing. This is tested in the AKT.
2. The ability to use that knowledge – for example, the trainee *knows how* to select those patients in whom the Combined Pill will be the best contraceptive choice. This is also tested in the AKT.

3. A demonstration that one can use that knowledge – the trainee *shows how* he takes a history and examines the patient before prescribing the Combined Pill. This is tested in the CSA.
4. The ability to use that knowledge in everyday practice – the trainee, in everyday, busy practice with patients of varying communication abilities and ages, *does* prescribe the Combined Pill safely and effectively. This is tested in the CbD.

CbD is a useful assessment because:

- it provides trainees with opportunities to demonstrate improvement in, and attainment of, the skill of professional judgement, over time and in a variety of contexts
- the assessment occurs as close as possible to the real situations in which doctors work
- it tests competency areas, particularly in many aspects of professionalism, that are difficult to test elsewhere, such as team working and how personal values affect decision making

Who carries out the CbD?

Hospital and GP trainers will prepare the questions, conduct the interviews, assess the trainees and provide feedback.

GP trainees will initiate or ask for the assessment when they have identified appropriate cases and ensure that the paperwork, or e-portfolio entry, is properly completed. Trainees should select children, mental health, cancer/palliative care and older adults, across varying contexts, i.e. surgery, home visits and out-of-hours contacts, to provide a representative case-mix.

How is CbD carried out?

When the ST1 or ST2 trainee decides to request a CbD, he will select two cases and present copies of the clinical entries and relevant records to the assessor one week before the discussion. The assessor selects one of the cases for discussion.

When the ST3 trainee requests a CbD, he selects four cases and present copies of the clinical entries and relevant records to the assessor one week before the discussion. The assessor selects one or two of the cases for each session, depending on time available. The assessor usually informs the trainee at least 24 hours in advance which case is selected for discussion.

The trainer prepares appropriate questions according to RCGP guidance as set out below (taken from http://www.rcgp.org.uk/docs/nMRCGP_CBD%20 Structured%20Question%20Guidance.doc [accessed July 2007]). Two or three competencies are tested in each CbD. For example, if 'practising holistically' is tested, trainees are mainly asked the questions from the first section:

Define[s] the problem
What are the issues raised in this case?
What conflicts are you trying to resolve?
Why did you find it difficult/challenging?

Integrate[s] information
What relevant information had you available?
Why was this relevant?
How did the data/information/evidence you had available help you to make your decision?
How did you use the data/information/evidence available to you in this case?
What other information could have been useful?

Prioritize[s] options
What were your options? Which did you choose?
Why did you choose this one?
What are the advantages/disadvantages of your decision?
How do you balance them?

Consider[s] implications
What are the implications of your decision?
For whom? (e.g. patient/relatives/doctor/practice/society)
How might they feel about your choice?
How does this influence your decision?

Justifies decision
How do you justify your decision?
What evidence/information have you to support your choice?
Can you give me an example?
Are you aware of any model or framework that helps you to justify your decision?
How does it help you? Can you apply it to this case?
Some people might argue, how would you convince them of your point of view?
Why did you do this?

Practise[s] ethically
What ethical framework did you refer to in this case? How did you apply it?
How did it help you decide what to do?
How did you establish the patient's point of view?
What are their rights? How did this influence your handling of the case?

Work[s] in a team

Which colleagues did you involve in this case? Why?
How did you ensure you had effective communication with them?
Who could you have involved? What might they have been able to offer?
What is your role in this sort of situation?

Uphold[s] duties of a doctor
What are your responsibilities/duties? How do they apply to this case?
How did you make sure you observed them? Why are they important?'

The trainer is advised to:
- use the written records as a starting point
- make and record an assessment of the quality of these records
- use pre-prepared questions, such as those in the above list, to explore the professional judgement demonstrated by the trainee
- pay particular attention to situations in which uncertainty has arisen, or where a conflict of decision-making has arisen
- allow 20 minutes per case
- allow 10 minutes for feedback, with any recommendations for change
- record evidence elicited in the notes sheet. The current (July 2007) notes sheet below is taken from the RCGP website (see RCGP website for updated versions: http://www.rcgp.org.uk/nmrcgp_/nmrcgp/wpba_tools/cbd.aspx).

	Proposed questions	Evidence obtained
Practising holistically		
Data gathering and interpretation		
Making diagnoses/decisions		
Clinical management		
Managing medical complexity		
Primary care administration and IMT		
Working with colleagues and in teams		
Community orientation		
Maintaining an ethical approach to practice		
Fitness to practice		

- The trainer makes a judgement on the level of the trainee's performance against each competency area. At the end of each case, a judgement of the level of performance demonstrated by the trainee is recorded on the marking grid. The marking grid supplied below is adapted from the grid provided on the RCGP website (see RCGP website for any updates: http://www.rcgp.org.uk/docs/nMRCGP_Sample%20Form.doc [accessed July 2007]).

Professional competencies	Insufficient evidence	Needs further development	Competent	Excellent
Practising holistically				
Data gathering and interpretation				
Making diagnosis/decisions				
Clinical management				
Managing medical complexity				
Primary care administration and IMT				
Working with colleagues and in teams				
Community orientation				
Maintaining an ethical approach				
Fitness to practice				

Feedback on areas for further development

What each competency means

The explanatory notes from the RCGP website are quoted below in full (http://www.rcgp.org.uk/Docs/nMRCGP_Clinical%20supervisors%20structured %20report%20v3.doc [accessed July 2007]).

Practising holistically: this competency is about the ability of the doctor to consider physical, psychological, socioeconomic and cultural aspects, taking into account feelings as well as thoughts. *Behaviours you may wish to consider: exploring the way in which the problem affects the patient's life, exploring the impact of the problem on the patient's family/carers.*

Data gathering and interpretation: this competency is about the gathering and use of data for clinical judgement, the choice of examination and investigations and their interpretation. *Behaviours you may wish to consider: systematically gathering information, using questions that are appropriately focused, making use of existing information, choosing physical examinations and targeting investigations appropriately, making appropriate inferences from the findings and results.*

Making diagnosis/ decisions: this competency is about a deliberate, structured approach to decision-making. *Behaviours you may wish to consider: clarifying the decision that is required, integrating information to aid pattern recognition, using probability to decide what is likely, revising hypotheses in the light of further information, thinking flexibly around the problem.*

Clinical management: this competency is about the recognition and management of medical conditions. *Behaviours you may wish to consider: recognizing common presentations, utilizing the natural history in management decisions, using simple measures when appropriate, varying management options when required, prescribing appropriately, referring appropriately and coordinating care with other colleagues, responding quickly and skilfully in emergencies.*

Managing medical complexity: this competency is about aspects of care beyond managing straightforward problems, including the management of co-morbidity, uncertainty, risk and thinking about health rather than just illness. *Behaviours you may wish to consider: simultaneously managing the patient's health problems both acute and chronic, tolerating uncertainty where this is unavoidable, explaining risks associated with management to the patients, encouraging patients to have a positive approach to their health.*

Primary care administration and IMT: this competency is about the appropriate use of primary care administration systems, effective record-keeping and information technology for the benefit of patient care. *Behaviours you may wish to consider: using administrative and computer systems appropriately, keeping good clinical records (timely, coded, sufficiently comprehensive).*

Working with colleagues and in teams: this competency is about working effectively with other professionals to ensure patient care, including the sharing of information with colleagues. *Behaviours you may wish to consider: being available to colleagues, working cooperatively, sharing information with others involved in the patient's care, using appropriate methods of communication according to the circumstances.*

Community orientation: this competency is about the management of the health and social care of patients in the local community. *Behaviours you may wish to consider: identifying important characteristics of the local community that might impact upon patient care, particularly the epidemiological, social, economic and ethnic features, using this understanding to improve patient management, identifying resources in the community, encouraging patients to access available resources, using health care resources effectively, e.g. through cost-effective prescribing.*

Maintaining an ethical approach: this competency is about practising ethically with integrity and a respect for diversity. *Behaviours you may wish to consider: identifying and discussing ethical issues in clinical practice, treating patients, colleagues and others fairly and with respect for their beliefs, preferences, dignity and rights, valuing differences between people and avoiding prejudice.*

Fitness to practice: this competency is about the doctor's awareness of when his/her own performance, conduct or health, or that of others might put patients at risk and the action taken to protect patients. *Behaviours you may wish to consider: observing the accepted codes of professional practice, allowing scrutiny and justifying professional behaviour to colleagues, achieving a healthy balance between professional and personal demands, seeking advice and engaging in remedial action where personal performance is an issue.*

How to use this book to prepare for CbD

This book includes:
- a CbD section – cases 1 to 10
- a concepts section

The CbD section – cases 1 to 10 will:
- provide a summary of the case being discussed
- introduce the discussion by considering the issues that the trainee may want to raise
- outline the two competencies that the trainer has chosen to test
- provide the actual questions the trainer has prepared to assess the chosen competencies
- provide a question and answer session
- offer answers which use various models to generate a number of options, and discuss the advantages and disadvantages of each option; the answers discuss the steps in the trainee's decision-making process; the trainee bases his decisions on ethical and evidence-based reasoning

In addition, background knowledge is required to:
- ○ choose a model to generate the options – these may be consultation models, change management models or ethical frameworks
  - ○ provide the evidence base, where applicable, to justify the final decision
- The 'Additional information' section provides the background knowledge in greater detail – this is for candidates to reach a deeper understanding of the subject.
- The 'Relevant literature' section signposts candidates to the primary sources of information. The literature changes at a rapid pace, and web sources are usually a good source of updated information and so, where possible, useful websites are listed.

The Concepts section:
- discusses common themes, i.e. the generic, background knowledge and skills required for CbD and modern general practice are discussed.
- offers alternative models for analysing and informing decision-making. This enables trainees to approach any question in the CbD section from

alternative perspectives. What a trainee decides depends on the individual doctor and the context; hence different choices may be more appropriate in different contexts.

Relevant literature

Miller GE. (1990) The assessment of clinical skills/competence/performance. *Academic Medicine*, **65**: 563–67.
RCGP (2007) www.rcgp.org.uk.
Simpson RG. (2004) Preparing for the oral module. *The Practitioner*, **248**: 287–289.

14 year old requests contraception

Case summary

WH is a 14 year old fit and healthy girl. She attends with her mum. WH requests a prescription for Microgynon, for contraceptive purposes. She specifically asks for Microgynon – her mum and her friends are on this Pill. You assess WH as Fraser competent. She has no contraindications to the Pill. She is slightly spotty. While you are happy to prescribe a combined oral contraceptive (the Pill), you suggest that a third generation Pill such as Marvelon may be better for her spotty skin. Mum replies that she remembers Marvelon from the Pill scare in the late 1990s. By this time, you have run late, so you assess Fraser competence, prescribe a three-month supply of Microgynon and advise WH to see you sooner if problems arise.

Opening question:

What issues or challenges does this case raise for you, the trainee?
- You are concerned about the limited time you had in which to deal with the large number of issues this case raised.
- Did you address the most important issues adequately?
- How could you safely shorten the consultation so as not to have clinics that over-run?

In this case, the trainer may decide to focus predominantly on two domains:
- **data gathering and interpretation** – gathering and using data for clinical judgment
- **clinical management** – recognizing and managing common medical conditions

To achieve sufficient depth of questioning in the above domains, the trainer may prepare the following questions:
- how did you assess Fraser competence?
- did you need to assess Fraser competence?
- you said that WH had no contraindications to the Pill – what information did you specially seek from her to arrive at this decision?
- why did you believe that Marvelon would have been a better choice for WH than Microgynon?
- was it important to explore mum's ideas regarding Marvelon and the Pill scare? Justify your reasoning.
- did you discuss alternative methods of contraception with WH? Justify your decision-making.
- did you discuss sexual health and child protection issues? Justify your reasoning.

How did you assess Fraser competence?

Lord Fraser's five criteria for a minor to consent to contraception without the consent of her parents are:

1. she understands the advice and is competent to consent to treatment
2. she is encouraged to inform her parents or guardians
3. she is likely to commence or continue sexual activity with or without contraception
4. her physical or mental health will suffer if she does not receive contraceptive advice or supplies
5. providing contraception is in her best interests

Why did you need to assess Fraser competence?

WH is 14 years old. The guidance applies to the under 16s. I applied the guidance because I believe that it is good guidance rooted in social reality.

If WH attended with her mother, then she is hardly seeking treatment without parental consent – are the Fraser guidelines applicable to the case?

In retrospect, it is probably more applicable if WH attended without her mother. However, the first part of the guidance is useful – it is important to assess that teenagers understand the advice given to them when considering issues of compliance. (*The discussion has uncovered a learning need, that is, 'When is Fraser guidance applicable?' See Additional information section below for an approach to continuing professional development.*)

You said that had WH presented alone, it would have been useful to apply Fraser guidance – what is useful about the Fraser guidance?

According to the Sexual Offences Amendment Act (2000), young people can only legally consent to heterosexual and homosexual sex from the age of 16 years. However, one in four women and one in three men say they had sexual intercourse before the age of 16 (Wellings *et al.*, 2001). The legal position does not mirror the social reality. The Fraser guidance is useful because it reflects social reality.

Because the guidance is pragmatic, I find it really useful when I am confronted with issues on teenage consent. I feel that my refusal to supply contraception to minors is unlikely to deter those who want sexual intercourse. By supplying contraceptives to a girl under the age of 16 without parental consent, I see myself as performing a duty to society.

I also find the Fraser guidance useful because it advises doctors to encourage their teenage patients to inform their parents of their treatments, which is sensible because parents have a right to know what is happening to their children to provide them with proper care.

You said that WH had no contraindications to the Pill – what information did you specially seek from her to arrive at this decision?

I asked WH whether:
- she suffered from focal migraines?

- she smoked?
- she had a significant family history of breast cancer or deep vein thrombosis?
- she was taking any prescribed or over-the-counter medication that may interact with the Pill rendering it less efficacious

I weighed and measured WH, and calculated her BMI. I took her BP. Had I elicited any contraindications to the Pill, I would have classified them into relative or absolute contraindications using the medical eligibility criteria (UKMEC) for combined oral contraceptive use or the WHO criteria, which is available on the internet: http://www.who.int/reproductive-health/publications/mec/index.htm.

Why did you believe that Marvelon would have been a better choice for WH than Microgynon?

- Marvelon is a 3rd generation Pill and these are said to have fewer minor side effects, such as greasy skin or acne, when compared to 2nd generation pills such as Microgynon.
- Pills are also classified as oestrogen-dominant (Marvelon) or progestogen-dominant (Microgynon). Oestrogen-dominant pills are better for greasy skin.

Therefore, for girls like WH with spotty skin, a 3rd generation, oestrogen-dominant pill seemed a better choice.

Was it important to explore mum's ideas regarding Marvelon and the Pill scare? Justify your reasoning

I think it was important to explore mum's ideas because the information she gives is very likely to influence her daughter's choice of Pill. WH is less likely to choose Marvelon if she believes this to be an unsafe Pill. Mum's concerns about the safety of 3rd generation Pills can be addressed by giving her up-to-date information about the likelihood of venous thrombo-embolism (VTE) on combined Pills.

2nd generation pills such as Microgynon have been used safely for a long time whereas 3rd generation Pills such as Marvelon were given a bad press in the 1995 Pill scare. The judgment in the group action against the manufacturers of 3rd generation Pills concluded that there was no increased relative risk of VTE from the third-generation oral contraceptives.

Data sheets of gestodene and desogestrel-containing Pills in the UK were changed in 1998 to say that they have a risk of VTE of about 25 per 100 000 women per year, while for 2nd generation Pills the risk is about 15 per 100 000 women per year.

Two studies (Lawrenceson *et al.*, 1999 and Farmer *et al.*, 2000) looked at VTE rates in 2nd and 3rd generation Pills and found an overall incidence of 38 per 100 000 women per year for both types of Pill. Therefore, women should be informed about the risk of VTE with combined Pills and be offered non-oestrogenic forms of contraception if they do not wish to take that risk.

Did you discuss alternative methods of contraception with WH? Justify your decision-making

I briefly discussed the Implanon implant and gave her a family planning leaflet which outlined alternative methods – WH needs to be aware of her contraceptive options in order to make an informed choice. The table below outlines all her contraceptive options. However, many of the methods mentioned will be unsuitable or unacceptable to a 14 year old.

Hormonal contraceptive methods	*Non-hormonal contraceptive methods*
The combined oral contraceptive: • Pill • patch (Evra)	Barrier contraception: • male condoms • female condoms (Femidom)
Progestogen only methods: • progestogen only pill (POP) • depo injection (depo-provera) • implant (Implanon)	The copper intra-uterine device The cap / diaphragm
Mirena intra-uterine system containing progestogen	Spermicide: • sponge (a carrier for the spermicide) • foam (Delfen)
	Sterilization (male or female)
	Natural family planning (including Persona)
	The withdrawal method

Depo-provera is not the first choice in teenagers because its use in the under-19s is associated with a reduction in the bone mass density (BMD) at a time when the BMD should be increasing. It is not known whether the reduction in BMD recovers completely when the teenager switches to alternative methods (DoH, 2004).

On balance, I thought the combined Pill was a good contraceptive choice because of its efficacy, ease of use and easy return to fertility on discontinuation, provided WH gets into an organized Pill-taking regime.

Did you discuss sexual health and child protection issues? Justify your reasoning

I did not discuss these issues for several reasons.

- There were many important issues in this consultation. I prioritized the issues and dealt with what I considered to be the top priority, that is, meeting WH's agenda, risk-assessing WH's suitability for oral contraception, and explaining to her how to take the Pill correctly.
- If I establish a good relationship with WH, she is very likely to consult me in future and I could address the sexual health agenda at this later stage. Her mum, the school nurse or internet websites, could already have provided this information.

- Had I, based on verbal and non-verbal cues during the consultation, strongly suspected abuse, I would definitely have broached the subject. Under these circumstances, I have a moral duty to WH to raise the issue and to act if necessary. My professional obligation under the GMC's *Good Medical Practice* is to make the care of the patient my first concern, particularly when protecting vulnerable people, such as minors. If I believed WH was at risk, I would follow child protection guidelines.

Additional information

Child protection and confidentiality

'Doctors dealing with child protection issues are frequently confronted by conflicts between the need to share information and the rules governing confidentiality, and their professional duties to different patients often within the same family.

- The doctor's first duty is to act in the best interests of the child. Where there is a conflict between parents and child and the child and others, the child's needs are paramount.
- Where there are reasonable grounds to believe a child is at risk of significant harm, the facts should be reported to Social Services.
- Primary Care Trusts, NHS Trusts and health authorities have a statutory duty, effected through their employees, to assist Social Services, making enquiries under the Children Act.
- Where consent to disclosure is refused by an apparently competent child, disclosure may still be appropriate if refusal results from duress, fear or the circumstantial pressures upon the child.

Where consent to disclosure is refused by an adult, relevant disclosure may be necessary in order to protect the best interests of the child and may be justifiable on those grounds. All decisions and the reasoning behind them should be thoroughly documented.'

Taken from: http://www.medicalprotection.org/Medical/United_Kingdom/ Publications/Factsheets/factsheet_child.aspx [accessed Nov 2004].

In the above discussion, you identified **learning needs**. Your trainer may ask you how you identify and address your learning needs, in which case you need to have a structured approach to continuing professional development.

There are five stages to the **continuing professional development** (CPD) cycle:

- assessment of individual and organizational needs
- making personal development plans
- implementation
- re-inforcement and dissemination
- review of the effectiveness of the CPD intervention

An assessment of learning needs

Learning needs can be conceptualized as the discrepancy between the starting point ('where are you now') and the end point ('where do you want to be') (Kaufman and English, 1979). Learning needs can be identified from personal review, clinical practice, from patients and from colleagues with whom you work.

From personal review
- Personal reading, internet and media, lectures and meetings, further study (e.g. diplomas) and research.
- Formal testing, e.g. quizzes in medical magazines; PEP – CDs; *BMJ* – learning modules; SWOT – analysis where the doctor identifies the strengths and weaknesses of his practice and the opportunities and threats to his progress; and Manchester Rating Scales.
- Reflection on challenging consultations or interactions (what happened; why did it happen; what can I do differently next time to alter the outcome).
- Videos of consultations / joint surgeries: actual performance is reviewed by the doctor or by a peer to see if the desired behaviours are present, e.g. did the doctor demonstrate empathy.

From clinical practice
- Audits: audit is a measurement of quality. It compares the actual level of performance against clearly defined, explicit standards. Changes are made and their effect is re-measured to see if they had the desired outcome. There should be self-improvement through standard setting, measurement, change and reassessment.
- MAAG audits (Medical Audit Advisory Group): compares the performance of the practice with other local practices; prioritizes areas of clinical practice that need improvement (e.g. diabetic care); and shares ideas for improvement.
- Significant event analysis (SEA): a critical review of important events, it includes both positive and negative events. The team reviews the strengths and weaknesses of the management and identifies ways in which things could be done differently. The aim is for the entire team to learn from the event and to apply the lessons learnt.
- Feedback from patient groups: the groups' views are incorporated in the practice plan.

From patients
- PUNS and DENS (patient's unmet needs and doctor's educational needs). Patients may ask doctors questions to which they do not know the answer. Doctors have to find the answer so meeting their educational needs.
- Complaints
- Patient satisfaction surveys and questionnaires: in addition to providing feedback on their overall experience of the practice, they also comment on the doctor's timekeeping and attitudes. The RCGP advises that patient surveys be done on an annual basis.

From the team
- Staff feedback: either informally though practice meetings or formally through 360 degree feedback. 360 degree feedback involves handing out a questionnaire to a cross-section of the PHCT (everyone from receptionist to senior partner). The information is collected anonymously by a 3rd party who analyses and feeds back to the individual so that he becomes aware of how others see him – Johari's window.
- Practice appraisals: the practice may be inspected by the PCT, the Committee for Health Improvement, and the deanery (if it is a training practice).
- PACT: prescribing trends within the practice compared to others regionally.

From others sources
- Guidelines: e.g. hypertension guidelines, or management of dyspepsia.
- Visits to other practices / teams, e.g. visiting the local drugs and rehab. team.

Grant (2002) identified 46 formal and informal methods of needs assessment.

The personal development plan (PDP)
All doctors were expected to have a PDP by April 2000. The PDP should contain the following information:
1. what the planned CPD activity is
2. its intended date of completion
3. how the educational need was identified
4. the changes to practice that will occur on completion of the CPD
5. the dates for completion of the changes detailed in (4).

For example, a locum doctor may identify from his PUNs and DENs a knowledge gap regarding the treatment of drug addicts in primary care.
1. The planned CPD may be to review the practice's protocol and discuss it with a partner who has an interest in addiction management.
2. It may take 2–3 hours (perhaps a few lunch hours) to read the protocol and email the interested partner to clarify matters.
3. The need was identified by being unable to manage the clinical needs of a drug addict in surgery.
4. In future, when working at practices that manage drug addiction, the locum will be able to write out the correct prescriptions and feel more confident about managing addiction.
5. Over the next two months, the locum doctor can keep a list of five addiction patients that he managed and review their records to see if follow-up consultations agreed with his management plans.

He can disseminate the information he has learnt to other locums when they meet at non-principals groups. The information can be shared, discussed and analysed, thus reinforcing his learning. The doctor may read the clinical governance report that the practice has produced – this should give him information about the effectiveness of his practice.

Personal preparation

Lewin's model of change (Iles and Sutherland, 2001) can be used to help in preparation and can be summarised as follows:

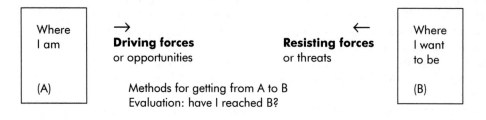

Step-wise preparation

The doctor can get direction from *Good Medical Practice for General Practitioners*. This describes the criteria for an 'excellent' GP.

- Using standards from *Good Medical Practice for General Practitioners*, the doctor writes down his goals ('where he wants to be').
- By reviewing his current practice, he identifies 'where he is'. He completes a needs assessment.
- He identifies the gaps between where he is and where he wants to be, and prioritizes his learning needs. The prioritization takes into account the needs of the practice (from the Practice Development Plan), the patients and the PCT (who may be offering incentives for change).
- The doctor identifies the tools or methods for addressing these needs. This includes self-directed learning, attending study days (e.g. how to set up a diabetic clinic), and meeting with other professionals (study groups / Balint groups).

The doctor evaluates whether he achieved his goals and provides evidence to this effect. This may include personal reflection, changes made to practice protocols, evidence from re-auditing, and a second round of patient and peer surveys.

Relevant literature

Department of Health (2001) The Health and Social Care Act 2001: Section 60 and 61. Background information, *Patient Confidentiality*.

Farmer RTD, et al. (2000) Effect of 1995 pill scare on rates of venous thromboembolism among women taking combined oral contraceptives: analysis of General Practice Research Database. *BMJ*, **321**: 477–479.

General Medical Council (2000) *Protecting and Providing Information*, paragraphs 34 and 35. London: BMA.

Grant J (2002) Learning needs assessment: assessing the need. *BMJ*, **324**: 156–159.

Iles V and Sutherland K (2001) *Organisational Change: managing change in the NHS*. NHS SDO RandD Program. London.

Kaufman R and English FW (1979) *Needs Assessment: Concept and Application*. Englewood Cliffs, NJ: Educational Technology Publications

Lawrenceson RA, *et al*. (1999) DoH seems to have underestimated incidence of venous thromboembolism in users of combined oral contraceptives. *BMJ*, **319:** 387.

Wellings K, *et al*. (2001) Sexual behaviour in Britain: early heterosexual experience, *Lancet*, **358:** 1843–1850.

www.info.doh.gov.uk/tpu/tpu.nsf

www.who.int/reproductive-ealth/publications/RHR_00_2_medical_eligibility_criteria_ second_edition/rhr_00_02_cocs.html

Earache and antibiotics

Case summary
Mr G brought his 5 year old son, DG, to see me in my Friday morning clinic. DG had had an earache for 12 hours and was up intermittently throughout the night. The family was due to leave on a holiday to France and Mr G requested antibiotics. During the consultation, DG did not look particularly ill or distressed, and both eardrums looked slightly pink. When I tried to explain that antibiotics were not indicated, Mr G became quite short-tempered saying that he was given a similar spiel with his older son who went on to develop a perforated drum. I gave DG a script for amoxicillin even though I thought antibiotics were not clinically indicated.

Opening question:

What issues or challenges does this case raise for you, the trainee?
- My concerns are whether I upset Mr G – could I have phrased things more diplomatically and achieved better rapport?
- Will the next doctor who sees DG think that I am not practising evidence-based medicine?

In this case, the trainer may decide to focus predominantly on two domains:
- **managing medical complexity** – to adopt appropriate working principles (e.g. incremental investigation, using time as a tool), to tolerate uncertainty, and to manage conditions that may present early and in an undifferentiated way, in partnership with the patient
- **community orientation** – to reconcile the health needs of individual patients and the health needs of the community in which they live, balancing these with available resources

To achieve sufficient depth of questioning in the above domains, the trainer may prepare the following questions:
- how did you establish Mr G's point of view? What consultation skills did you use to do this?
- what were the differences in Mr G's agenda and your agenda?
- how did you tackle the differences in agenda? How did you try to merge agendas?
- what made this case particularly difficult? How did you resolve the difficulties?
- what are the implications of your treatment on the patient and on society?

How did you establish Mr G's point of view? What consultation skills did you use to do this?
My aim was to establish Mr G's reason for presenting with his son, that is, his ideas regarding the problem; his concerns about the progression of illness; and his expectations of the consultation. Therefore, to clarify his agenda:

- I asked open questions, such as 'what can I do for you today?'
- I actively listened to his description of DG's symptoms. I asked him about what treatments he had tried and whether they had been useful
- when he asked for antibiotics, I asked him why he thought antibiotics would be useful; I did not make any suggestions for treatment until I had established the reasons for his attendance and his health beliefs

I used several consultation skills:
- active listening – I paid attention to what Mr G said to gain an understanding of the situation, and to acknowledge his perspective and feelings
- non-verbal communication – I looked at him when he spoke and occasionally glanced at DG. I sat facing them and made good eye contact. I nodded to show understanding and made appropriate facial gestures
- connecting – when I started talking, I used appropriate language, for example, 'DG's ear drum is red' rather than, 'his tympanic membrane is erythematous'; throughout my consultation, I looked for signs that Mr G was accepting of what I was doing and saying
- summarizing – after Mr G told me the history, I said, 'Am I correct in thinking that you believe DG has an ear infection and that antibiotics will cure the symptoms?'

My aim in using these skills was to achieve patient-centred consulting.

What do you mean by patient-centred consulting?
Patient-centredness can be defined as the extent to which the consultation's agenda, process, and outcome are determined by the patient (Neighbour, 2004). The important features of patient-centred consulting are:
- understanding the 'whole' person – having an holistic perspective
- exploring the patient's wants, needs and health beliefs
- based on a shared understanding of the illness, negotiating a mutually acceptable treatment plan with the patient to achieve concordance

Why is patient-centred consulting important?
- Some people argue that it is fashionable.
- It is part of a national policy as detailed in *Patient partnership: building a collaborative strategy* (NHS Executive, 1996).
- In patient-centred consultations, fewer investigations and referrals are generated (Stewart, 1984).
- Patient-centred consulting achieves better treatment outcomes in the management of chronic diseases (Kaplan, 1989).
- Patient-centred consulting improves patient satisfaction – the patients like it! (Howie, 1999).
- Patient-centred consulting is achievable – doctors can be trained to consult in this way.

What were the differences in Mr G's agenda and your agenda?

- Mr G wanted antibiotics believing that if DG took antibiotics the condition would resolve, his son would get better, clinical complications such as tympanic perforation would be avoided, and the family holiday would be undisturbed.
- My agenda was to treat DG's pain and await self-resolution of the otitis media. I had this agenda because challenging unnecessary antibiotic prescribing would encourage future self-treatment of the illness, discourage re-attendance for future episodes, and reduce antibiotic resistance. I would also be practising evidence-based medicine in line with current national guidelines thereby earning the respect of my colleagues.

How did you tackle the differences in agenda? How did you try to merge agendas?

I tried to maintain rapport and establish credibility. I tried to merge agendas by negotiating a shared understanding of the problem.

- To maintain rapport, I tried to remain approachable, easy to talk to and sympathetic. I didn't try to talk over the patient.
- To establish credibility, I tried to conduct a professionally sound examination with the least possible discomfort to DG. I also tried to show Mr G that I knew what I was talking about by presenting him with the findings of the medical research. For example, I knew that del Mar *et al.* (1997) showed that antibiotics only benefit 14% of children who are still in pain 24 hours after presentation. However, antibiotics double the risk of vomiting, diarrhoea and rashes. My message to Mr G was that most children with acute otitis media do not suffer adverse sequelae without antibiotics. The average number needed to treat (NNT) for 1 child to benefit (resolution of symptoms 1 day sooner on average) from initial antibiotic therapy is 13 (http://www.emedicine.com/emerg/topic393.htm).
- To negotiate a shared understanding, I simply explained the research findings. I expected Mr G to accept the findings and change his beliefs about the effectives of antibiotics in otitis media. I was surprised when he didn't change his beliefs. (*This is the trainee's learning need*).

What made this case particularly difficult? How did you resolve the difficulties?

Two things made this case difficult.

- When he told me his other son suffered a perforated eardrum, I felt anxious. Even though I knew that the chances of DG perforating his drum were very small, I felt that if he did, I would probably receive a complaint or I'd be sued. In the face of clinical uncertainty, I felt anxious and behaved defensively.
- When Mr G became short-tempered, I realized I'd failed to change his beliefs and we'd lost rapport. I wanted to maintain a relationship with Mr G but I felt further discussion was likely to become increasingly confrontational.

I tried to resolve the situation by prescribing antibiotics on this occasion. I felt that a one-off unnecessary prescription for antibiotics might be the price to pay for maintaining a harmonious doctor–patient relationship. However, I do realize that such prescribing behaviour may reinforce Mr Gibson's health beliefs regarding antibiotics and promote dependence on unnecessary prescribing.

What are the implications of your treatment on the patient and on society?
On the patient: there is a slim (1 in 7 to 20) chance that giving DG antibiotics shortens the duration of his symptoms by 24 hours. On the other hand, antibiotics double the risk of vomiting, diarrhoea and rashes. Had I persuaded Mr G to accept alternative treatments, I would have avoided this risk. Alternatives include the provision of a delayed script for antibiotics, use of appropriate analgesia and the provision of self-help leaflets.
- Provision of a delayed script – the strategy of the patient collecting the script for antibiotics if their symptoms have not improved in 48 hours is effective (Little *et al.*, 1997).
- Non-steroidal anti-inflammatories are superior to placebo in the treatment of earache.
- McFarlane *et al.* (1997) found that patient information leaflets are effective at reducing reconsultation rates and increasing patient satisfaction.

On society: doctors try to distribute limited resources (time, money, and expensive treatments) fairly.
- On average, a GP expects to see 100 cases of otitis media a year, amounting to 1.5 million episodes in England and Wales each year. This could add up to a lot of time being spent and a lot of antibiotics being prescribed for a potentially self-treatable illness.
- Spending a great deal of time with one patient over a self-limiting minor illness, especially in the middle of a busy surgery, may cause doctors to run late and consultations with less assertive, sicker patients may be compromised.
- On the other hand, a long consultation in which doctors strive to negotiate agendas may improve the doctor–patient relationship and reduce the frequency of consulting.

Additional information

Your trainer could ask you about complaints: you said you were afraid of receiving a complaint if you didn't prescribe antibiotics. Tell me about the practice's complaints procedure.

The complaints procedure
The practice complaints procedure is readily available in the practice information leaflet. It details:
- how the complaint will be dealt with

- the purpose of the procedure
- an anticipated time-table – the practice acknowledges receipt of the complaint within 2 days in writing; the practice discusses the issues and responds to the complaint within 10 days; a complaint should be made within six months of the incident
- assurance of confidentiality
- possible outcomes of the procedures:
  ○ resolution – a meeting between the complainant and practitioner is held only if both parties genuinely want this and the meeting has a clear purpose
  ○ if the issue remains unresolved, the PCT manager can act as an in-house intermediary; the conciliators do not report details of the case to the PCT – their job is to facilitate discussion
  ○ the complaint will formally pass to the PCT; the patient can contact the PCT convener to organize an independent review panel. The convener will review the details of the complaint and may decide to take no further action. A panel may be convened – the aim is to resolve the grievance in a conciliatory manner. Disciplinary action is not taken.

In 1996 a new NHS complaints procedure was introduced, with two important aims.
- It separated complaints from disciplinary procedures. The new complaints procedure sought to bring about a conciliation of the damaged relationship. Most people who complain want an apology and a clear explanation in lay language of the incident with reassurance that preventative action will be taken to ensure that there is no repetition of the incident. This is contrary to the popular belief that patients are only seeking financial compensation.
- Complaints should be dealt with informally and locally. In 1996, more than 90% of complaints were dismissed or resolved.

How can the practice learn from the complaint?
The complaint should be discussed at the next Significant Event Audit (SEA). The PHCT should identify areas for improvement and take actions to prevent similar occurrences. The doctor should reflect on the incident and note it in his PDP for discussion at his appraisal.

How can the practice avoid complaints?
Pre-empt a complaint. If the doctor recognizes that he has had a dysfunctional consultation, a quick telephone call may head off a complaint. If a doctor makes an incorrect or delayed diagnosis, the GMC advises that a full and honest explanation with an apology should be provided. Good communication reduces complaints (Beckman et al.,1994).

What are the common complaints made in general practice?
Common complaints (1998 data from County Durham):
- the patient disliked the attitude of the GP and there was a break-down in communication (including failure to visit or refer) – 30%

- delayed or incorrect diagnoses – 28%
- complaints about staff or the premises – 21%
- problems with the practice management – 18%
- others (including removal from list) – 3%

Why are complaints stressful to doctors?
- Doctors feel that patients who complain have power over them, making them feel helpless and uncertain.
- Doctors feel that they are working hard for people who have very high expectations, are not particularly grateful and very quick to blame them for anything that goes wrong with their care.
- Doctors feel devalued by the increasing consumerism of patients and very rarely separate complaints from litigation in their thoughts.

Guidelines, such as those produced by NICE, may assist doctors to making difficult decisions about the equitable distribution of limited resources. Do guidelines change doctors' prescribing patterns?

Wathen and Dean (2004) looked at this issue with regard to how GP prescribing behaviour was affected by the NICE guidance. In their qualitative study, they sent a postal questionnaire, developed from semi-structured interviews, to all GPs within a North Devon PCT. They wanted to explore factors that were encouraging or discouraging adherence to NICE guidance. There was an 83% response rate. This study concluded that:
- NICE guidance in isolation had little impact on GP prescribing
- where the guidance coincided with information from other sources, or personal experience, there was some evidence that technology appraisals triggered an increase in prescribing, but that this was not always sustained
- the recommendations of NICE concerning zanamivir were universally rejected and there was evidence that this had undermined confidence in NICE recommendations in general.

Why don't doctors follow guidelines?
Lipman (2004) discussed this issue. He concluded that the 'reductionist assumptions underlying the construction of evidence-based guidelines from systematic reviews lead to inflexible recommendations on the management of disease. Anthropologists and sociologists make an important distinction between scientifically defined diseases and the culturally constructed experience of illness. Because GPs deal with patients suffering illness that may or may not result from disease, disease-centred guidelines often conflict with their needs and wishes. The development of evidence-based medicine was intended as a tool to help doctors make sense of evidence in the context of individual patients' problems. Few GPs are skilled in it, and it has been appropriated by powerful expert groups such as guidelines developers and the pharmaceutical industry.' Lipman suggested that more understanding of evidence-based medicine by GPs leads to better informed decision making by them and their patients.

Relevant literature

Beckman HB, Markakis KM, Suchman AL and Frankel RM (1994) The doctor-patient relationship and malpractice. Lessons from plaintiff depositions. *Archives of Internal Medicine*, **152**: 12.

Del Mar C, Glasziou P and Hayem M (1997) Are antibiotics indicated as initial treatment for children with acute otitis media? A meta-analysis. *BMJ*, **314**:1526–1529.

Howie JG (1999) Quality at general practice consultations: cross-sectional survey. *BMJ*, **319**: 738–743.

Kaplan SH (1989) Assessing the effects of physician–patient interactions on the outcomes of chronic disease. *Med Care*, **27**: S110–127.

Little P, Gould C and Williamson I (1997) Reattendance and complications in a randomised trial of prescribing strategies for sore throat; the medicalising effect of prescribing antibiotics. *BMJ*, **315**: 350–352.

Lipman T (2004) The doctor, his patient, and the computerized evidence-based guideline. *Journal of Evaluation in Clinical Practice*, **10**: 163–176.

Mcfarlane JT, Holmes WF and McFarlane RM (1997) Reducing reconsultations for acute lower respiratory tract illness with an information leaflet; a randomised controlled study of patients in primary care. *British Journal of General Practice*, **47**: 719–722.

Neighbour R (2004) *The Inner Consultation*. Radcliffe Publishing, Oxford.

NHS Executive (1996) *Patient partnership: building a collaborative strategy*. Department of Health.

Rollnick S, Seale C, Rees M, Butler C, Kinnersley P and Anderson E (2001) Inside the routine general practice consultation: an observational study of consultations for sore throats. *Family Practice*, **18**: 506–510.

Stewart MA (1984) What is a successful doctor–patient interview? A study of interactions and outcomes. *Soc Sci Med*, **19**: 167–175.

Wathen B and Dean T (2004) An evaluation of the impact of NICE guidance on GP prescribing. *British Journal of General Practice*, **54**: 103–107.

Acute otitis media:
http://www.clinicalevidence.com/ceweb/conditions/chd/0301/0301.jsp

American website on evidence based medicine:
http://www.emedicine.com/emerg/topic393.htm

Improve your communication skills:
http://www.skillscascade.com/handouts.htm; in particular, see
http://www.skillscascade.com/files/commresearch.htm and
http://www.skillscascade.com/files/research.htm

Request for a sick note

Case summary

Mrs GH, a 46 year old woman with well-controlled hypertension who rarely consults with minor illnesses, saw me on Monday to request a sick note. She was unable to work her Friday late night shift because she had a cold. By the time of consultation, the cold had resolved spontaneously and her examination was unremarkable. However, on her return to work, her boss demanded a sick-note. She was very apologetic for consulting saying that she didn't see me on Friday as she knew the cold would resolve spontaneously.

I informed Mrs GH that I could not issue a sick note. I explained that I could write a letter to her employer, for which the practice charges an administration fee. I wrote a letter along the lines of 'Mrs GH tells me she was unable to attend work because she had a viral illness.' When Mrs GH called for the letter later that day, she asked me to amend it to 'I certify that Mrs GH was unable to attend work because she had a viral illness'. She joked that if she was paying for the letter, she'd like it to be a good one. I didn't change the letter.

Opening question:

What issues or challenges does this case raise for you, the trainee?
- Should I have re-worded the letter and preserved the doctor–patient relationship?

In this case, the trainer may decide to focus predominantly on two domains:
- **maintaining an ethical approach to practice** – practising with integrity and being able to justify and clarify personal ethics
- **fitness to practice** – demonstrating an awareness of how your own attitudes and feelings are important determinants of how you practise, and having an understanding of the financial and legal frameworks in which health care is given at practice level

To achieve sufficient depth of questioning in the above domains, the trainer may prepare the following questions:
- what was your dilemma in the above case?
- what were your possible options?
- could you use a model to help you to make a decision when faced with such a dilemma in future?
- what are your responsibilities to Mrs GH and have you fulfilled them?

What was your dilemma in the above case?
In refusing to change the wording of my letter, I am being completely truthful – I am not testifying in a written statement that Mrs GH was ill three days ago. I cannot make this statement because I didn't see or examine her during her illness. On the other hand, I would be doing the best for my patient (acting beneficently) if I helped her with the difficulties she is having with her demanding employer.

The second dilemma is that the patient and I have different ideas on what she has paid for: I believe that she has paid a fee to cover the administrative cost of the letter, while she believes that she paid for the contents of the letter.

What were your possible options?
I could have amended the letter and charged the administrative fee:
- Mrs GH, and perhaps even her employer, would be happy
- I could have preserved my doctor–patient relationship with Mrs GH
- I would have had a quick non-confrontational consultation, which would have made me happy too

I could have refused to amend my letter and charged the administrative fee (the option I chose).
- I was honest in my letter. The charge was levied for the administrative services. Asking for a fee is not illegal – if an employee requires a 'sick note' for an illness of less than seven days' duration, then a private doctor's statement may be provided. The fee for this is £10, which is a set BMA rate, to be met either by the patient or the employer. I behaved ethically and defensibly.
- The message I was sending to Mrs GH and her manager was that it is inappropriate to ask GPs to provide sick notes to cover minor illness. The manager cannot expect GPs to police sickness absence. The NHS has a finite number of resources and stretching these resources to provide a cheap occupational health service to private companies reduces the time available for seeing and treating ill patients.

I could have issued my original letter, but not charged for it.
- I would have been honest. Mrs GH would not have felt she that was entitled to a 'better letter'. We would have retained our good doctor–patient relationship.
- However, providing a 'free' doctor's letter could encourage patients to attend for minor illness, thereby promoting inappropriate health-seeking behaviour. If letters are provided free of charge to patients with minor illness, the practice appointments could be inundated with patients requesting letters, which is an inappropriate use of resources.

I immediately rejected the option of providing an FMed 3.
- The FMed 3 is used to certify periods off work lasting greater than seven days. Mrs GH only had one day of sickness absence. In such cases, employers should provide a self-certification certificate (SC2) so that employees can declare their illness, although strictly they do not need to do this for their first three days of illness.
- The doctor needs to have examined the patient first and the Med3 is issued within a day of that clinical contact. Having seen Mrs GH three days after her illness, I could not have issued an FMed 3 retrospectively.

I immediately rejected the option of providing an FMed 5 because an FMed 5 is used for retrospective certification but only if:

- patients require a statement for a past period of illness during which they saw their doctor but for which no doctor's statement was issued at contact; or
- if doctors wish to advise patients, whom they have not examined, to refrain from work provided the doctors have received adequate written reports within the last month from another doctor.

Could you use a model to help you to make a decision when faced with such a dilemma in future?

I could apply an ethical model if faced with such a dilemma in future. There are several ethical models or theories, namely theories of duty-based ethics, utilitarianism and virtue ethics.

Duty based ethics (deontology): these state that an action is right if it is in accord with a moral rule or principle. Certain acts are wrong in themselves, independent of their foreseeable consequences.

With regard to the above scenario, lying is wrong, so I should not testify in a written statement that the patient was ill three days ago if I not had seen or examined her during her illness. Therefore, when I write that '*the patient tells me that she was ill three days ago*', I am being completely honest and behaving in a principled manner.

However, beneficence (doing good) and non-maleficence (not doing harm) also need to be considered.

- I would be doing the best for my patient (acting beneficently) if I issued a note to help her with the difficulties she is having with her demanding employer. After all, the patient acted appropriately. She knew that she had a minor ailment and took responsibility for her own health – her health-seeking behaviour was entirely appropriate. The problem with this course of action, even if it does my patient good, is that it does the NHS no good, because her employer's attitude is encouraging doctor-dependence and inappropriate presentations to an already overstretched health service.
- If I refuse to provide a note, this could be harmful to my patient and the health service (against the principle of non-maleficence).
  - My patient could get into trouble with her unreasonable boss. It's not her fault that he is unreasonable.
  - This course of action could be harmful to the health service because, if I refuse to provide a note on the grounds that I did not see her when she was ill, the patient may decide to present with minor symptoms on the next occasion. Refusing to provide a sick note, even if it is the principled thing to do, could, in the long-term, be promoting inappropriate health-seeking behaviour.

Utilitarianism ethics, particularly consequentialism: this principle states that an action is right if it promotes the best consequences – the greatest good or happiness for the greatest number. Those actions that promote, or intend to promote, more happiness are better than those that promote less happiness. A weakness of this theory is that it is not possible to measure happiness.

With regard to the scenario, not amending the letter, and having a robust sickness absence policy is more likely to have long-term benefit, and the happiness this brings to society as a whole, outweighs the short-term benefit to the patient, employer and doctor.

Virtue ethics: this principle states that an action is right if it is what a virtuous person would do in the circumstances. A virtuous person is someone of good moral character, i.e. he is kind, generous, and empathetic. With regard to the scenario, if I:

- amend my letter: I would be responding kindly to my patient's needs
- do not amend my letter: I would be acting responsibly and rationing limited resources, such as appointment times and administrative work, fairly

A weakness of this theory is that it is tied to cultural norms, so that an act, which seems virtuous today could be viewed as paternalistic tomorrow.

The behaviour that is expected of today's doctors is detailed in the GMC's *Good Medical Practice*, which states that it is the primary duty of doctors to make the care of their patients their first concern. Therefore, in the current cultural climate, it seems that the autonomy of patients takes precedence over the doctors' gatekeeper role – hence a virtuous doctor would make the happiness of his patient his first concern.

What are your responsibilities to Mrs GH and have you fulfilled them?
My responsibilities are to:

- *Make the care of my patient my first concern.* To me, this means that my primary duty is to focus on my patient's health. If I am faced with a dilemma such as saving the patient or advancing the interests of scientific research, then the former takes precedence. In the sick note scenario, the doctor's primary focus should to encourage appropriate health seeking behaviour. This overrides any duties to police sickness absence for the financial benefit of society.
- *Protect and promote the health of patients and the public.* I can only meet this responsibility if I have sufficient resources, such as appointment times. Where I have limited resources, then I need to take steps to ensure that these are distributed first to those patients with the greatest need. Therefore, to protect the health of my patients, I need to distribute my appointments appropriately. I would be failing in this duty if I permitted my surgeries to be cluttered with sick note requests for minor illnesses.
- *Treat patients as individuals and respect their dignity*
    - ○ Treat patients politely and considerately – it is appropriate for me to take steps to discourage sick notes requests. It is also appropriate to listen to Mrs GH and explain the appropriate use of sick notes. Getting angry, sarcastic, rude or offensive would be impolite and inconsiderate.
    - ○ Respect patients' right to confidentiality – discussing information gained from a doctor–patient relationship with other people, including employers, without the patient's express consent, is an abuse of my position.

- *Work in partnership with patients*
  - ○ Listen to patients and respond to their concerns and preferences – to me, acknowledging and responding to patients does not mean that I have to accede to their requests. For example, if Mrs GH asks for a sick note and I respond by explaining why it is not possible for me to provide one, then I have discharged my responsibilities in listening and responding to her concerns and preferences.
  - ○ Give patients the information they want or need in a way they can understand. For example, in responding to Mrs GH's request for a sick note, I need to alter the wording of my explanation to suit her level of understanding. If she fails to understand, then I have failed in my duty to communicate effectively. Understanding information is different to accepting or believing that information. My responsibility is getting her to understand the information. It is up to her whether she accepts and believes it.
- *Be honest and open and act with integrity*
  - ○ Never discriminate unfairly against patients or colleagues – it would be unfair of me to refuse to issue a sick note to Mrs GH but to issue one to another patient with whom I am friends or from whom I fear a complaint. The sick note policy should apply equally to all patients.
  - ○ Never abuse your patients' trust in you or the public's trust in the profession. For example, back-dating a sick note, or making up a reason for the patient's illness, is an abuse of the public's trust in the profession.

Relevant literature

GMC (2006) Good medical practice. http://www.gmc-uk.org/guidance/good_medical_ practice/duties_of_a_doctor.asp
Sokol DK and Bergson G (2006) Ethics made easy. *StudentBMJ*, **14**: 397–440.
For ethical frameworks and their application to cases, see:
    http://www.ethics-network.org.uk/reading/Guide/SectionC/sectionC.htm

Patient worries about chest pain

Case summary

Mrs RD is a 46 year old woman whom I have seen in the past for treatment of her familial hypercholesterolaemia; latest total cholesterol was 4.5 mmol/l. I also treated her last year for a depressive episode following a family bereavement.

She now presents with chest pain, located on the anterior and posterior aspects of her left chest, overlying her heart. The discomfort (3/10 at worst) occurs both at rest but also with exercise and is occasionally associated with palpitations. Her ECG last week was normal. Mrs RD's mum suffered a fatal MI at age 34 and her 40 year old brother had a triple bypass last year.

Mrs RD is happy in her marriage and looks forward to visiting her son in Japan next year. She recently tried to purchase a house but the sale fell though at the last minute; the entire process was stressful. Mrs RD feels tired and is frustrated by her lack of energy. She is usually quite a busy woman but at moment everything, including her hobbies (walking and gardening) seem to be an effort.

I advised her to start an exercise program with at least 25 minutes of exercise five times per week. The exercise may boost her energy levels. However, if she consistently develops chest pain, then she needs to re-attend for referral to cardiology to exclude angina. Mrs RD was happy with this plan.

Opening question:

What issues or challenges does this case raise for you, the trainee?
- My concern is whether Mrs RD requires further investigation for cardiac disease, specifically to exclude angina.
- I do not believe that Mrs RD is experiencing a recurrence of her depression. Could her symptoms be attributed to anxiety? If they are, what could I do for her?

In this case, the trainer may decide to focus predominantly on two domains:
- **practising holistically** – with attention to the physical, psychological, socio-economic and cultural dimensions of the case and taking into account the patient's feelings and thoughts
- **data gathering and interpretation** – gathering and using data for clinical judgment, and justifying the choice of examination, and the interpretation of the chosen investigations

To achieve sufficient depth of questioning in the above domains, the trainer may prepare the following questions:
- what do you think was the patient's agenda: what were her ideas, concerns and expectations? How did you elicit this?
- what effect did the symptoms have on her work, family and other parts of her life? (*illness vs. disease*)

- what prior knowledge of the patient did you have which affected the outcome of your consultation(s)?
- did you identify any ongoing problems that might have affected this particular complaint?
- your differential diagnosis was chest pain due to anxiety or to angina. What are the features of the chest pain that led you to this differential?
- what skills did you use to obtain the history in this case?

What do you think was the patient's agenda: what were her ideas, concerns and expectations?
- Her ideas: Mrs RD said she knew her body. In both her pregnancies, she knew straight away that she was pregnant. Now she was aware of the chest pain and she believed that her body was sending her a message that things were not right.
- Her concerns: Mrs RD was concerned about the cause of the chest pain. She was worried about cardiac disease because of her family history. She was also concerned that her recent stress over the house purchase may be the cause and if this was the case, she worried about experiencing a recurrence of depression.
- Her expectations: Mrs RD expected me to get to the bottom of her chest pain and to explain my reasoning to her. She did not expect blood tests as she had recently had these done. She did not ask for a referral.

How did you elicit this?
I used a mixture of open, closed and reflective questions.
- Asking open-ended questions allows me to understand what issues are important to patients. The way patients structure their answers also familiarises me with their style of communication. An example of an open-ended question I asked was 'what do you think is causing the chest pain?'.
- Close-ended questions allow yes, no, or some other fixed response – this is useful for clarying information and for getting agreement with the patient before moving on to the next step. For example, I asked, 'does the pain go away when you rest?'.
- Reflective statements help me to clarify my understanding, as well as the patient's understanding, of what is being communicated. 'You said stress – what do you mean by stress; what could have caused the stress?'
- I also made empathic statements that reflected the emotions expressed by Mrs RD. 'You seem worried because of your family history.'
- My nonverbal communication reinforced the message that I was approachable and attentive. I maintained eye contact, showed concerned facial expressions, nodded in agreement, where appropriate, and touched the patient for reassurance.

What effect did the symptoms have on her work, family and other parts of her life?

When I asked whether the chest pain was provoked by activity, she said she had attended a party last weekend and spent four hours dancing without getting chest pain. From this, I assumed that she remained socially active. I did not specifically ask if her symptoms prevented her from completing activities at work or whether the fear of provoking symptoms curtailed any social activities. In patients with chest pain, it may be useful to ask about sexual activity, as it may be an unvoiced concern for some patients who are too embarrassed to introduce the topic themselves. A learning need is identified.

What prior knowledge of the patient did you have which affected the outcome of your consultation(s)?

I had prior subjective and objective knowledge about the patient.

- Subjective: I treated Mrs RD last year so we already had a relationship and it was relatively easy to re-establish rapport.
- Objective: this presenting complaint was dealt with in two consultations, each a week apart. At the first consultation, I had her blood results to hand. I also had her BP readings, Framingham score and family history available on the problem summary page of her consultation notes. At the second consultation, I had the results of her ECG to hand.

My prior knowledge of this lady led me to believe that she wanted, on the basis of her family history, to explore her symptoms to reach an understanding of what was happening to her. Balint (1957) wrote about the mutual investment fund between doctors and long-term patients. This term describes the shared experiences and trust that GPs and patients accumulate over many years. Mrs RD and I have developed a relationship over time. By knowing what sort of character she is, I am in a position to assess whether her psychological problems (stress) are manifesting physically (as chest pain) or whether her physical disease (angina) is having its own psychological consequences (anxiety).

Did you identify any ongoing problems that might have affected this particular complaint?

There were two ongoing problems. First, she has risk factors (family history and hypercholosterolaemia) for angina. Secondly, since she broke her little toe three months ago, over the next six weeks she reduced her physical activity from walking three miles at least four times a week to gardening on weekends. Since then, she has felt tired and unmotivated.

Your differential diagnosis was chest pain due to anxiety or to angina. What are the features of the chest pain that lead you to this differential?

I suspected anxiety because:

- there was a precipitating life event, i.e. the stress associated with buying a house
- she also described feeing tired and easily fatigued.

Reasons for not suspecting anxiety disorder were:
- Mrs RD did not describe restlessness, poor concentration, irritability, trembling or twitching of the muscles, feeling shaky, muscle aches or soreness, disturbed sleep, nausea, diarrhoea, tachycardia, shortness of breath and dizziness.
- She is happily married. Being divorced, separated or living alone is a risk factor for anxiety.
- Although anxiety and depressive symptoms may co-exist, she did not have symptoms of depression either.

I suspected angina because:
- of the location of the pain. Angina pain is in the centre of the chest, over the whole praecordium or largely on the left. However, Mrs RD also said it was also located posteriorly and angina is uncommon in the back.
- Mrs RD has risk factors for coronary heart disease (CHD). If two or more of the risk factors (such as family history, cigarette smoking, diabetes mellitus, hyperlipidaemia, hypertension, obesity and lack of exercise) are present, the diagnosis is much more likely.

Reasons for not suspecting angina were:
- the nature of the pain: Mrs RD did not describe a crushing or pressing pain, nor did she describe the burning pain that can be seen with reflux
- the pain was not reliably brought on by exertion: the pain should be reproducible and patients can often anticipate the level of exertion that typically provokes the pain
- the pain should cease within five minutes of rest: Mrs RD sometimes had pain at rest. Unlike Prinzmetal angina, these episodes were not typically in the early hours of the morning.
- Mrs RD is a non-smoker, has a BMI of 26, and is neither hypertensive nor diabetic. She is 46 years old. The incidence of angina in women under the age of 64 is less than 5%.
- the 12-lead ECG did not show ischaemic changes. However, some patients with angina do have a normal resting ECG. Abnormalities on ECG imply a poorer prognosis.

What skills did you use to obtain the history in this case?
- *Active listening:* I concentrated on what Mrs RD was saying. Writing notes, or looking at the computer, or thinking about over-running my clinic did not distract me. My focus was on Mrs RD. I listened to what she said and how she phrased it. I checked for congruity with her non-verbal language – her facial expressions and body language.
- *Open, closed and reflective questioning:* open questioning allowed Mrs RD to talk and gave her the space to express her agenda. This, I believe, empowered her. Closed questions enabled me to obtain the specific details of her symptoms, which I needed to construct a differential diagnosis. Reflective questions, where I repeated the last few words of Mrs RD's sentence, encouraged her to expand on the issue.

- *I displayed empathy and warmth:* I tried to let Mrs RD know that I understood and accepted her feelings about the chest pain, i.e. that I had perceived her concern, curiosity, and uncertainty. In my discussion, I tried to express warmth by being approachable, responsive and helpful to her. I felt that if Mrs RD trusted me, we could use time and the proposed exercise regime as diagnostic tools rather than request stress ECGs and complete anxiety questionnaires. By choosing this management plan, I took a proactive approach and used the therapeutic relationship in the treatment of the patient. Balint (1957) described this as the doctor being used as a drug, that is, doctors taking a proactive approach and being instrumental in their treatment of patients.

Additional information

Working in partnership with patients
Patients want to make decisions in partnership with doctors. All patients are different and vary in their preference for:
- desiring information – some want direction to alternative sources of information, while others want to know what the doctor thinks is best
- needing assistance with interpreting the information – some internet users want help with understanding the outcomes of drug trials, while other patients simply want a clarification of what the hospital consultant said
- help with the final decision-making – some patients want active guidance from their doctors while others wish to make their decisions themselves

The essence of effective patient-centred consulting is to know the patient well and to facilitate their choices.

Using Neighbour's consultation model to achieve patient-centred
1. Connect
- Eye-contact; warm welcome; empathy – acknowledge the patient's feelings throughout the consultation; touch; privacy; appropriate use of silence.
- Remark upon the patient's expression/movements/state of agitation (non-verbal cues), for example, 'Mrs RD, you look concerned today'.
- Ask open questions to establish her agenda. Has she come to confirm her fears that she has angina, that is, establish her ideas, concerns and expectations.
- Establish what she understands, and what she wants to know. The vast majority of patients want to know their prognosis, even if it is poor. Disclosure allows the patient to make informed decisions.

2. Summarize
- Use language the patient understands (jargon-free).
- Use the patient's own words. 'Your chest palpitations may be caused by the stress you are experiencing'.
- Use simple language, be tactful, sensitive, but be honest.

3. Handover

- Confirm that she has understood the diagnosis and management plan.
- Ask her to summarize the information back to you.
- Give her permission to return with further questions: 'People often walk out of a doctor's surgery and think of all sorts of questions that they should have asked. If this happens to you, please come back and ask me these questions'.

4. Safety net

- Arrange follow-up, either formally, or leave it up to the patient.
- For example, 'Mrs RD, I suspect these muscular pains will improve as you become fitter. If you start getting chest pain regularly with exercise, please come back and see me for further tests'.

5. Housekeeping

- Acknowledge your own feelings: a long consultation in which you deal with anxiety may leave you feeling anxious and uncertain.

Negotiating a treatment plan to achieve concordance

Concordance is a shared treatment contract between the prescriber and the patient – the two parties share the power. It differs from compliance where the balance of power lies with the prescriber; the patient being the passive recipient of a treatment plan which is devised by the prescriber in the patient's best interests. The pendulum has now swung away from medical paternalism towards a respect for patient autonomy. In Berne terminology, the relationship is more one of adult–adult than parent–child.

From **Gamey G** (2000) Looking after patients who won't look after themselves. *StudentBMJ*, **8:** 13–15. http://www.studentbmj.com/back_issues/0200/education/ 17.html [accessed July 2007]

Gamey writes: 'As doctors, we tend to like those patients who do what they are told. Such patients are "complying" with our advice. But this kind of paternalistic relationship is outdated and unhelpful. The patient's view of the world – based on experience, culture, family history, and personality – may be different from ours. If we see this as an obstacle to be overcome at all costs we will alienate our patients and they will continue to make unhealthy choices. Encounters between doctors and patients entail the bringing together of often conflicting explanatory systems about illness and health, and negotiation is the key to a "successful" outcome. We should try to build an honest and open therapeutic alliance with our patients, sharing our own thoughts and beliefs with them, to reach a mutually respectful agreement. This model of working is called "concordance" and it has replaced the term "compliance".'

Sometimes patients who consult frequently for minor ailments and who don't take the doctors' advice are called heart-sink patients. What is meant by heart-sinks?

O'Dowd (1988) used the term heart-sink patients to describe patients who:

- consult frequently

- have features of psychosomatic illness, with underlying depression or anxiety into which they have no insight
- invoke feelings of anger, resentment and despair in the doctor

The patients tend to be:
- female
- of lower socio-economic class
- older (over 40 years)
- and have thick medical notes (with lots of previous medical interventions and referrals)

Good says that heart-sinks look at medicine as a salvation – medicine influences and suggests, or in some cases, wholly supplies the character and identity of some individuals' personal suffering and is the apparent source of their salvation or redemption.

Gerrard and Riddell said that one doctor's set of heart-sinks is not the same as another's, implying that the problem does not lie solely with the patient – the patient–doctor relationship is dysfunctional. Conflict arises because the patient and doctor approach the problem from different angles. The patient is looking to medicine to improve their happiness (soteriological health beliefs). The doctor has a limited model of medicine, usually a biological, disease-focused model, and lacks an holistic approach.

Mathers *et al.* (1995) found that doctors who have heart-sinks are more likely to be:
- inexperienced
- have a greater perceived workload and lower job satisfaction
- lacking in postgraduate qualifications and communication skills

Groves (1951) defined four types of difficult patient.
1. *Dependant clinger:* they make repeated requests for reassurance and have an inexhaustible need for love and attention, provoking resentment in the doctor. The game they play is 'Poor me!'.
2. *Entitled demander:* complains about imagined shortcomings in the service provided. They try to manipulate the doctor through the use of intimidation and provoke feeling of guilt and anxiety. This is a reflection of their own fear and insecurity. The game they play is 'I'm going to take this further!'.
3. *Manipulative health rejector:* they constantly return complaining that their treatment is not working. They seek attention rather than relief from their symptoms and tend to play the 'Yes, but....' game.
4. *Self-destructive denier:* refuses to accept that their behaviour affects their illness, and will not modify their habits, hence self-harming to the point of destruction. These include the incurable alcoholics and non-compliant diabetics. They provoke rejection in the doctor. The game they play is 'Kick me!'.

What are your coping strategies for dealing with heart-sinks?
A useful management strategy was outlined by Barsky and Borus (1995). Rule out the presence of diagnosable medical disease:

- Review the notes. Be careful about ordering investigations and referring the patient – this fosters the sick role and negative tests usually heighten the patient's anxiety.
- Search for psychiatric disorders: look for depression, anxiety and panic disorders as these may present with physical symptoms.
- Build a collaborative alliance with the patient: acknowledge the patient's suffering but be careful not to encourage the sick role. See one doctor for regular, planned follow-up and avoid examinations unless new symptoms develop.
- Listening to the patient can be therapeutic for the patient – this is called 'holding' the patient's anxieties. However, recognize that these patients are manipulative and demanding, so set out boundaries such as the frequency of meetings and the 'rules of engagement'.
- Set goals for treatment:
   o reduction in severity or frequency of symptoms and improvement in function – help the patient cope rather than searching for a cure
   o patients should be actively involved in their management decisions – they should not assume a passive role
   o realistic, incremental goals should be set, e.g. graduated exercise programmes
- Providing limited reassurance: patients need to be told that lethal or progressive disease has been excluded and an exhaustive search for the root cause is not indicated. Rather, it would be more productive to concentrate on reducing symptoms – this acknowledges their symptomatology and refocuses their goals.
- Prescribing cognitive behavioural therapy (CBT) +/- antidepressants if patients do not respond to the previous five steps: CBT is shown to be effective in the treatment of medically unexplained symptoms such as IBS, fibromyalgia and chronic fatigue syndrome. CBT helps patients to find alternative explanations for their symptoms – they alter their health beliefs and change their illness behaviour. A meta-analysis involving 6500 patients showed that anti-depressants can provide useful symptomatic relief whether depression is present or not (NNT 3). Benefit is seen within 1–7 days.

What are the strategies doctors can use to cope with heart-sinks?
- Doctors should recognize the feelings provoked by heart-sinks. Those who are more self-aware and have better consulting and counselling skills cope better.
- Heart-sinks do occur. However, the emotional burden can be reduced by:
   o improving the doctor's working environment – allow longer consulting by having flexible appointment lengths
   o discussing in peer/Balint groups
   o housekeeping (Neighbour) – deal honestly with the emotions invoked by the demanding patient

From **Ring A,** *et al.* (2004) Do patients with unexplained physical symptoms pressurise general practitioners for somatic treatment?: a qualitative study. *BMJ*, **328:** 1057–1060.

This study looked at seven general practices in Merseyside, England – 36 patients with medically unexplained symptoms from 21 general practices had their consultations audio-taped. The study concluded that most patients with unexplained symptoms received somatic interventions from their GPs but had not requested them. Though such patients apparently seek to engage the GP by conveying the reality of their suffering, GPs respond by treating their symptoms.

From **Dowrick FC,** *et al.* (2004) Normalisation of unexplained symptoms by general practitioners: a functional typology. *British Journal of General Practice*, **54:** 165–170.

This study concluded that:
- normalization without explanation, i.e. rudimentary reassurance and the authority of a negative test result, rendered somatic management more likely.
- normalization with ineffective explanation provided a tangible physical explanation for symptoms, unrelated to patient's expressed concerns – this was also counterproductive
- normalization with effective explanation provided tangible mechanisms grounded in patients' concerns, often linking physical and psychological factors. These explanations were accepted by patients; those linking physical and psychological factors contributed to psychosocial management outcomes.

These findings can inform the development of well-grounded educational interventions for GPs.

From **Woivalin T,** *et al.* (2004) Medically unexplained symptoms: perceptions of physicians in primary health care. *Family Practice*, **21:** 199–203.

The aim of this Swedish study was to explore GPs' perceptions and ways of managing patients with medically unexplained symptoms (MUS). The GPs described how they used four different approaches to manage patients with MUS:
- biomedical
- psychological
- educational
- psychosocial

Different approaches were used, depending on the patient and the situation, and the GPs even switched approach when working with the same patient. The study concluded that in their work with patients with MUS, GPs need support and further training to improve the way the biomedical frame of reference is integrated with the humanistic perspective.

From **Morgan ED,** *et al.* (2004) Continuity of care and patient satisfaction in a family practice clinic. *Journal of the American Board of Family Practice*, **17:** 341–346.

Continuity of care is important to general practice. This American study surveyed the patients of a military practice over a period of one week. The response rate was 68.3%. Responders were not more likely to be seeing their own doctor. Regression analysis revealed that:

- 12% of patient satisfaction was associated with long-term continuity rates
- 23% by satisfaction with the doctor
- 17% by how easy it was to make the appointment
- a subset of patients (13%) valued choice of appointment time or choice of other doctors over continuity of care

Conclusions: patient satisfaction is associated with continuity, especially for high clinic users. Although continuity is important, a subset of patients values the ability to see other doctors and to change doctors.

Relevant literature

Balint M (1957) *The doctor, the patient and the illness*. Pitman, London.
Barsky AJ, Borus JB (1995) Somatization and medicalization in the era of managed care. JAMA, **274:** 1931–1934.
Gerrard TJ, Riddell JD (1988) Difficult patients: black holes and secrets. *BMJ*, **297:** 530–532.
Groves JE (1978) Taking care of the hateful patient. *N Engl J Med*, **298:** 883–887.
O'Dowd TC (1988) Five years of heartsink patients in general practice. *BMJ*, **297:** 528–530.
Mathers N, Jones N, Hannay D (1995) Heartsink patients: a study of their general practitioners. *Br J Gen Pract*, **45:** 293–296.
The Bath VTS website provides a comprehensive summary on patients with medically unexplained symptoms and has an excellent survival guide on how to deal with heart-sinks (see http://www.gppro.co.uk/newgpr/spring03/heartsin.htm).

Patient declines smear test

Case summary

Miss JF is a 28 year old woman who is usually fit and healthy. She presented to your afternoon clinic last week complaining of uncomfortable, runny eyes. You made a diagnosis of conjunctivitis and the two of you agreed to await self-resolution of this minor illness rather than use topical chloramphenicol.

During your consultation, you notice that despite several invites, Miss JF has repeatedly declined a smear test. When you offer to book her a test, she declines saying smears are uncomfortable and make her anxious. Despite your attempts to praise the skill of your practice nurse, Miss JF declines again. You accept and document her decision and the consultation ends amicably.

Opening question:

What issues or challenges does this case raise for you, the trainee?

- Your concern is whether you should have offered to do the smear for Miss JF at time of your appointment. This could possibly have saved her anxiety about waiting for a nurse appointment, but you would have run late and made other patients late.
- To what extent should you encourage Miss JF to have a smear? She seemed quite firm in her response and you didn't want to antagonize her.

In this case, the trainer may decide to focus predominantly on two domains:

- **maintaining an ethical approach to practice** – practising with integrity and respecting diversity
- **primary care administration** – effective recordkeeping to aid and improve patient care.

To achieve sufficient depth of questioning in the above domains, the trainer may prepare the following questions:

- what was your dilemma in the case?
- what were your possible options?
- could you use a model to help you to make a decision when faced with such a dilemma in future?
- your colleague says that you should have scared her into having a smear – how do you respond?
- what are your responsibilities to this patient and have you fulfilled them?
- you free-texted in your consultation notes that the patient declined a smear test – could you record this differently? In your consultation with this patient, what are the advantages and disadvantages of free-texting?

What was your dilemma in the case?

I think that having regular smears detects cervical dysplasia at an earlier stage when less invasive treatments can be offered – that is, it is a useful screening test that has the potential to reduce later morbidity and mortality. Given the usefulness of the test, I find it difficult to accept a patient's refusal because of the perceived discomfort or anxiety associated with the procedure. However, patients can refuse treatment. My dilemma is knowing the difference between 'encouraging' and 'coercing' patients to undertake cervical screening.

Besides the option you chose, what were your alternatives:
- Not discuss the smear issue at all. The advantage with this approach is that I run to time, I don't keep other patients waiting, and I have more time to give to people who actually want the treatment I have to offer. The disadvantage of this is that I may miss an opportunity to discuss Miss JF's ideas about smears and address any specific concerns she may have. Also, if I ignore patients who initially do not understand why certain tests are done, I create a system by which the educated and informed get the resources at the expense of the less well informed.
- Offer Miss JF the test but do not take the opportunity to address her ideas and concerns. The advantage with this approach is that I made an effort that I can then document in her notes – I have practised defensible medicine. By letting the matter go for now, I don't antagonize the patient. I also know that the practice will send yearly reminders to Miss JF, providing her with updated information and an opportunity for testing should she change her mind. The disadvantage with this is that I may not have given Miss JF sufficient information by which to make an informed decision.
- Offer the test and address Miss JF's specific ideas and concerns. The advantage with this approach is that I have empowered the patient by providing adequate information, in language she can understand, about the procedure and the advantages and disadvantages of screening. The disadvantage is that I may run late. Also I may be accused of doing a 'hard sell', that is, I may be suspected of 'pushing' the smear to reach QoF targets. I may be accused of wanting the financial reward rather than be thanked for enabling women to make an informed choice on whether or not they want to be screened. Since target payments for cervical screening were introduced in the UK in 1990, coverage increased from 53% in 1990 to more than 80% since 1993. Some argue that the financial incentive may subconsciously influence GPs to provide biased patient information which emphasizes the benefits of screening whilst glossing over the risks and side effects.

Could you use a model to help you to make a decision when faced with such a dilemma in future?
I could use an ethical model to inform my decision-making.

Autonomy: a patient can refuse to have a smear. A health professional needs to explain the reasons for the smear, the advantages (i.e. picking up early dysplasia and cancer) and the disadvantages (discomfort, false positives and negatives). The patient can refuse the treatment and the reasons for her refusal need not be sensible, rational or even well considered. Being of sound mind, and not being unduly influenced by other parties, she has the right to decide for herself.

Beneficence: a smear, by detecting cervical dysplasia at an earlier stage has great potential to improve her health outcomes. Screening prevents 1000–4000 deaths per year in the UK from squamous cell carcinoma (www.cancerscreening.nhs.uk/cervical/index.html).

Non-maleficence: the Bristol study involving approximately 226 000 women (Raffle *et al.*, 1995) showed that new abnormalities were found in 7% of women; 2.5% had colposcopy. The specificity of cervical screening was not optimal – there was considerable harm from screening. The patient could have weighed up the risk:benefit ratio and decided against screening. The psychological and social impact of a false positive smear cannot be underestimated.

Your colleague says that you should have scared her into having a smear. How do you respond?
- The colleague may justify this reasoning by saying that the new GMS contract awards 11 Q and O points to practices which achieve 80% coverage. The income generated (approximately £1375 in 2005) can be used to develop further services within the practice for the benefit of all the patients. By scaring the patient into having a smear to achieve target payments, I will be doing the greatest good for the greatest number of patients – using a utilitarianism argument.
- I could respond by saying that this is not a course of action likely to be supported by the GMC and RCGP. Therefore, I would prefer to respect the patient's autonomy (her right to make informed decisions) over the principle of utilitarianism. The new GMS contract recognizes the right of patients to decline screening and awards some Q and O points accordingly. The 2005/06 exemption reporting rate for practices in England for cervical screening was 4.6% (RCGP, March 2007).

What are your responsibilities to this patient and have you fulfilled them?
The GMC's *Good Medical Practice* states that the care of the patient is the doctor's first concern (patient primacy).
- I feel that by providing Miss JF with adequate information, in language she understands, about the procedure and the benefits and shortcomings of screening, I have fulfilled my responsibilities to her.
- I have also respected her decision to refuse screening.
- I have not tried to coerce her into changing her mind.

Doctors also have a duty to keep up-to-date. By reflecting on this case, I can identify my learning needs and strive to improve my practice. I could audit the percentage of women who decline the offer of a smear and compare this to the local and

Case-based Discussion

national average. Is there something about my practice that is causing women to decline? I could audit the percentage of inadequate smears within the practice – are women declining because our practice offers a less than optimal service? Do any smear takers need retraining? I could look at the type of patient information that is sent out and ensure that it is simply written, unbiased and up-to-date.

You free-texted in your consultation notes that the patient declined a smear test. Could you record this differently?
- I could have Read-coded her refusal of a smear. However, I am not aware of the correct Read-code.
- I could speak to the nurse who runs the smear recall about which is the most appropriate Read-code to use.

In your consultation with this patient, what are the advantages and disadvantages of free-texting?
- Advantages: I have sufficient space in which to document the patient's particular reasons for refusal. This information will then be available for future consultations during which there may be more time in which to address specific concerns. The more detailed the recording, the better the quality of information available for subsequent discussion – this may enable better continuity of care. Some doctors argue that if they are only able to remember a finite number of facts, it may be in the patient's interests to remember medical facts rather than details about Read-codes.
- Disadvantages: future audits and searches rely on appropriate and agreed Read-coding. Unlike free-texting, Read-codes ensure that patients are recalled appropriately. Auditing, which is an important tool for improving the quality of clinical practice, relies on good quality data entry.

Additional information

Your trainer may wish to extend the assessment to include questions on undertaking audit in primary care.

Why is audit important in primary care?
Audit is an important clinical governance (CG) activity. The aim of CG is to explicitly demonstrate that good quality care is being delivered and that continual improvements in care are being made. Clinical audit aims to lead to an improvement in the quality of health service so that:
- patient care is improved
- the professionalism of staff is enhanced
- resources are used efficiently
- continuing education is focused
- administration is efficient
- accountability is demonstrated

Under the new GMS contract, doctors are remunerated for providing evidence of good quality care. The evidence usually derives from practice audits. To attain these points, audit activity must occur in the practice.

In our practice, Nurse X is interested in undertaking audit. Explain to him the basic principles of audit.
Auditing is a systematic process, starting with an idea for the audit.

Ideas: based on Nurse X's interests, I would discuss possible ideas for audit and allow him to choose an example, such as 'Patients on thyroxine should have their TSH checked every 15 months'.

Justification for the audit: he would need to justify why he is checking the TSH every 15 months – is this recommendation based on good research or local protocols? He needs to quote the source of the recommendation. In some cases, he may need to search the literature and appraise the evidence.

Criteria chosen: criteria should be SMART (specific, measurable, achievable, reliable, timely) measures of quality.
With regard to thyroxine:
- Specific: was the TSH checked – yes or no.
- Measurable: the number of patients who had their TSH checked can be counted.
- Achievable: the audit is not beyond the scope of general practice and is suitable for a beginner. There are a limited number of Read-codes in the search.
- Reliable: the search is measuring what you actually want it to measure and you can use this result to improve patient care. For example, you want to identify patients who have not had their TSH measured so that you can offer them a test.
- Timely: the practice has a limited number of patients on thyroxine so the audit should be quick and easy to do even with manual note checks.

Standards set: standards are the levels of care you are prepared to accept. The new GMS contract awards six points if 90% of patients on thyroxine have their TSH measured in the last 15 months. After discussion with the PHCT, you may wish to set a higher percentage or stricter time frame to allow a safety margin.

Data collection: discuss with the audit lead how best to 'catch' all patients on thyroxine. Which Read-codes are needed? Does everybody Read-code appropriately and how would you identify patients whose diagnosis and results were free-texted?

Results and changes: discuss the results of the initial data collection. Present the results to the PHCT in a simple format. Agree changes and identify persons responsible for implementing the changes.

Second data collection: after implementing the change, the practice needs to re-audit. Have the changes resulted in the standards being met? If not, further action needs to be taken with a planned review date, i.e. go around the audit cycle again.

Conclusions: is the practice delivering high quality care to hypothyroid patients? What evidence is there to support this?

Relevant literature

Muir Gray JA (2004) New concepts in screening. *Br J Gen Pract,* **54:** 292–298.
Raffle AE, *et al.* (1995) Detection rates for abnormal cervical smears: what are we screening for? *Lancet,* **345:**1469–1473.
The Bath VTS website provides an excellent step by step 'how to do an audit' for those who have little or no experience of clinical audit in a general practice setting. See: http://www.mharris.eurobell.co.uk/contents.htm.

Patient requests an advance directive

Case summary

Mr J is 76 years old and has end-stage heart failure. He has been admitted to hospital six times in the past year with acute exacerbations. He came to see me for advice on drawing up a living will. During our first consultation, I assessed what he knew about living wills and his family's views. Before I saw him again, I spoke to his *'named'* doctor whom he had not seen in the last eight months. His named doctor said that he was not surprised at Mr J's wish to draw up an advance directive. Both his children had emigrated to Australia and Mr J did not want to burden his wife in his final years. Mr J had always made the decisions in the family and Mrs J was a slightly nervous woman who appeared to rely on her husband's advice. Mr and Mrs J attended the second consultation. I provided them with further information. They agreed to bring a final copy of the advance directive, once their solicitor had looked at it, to the surgery for enclosure in Mr J's notes.

Opening question:

What issues or challenges does this case raise for you, the trainee?

- I do not have prior experience in advising patients on how to go about organizing advance directives. I am concerned whether I gave the correct advice and involved all the parties that needed to be involved.

In this case, the trainer may decide to focus predominantly on two domains:

- **making diagnoses and decisions** – having a conscious, structured approach to decision making, to provide a person-centred approach that is appropriate to patient's circumstances
- **working with colleagues** – working effectively and sharing information with colleagues, coordinating care with other professionals, to provide long-term continuity of care as determined by the needs of the patient

To achieve sufficient depth of questioning in the above domains, the trainer may prepare the following questions:

- what were you particularly worried about in this case?
- how did you come to your final decision?
- did you use any guidelines to help you?
- did you consider the implications of your decision for the relatives/ practice/society? Tell me more about how they might feel. How did this influence your final decision?
- did you involve anyone else in this case? Why? How did they help?
- how did you ensure that you had effective communication with others involved in this case?

What were you particularly worried about in this case?

An advance directive is a legally binding document drawn up in advance by a patient. It allows them to consent to or refuse specific medical treatments when they are too ill to communicate their decisions for themselves. Most people perceive advance directives as expressing a refusal of treatment, however, it may equally authorize that life prolonging measures be maintained. I am worried about the advice I gave to Mr J in drawing up this legal document. Was my advice and assessment complete, or did I overlook anything that could affect the validity of the document?

What advice did you give?

I advised Mr J that he can chose between six types of advance statements.

1. He can request the type(s) of treatment he would prefer in certain circumstances, e.g. if admitted with confusion, he could chose not to have antibiotics.
2. He can state his general values and beliefs, e.g. he prefers not to have a blood transfusion because he is a Jehovah's witness.
3. He can name a proxy who knows him well enough so that he or she can express the patient's wishes in the event of a life-threatening illness.
4. He can give instructions (directives) regarding his future treatment, e.g. he prefers not to be admitted to the district hospital, but is happy to be treated at home or in the hospice.
5. He can specify that life-sustaining treatment can be withheld when he deteriorates irreversibly, e.g. if confused and restless, he would like to be made comfortable, but he prefers not to have cardio-pulmonary resuscitation.
6. He can specify a combination of all the above.

I also advised Mr J that advance directives should be drawn up with the aid of legal advice. Formatted versions are available from the Terence Higgins Trust or the Voluntary Euthanasia Society. The directive should contain the following information:

- Mr J's full name and address
- name and address of his GP
- the date on which the document was drawn up
- the date on which the document will be reviewed (usually when circumstances change or in five years)
- a statement indicating that advice was obtained from health professionals
- a clear statement of his wishes
- the contact details of the nominated proxy

Once completed, the living will should be witnessed and signed by Mr J, his GP, his solicitor and the nominated proxy.

I informed Mr J that he, his solicitor, his GP and the hospital should keep a copy of the advance directive. Mr J could also wear a medic-alert bracelet so that the emergency services are also informed.

You said you made an assessment of Mr J. What did you assess?

I assessed whether:

- Mr J was mentally competent at presentation
- he had adequate information so that he could make an informed decision and whether he understood the consequences of his decisions
- he was being coerced

How did you come to your final decision?

I came to my decision by testing Mr J's competence, because for his living will to be valid, he must be competent. To meet the test of competence, Mr J must:

- **comprehend** and retain the necessary information. During our conversation, I periodically tested his comprehension by checking his understanding of the information I'd given.
- **believe** the information. Checking for belief is subtler; I excluded conditions that would cause Mr J to have 'altered thinking', such as depression, psychosis or anorexia. If Mr J has depression with psychotic features, then he is unlikely to believe the information regarding his treatment and thereby fails the test of competence.
- **weigh** up the information, balancing risks and needs, to arrive at a true choice. I gave Mr J adequate information regarding his treatments and also time, between the consultations, to make a reasoned judgement. A true choice is one that he makes without coercion. This is why I wanted to meet his wife and why I wanted to get a second opinion on the family circumstances from his named GP who knew the family for many years.

Did you use any guidelines to help you?

Advance directives allow patients to consent to or refuse treatments when they are incapacitated. I used the GMC's guidance on consent from which I learnt that for consent to be valid:

- the patient must be sufficiently informed
- the patient must be competent
- consent must be given voluntarily

I also looked at the GMC's guidance on seeking patients' consent.

Did you consider the implications of your decision for the relatives/practice/society? Tell me more about how they might feel. How did this influence your final decision?

Regarding his relatives: Mr J needs to nominate a proxy, that is, a surrogate who will have continuing power of attorney. The proxy should be emotionally stable and should be able to make reasoned judgements based on adequate information in the patient's best interests.

- The person selected may feel burdened by the enormity of the task.
- The proxy may feel that they do not know the patient well enough to make the same decisions the patient would have chosen in similar circumstances.
- Relatives may be distressed if previously unaware of the living will's existence.
- On the other hand, an advance directive has the potential to make everybody aware in advance of the patient's wishes. It may reduce confusion arising

during stressful situations and provide relief to family and friends by unburdening them from the difficult decisions regarding treatment.

Regarding the practice/hospital:
- The living wills may lack sufficient information – they are left open to interpretation and different doctors may make different interpretations.
- The living wills may be too specific – they may not cover every eventuality. For example, a patient may state that surgery must not be performed if terminal cancer is present, but palliative surgery may be indicated in terminal bowel cancer, not to prolong life, but to relieve the distressing symptoms associated with unrelieved bowel obstruction. In such a case, a legally binding advance directive will prohibit doctors from providing the most appropriate palliative care available (Jarmulowicz, 2000).
- Patients cannot refuse basic care, but in providing hygiene, pain relief and the offer of oral nutrition and hydration, relatives may see the medical profession as not respecting the advance directive.
- Finally, various health care professions may look after the patient – many of them may be unaware of the document's existence. Surveys show that not all hospital trusts had policies for advance directives (Hoffenberg, 2006).

Regarding society:
- The patient's autonomy is recognized and respected. This is a reassuring move away from the medical profession's paternalistic position of *'doctor knows best'* to one in which the patient gives informed consent.
- On the other hand, refusal of treatment can be valid only if the specific facts pertaining to the current situation are available. Living wills will be made many years in advance when all the details of the conditions and its possible treatments cannot be foreseen. If the directive is not specific, it is open to interpretation. If it is too specific, it is unable to cover every eventuality. The legality of the document can then be questioned.

How did these considerations influence your final decision?
I asked Mr J how he would draw up his advance directive so that his nominated proxy, his relatives, his GP, his solicitor, the hospital and emergency services are all made aware of his wishes and decisions. I asked if he had:
- nominated a proxy
- decided which directives he would like to exercise
- informed his family, his proxy and his solicitor
- drawn the document up correctly

Did you involve anyone else in this case? Why? How did they help?
I saw Mr and Mrs J in a joint consultation. Mrs J understood what her husband was trying to achieve in drawing up a living will. If Mrs J was not party to the discussion,
- if asked to be the proxy, she may find it difficult to understand what is expected of her

- if not asked to be proxy, and if Mr J had drawn up the living will without her knowledge, she may have been distressed by its existence when it is evoked in the future

I spoke to Mr J's named GP, who knew the family for many years, to get his perpective on Mr J's mental state, character and family circumstances. This helped me to interpret Mr J's request and aided in my assessment of his competence to consent.

I also advised Mr J to speak to his solicitors but I chose not to speak to them myself. I assumed that they would contact me, after seeking consent from Mr J, if they wanted further information.

I intended to send a copy of the completed advance directive to Mr J's consultant for enclosure in his hospital notes. I did not advise Mr J to speak to the consultant before drawing up his advance directive because I felt Mr J had been given sufficient information by which to make informed decisions. *This point is debatable and the trainer may go on to ask for which patients you would get a consultant opinion.*

How did you ensure that you had effective communication with others involved in this case?

I wanted Mr J's named GP (Dr X) to give me his opinion of the patient's decision to draw up a living will. For this to occur, I thought Dr X would want to know why I wanted the information and how I intended using the information. Therefore, to clarify my agenda to Dr X, I sent him a short email and asked when it would be best to speak to him. I felt that this approach gave Dr X time to look over the case notes, if needed. By setting a time for the conversation, I felt I would be able to get Dr X's full attention and informed opinion rather than snatch a quick opinion in the corridor between patients. I actively listened to Dr X's opinions without interruption and in turn aired my thoughts openly and frankly. I was constructive in my discussion – I presented the problem at hand and asked for help in finding a solution. At the same time, I made Dr X aware that I took responsibility for my patient and the decisions I made.

Additional information

You said that you consulted the GMC's guidance on consent. What did you learn from this guidance?

From **General Medical Council** (1998) *Seeking patients' consent: the ethical considerations.* GMC, London.

I ascertained that the information which patients want or ought to know, before deciding whether to consent to treatment or an investigation, may include:
- details of the diagnosis, and prognosis, and the likely prognosis if the condition is left untreated
- uncertainties about the diagnosis including options for further investigation prior to treatment

- options for treatment or management of the condition, including the option not to treat
- the purpose of a proposed investigation or treatment; details of the procedures or therapies involved, including subsidiary treatment such as methods of pain relief; how the patient should prepare for the procedure; and details of what the patient might experience during or after the procedure including common and serious side effects
- for each option, explanations of the likely benefits and the probabilities of success; and discussion of any serious or frequently occurring risks, and of any lifestyle changes which may be caused by, or necessitated by, the treatment
- advice about whether a proposed treatment is experimental
- how and when the patient's condition and any side effects will be monitored or re-assessed
- the name of the doctor who will have overall responsibility for the treatment and, where appropriate, names of the senior members of his or her team
- whether doctors in training will be involved, and the extent to which students may be involved in an investigation or treatment
- a reminder that patients can change their minds about a decision at any time
- a reminder that patients have a right to seek a second opinion
- where applicable, details of costs or charges which the patient may have to meet

You said that you communicated with Dr X in writing and verbally. How would you assess whether you had good communication with Dr X?

From **Kersley S** (2002) Do your colleagues understand you. *BMJ Career Focus*, **324:** S117 (see http://careerfocus.bmj.com/cgi/content/full/324/7342/S117).

- Do you have your say, and is your opinion acknowledged and considered?
- Do you feel heard?
- Do you listen as much as you talk? We have two ears and one mouth for this reason: listen twice as much as you talk.
- What are you prepared and not prepared to do?
- Have you talked to your colleagues?
- Have you listened to them?
- Are you clear on what your colleagues expect of you? Do you have a specific role different from those of your colleagues?
- How flexible are you prepared to be?
- What will you say no to?
- What are your standards?

You communicated with Mr and Mrs J and Dr X. It looks as if you established good rapport with them. What steps did you take to establish rapport?

From **Walter J and Bayat A** (2003) Neurolinguistic programming: verbal communication. *StudentBMJ*, **11:** 131–174 (see (http://student.bmj.com/issues/03/05/life/163.php).

With regard to NLP, Walter and Bayat say 'Communication is made up of words or linguistics (7%), tonality or how the voice sounds (38%), and physiology or body language (55%)...

Communication by our physiology or body language relates to posture, gestures, facial expressions (including blinking), and breathing. The remainder of our communication, being tonality, relates to the tone (pitch), tempo, timbre (quality), and volume of our voice. We can use these forms of communication by trying to match some of these qualities in the person with whom we are trying to communicate. This is known as establishing rapport and works on the principle that people like people who are similar to them. The two ways of establishing rapport are known as matching and mirroring. With matching, you copy one or more aspects of the non-verbal communication exactly. With mirroring you copy, but in such a way as to create a mirror image of the action.'

You emailed Dr X before discussing the case with him. Would you have discussed the case in the same way if you had been consulting with Dr Y, a slightly brusque senior partner?

Personality types and communication
Houghton and Allen (2005) discuss how personality type affect communication styles, and how our behaviour can alter when we are stressed. A doctor who usually has a preference for Extraversion, Intuition, and Feeling, may under stressful conditions, adopt a contained (Introversion), relatively impersonal (Thinking), and focused on hearing the details (Sensing) style.

Relevant literature

BMA (1995) *Advance statements about medical treatment – code of practice report of the BMA.*
BMA (1999) *Withholding and withdrawing life-prolonging treatment.*
GMC (1998) *Seeking patients' consent: the ethical considerations.* www.gmc-uk.org
GMC (2002) *Withholding and withdrawing life-prolonging treatments. Good practice in decision making.* www.gmc-uk.org
Hoffenberg R (2006) Advance healthcare directives. *Clin Med,* **6:** 231–233.
Houghton A and Allen J (2005) Understanding personality type. *BMJ Career Focus,* **330:** 36–37. See http://careerfocus.bmj.com/cgi/content/full/330/7484/36 to read more about personality types and communication.
Jarmulowicz M (2000) Advance directives: questionnaire survey of NHS trusts. *BMJ,* **320:** 24–25.
Kessel AS and Meran J (1998) Advance directives in the UK: legal, ethical, and practical considerations for doctors. *British Journal of General Practice,* **48:** 1263–1266.
A very good summary on advance directives is available from the British Geriatrics Society website: http://www.bgs.org.uk/compendium/compg2.htm.
Best practice is outlined in an easy to read Australian document entitled 'Using advance care directives': http://www.health.nsw.gov.au/pubs/2004/pdf/adcare_directive.pdf.

Withholding life-prolonging treatment

Case summary

77-year-old Mr J with end-stage heart failure saw me a few months ago to draw up a living will stating that he did not want to be admitted to hospital or be given life-saving treatment in the event of irreversible deterioration. Two months ago he suffered a stroke and is now demented and bed-bound. Three days ago, his wife, who cares for him at home, requested a visit. After examining him, I suspected that he had pneumonia. His wife, who is also his proxy, wanted me to prescribe antibiotics. I faced a dilemma:
- if I gave antibiotics, I felt I would not respecting Mr J's living will, but I would act as Mrs J wanted
- if I didn't give antibiotics, I felt I would be respecting Mr J's autonomy, as protected by the living will, but Mrs J may feel that I was allowing her husband to suffer needlessly

Eventually, I prescribed the antibiotics, in liquid form. Mr J is still alive and being cared for at home.

Opening question:

What issues or challenges does this case raise for you, the trainee?
- Did I do the right thing by giving the antibiotics or did I disrespect Mr J's advance directive?

In this case, the trainer may decide to focus predominantly on two domains:
- **working with colleagues** – working effectively and sharing information with colleagues, to manage and coordinate palliation
- **fitness to practice** – showing an awareness of your own performance, conduct or health and taking action to protect patients; being aware of your own capabilities and values

To achieve sufficient depth of questioning in the above domains, the trainer may prepare the following questions:
- did you involve anyone else in this case? For what purpose?
- if many people are involved in this case, what do you see as your role?
- do you think that what you have already documented and discussed with other members of the Primary Health Care Team is adequate for a seamless transfer of care, say in the event of you being unavailable and not contactable in the next few days?
- what did you advise Mrs J to do if her husband deteriorated overnight?
- what do you feel are your responsibilities to patients with regard to withholding and withdrawing life-prolonging treatment? How did you make sure you observed them in this case?

Did you involve anyone else in this case? For what purpose?
I involved several people: Mrs J, Mr J's named GP at the practice, the district nurses and a consultant in elderly care.

Mr J's named GP (Dr X): I checked with Dr X that the current situation is one to which the advance directive is applicable. He advised me that a living will is a legally binding document that expresses the patient's autonomy. It is valid if:
- Mr J was competent at the time the decisions were made. I assessed his competence at the time he drew up the document.
- he was given sufficient information to understand the consequences of his choices. At the time, I gave him this information and he spoke to his solicitors.
- he was not coerced into making the advance directive. I was involved in the drawing up of the document and I know that he made up his own mind.
- the directive is applicable to his current situation. His directive states he did not want admission to hospital and he would prefer that life-sustaining treatment be withheld should he deteriorate irreversibly. This is the dilemma: I thought that antibiotics for a chest infection fell under the category of life-sustaining treatment, but Mrs J wants antibiotics at home to prevent pain and suffering – she regards antibiotics as palliative rather than life-saving. Dr X advised me to speak with the family to reach a consensus on whether to give antibiotics.

The family: Mrs J is the main carer and also the patient's nominated proxy in his living will. The proxy is usually the person who knows the patient well to see that his wishes are carried out in the current circumstances. I needed to know if:
- Mr J would want to be kept alive in his current bed-bound demented state?
- the directive is too vague: by life-sustaining treatment, was Mr J referring to cardio-pulmonary resuscitation as well as antibiotics?
- would he have considered his current state to be a burden on his family?

I clarified with Mrs J her reasons for wanting antibiotics. She did not consider antibiotics to be 'life-saving' in the same way as CPR or ventilation in ITU. I took this to indicate that her husband was likely to hold this view as well.

Her sons live in Australia and she regularly speaks to them on the telephone. I offered to speak to them to answer any queries they may have. Mrs J did not take up this offer and I respected her wishes. I did not want to appear to undermine her wishes by insisting on speaking to her sons. If other relatives were present, I would have consulted with them to reach a consensus on whether to give antibiotics.

The district nurses: I spoke to the district nurses for two reasons: first, to get their opinion on the best course of action. Their opinions are formed from regular contact with Mr and Mrs J. Secondly, the family may already have discussed with them issues such as Mr J's quality of life should he survive this episode. I did not want my discussion with the family to duplicate ground already covered by other members of the PHCT.

The consultant in elderly care: this discussion was to address my learning needs – was I balancing the conflicting principles of autonomy (i.e. respecting the living will) and non-maleficence (i.e. first doing no harm) in a justifiable manner. I assumed that the consultant had lots of experience with these issues and that if I talked through the case with him, I would become consciously aware of each step of my decision-making. I learn better by talking things through with people rather than reading the GMC guidance only. Therefore for me to learn from this case, I needed to discuss it. I think that having learnt from this case, I am less likely to ask for his opinion if faced with a similar situation in the future. (See 'Learning styles' below.)

If many people are involved in this case, what do you see as your role?
As the GP registrar who has looked after Mr J since I joined the practice, I see myself as having the responsibilities of his GP. As such, I see myself as being his advocate and the coordinator of any holistic care he may require. I am also the person who refers him for further care to other medical teams, namely palliative, hospice, or the hospital-based services if I assess these are appropriate. The latter gives me a gate-keeper function which sometimes conflicts with my role as his advocate.

However, as the GP registrar within a training practice, I have been delegated responsibility for patient care by the named doctors on whose 'lists' patients appear. Therefore, I also have a responsibility to the named doctors, to whom I will return care when I leave the practice, to share information and decisions about patients, particularly in sensitive cases where there are medico-legal issues. Having said this, I feel that ultimately, the care of the patient is my first responsibility, as per the GMC's *The Duties of a Doctor* (2006).

In this case, Mr and Mrs J have chosen to see me over a ten month period. I see it as my duty to look after Mr J in what could be his terminal illness, to provide advice, prescribe appropriately and support the family. Therefore, while I share information and take advice from colleagues, the ultimate decision to prescribe antibiotics, or not, lies with me, unless the patient, the named GP or I expressly transfer care to a named professional.

Do you think that what you have already documented and discussed with other members of the Primary Health Care Team is adequate for a seamless transfer of care, say in the event of you being unavailable and not contactable in the next few days?
As can be seen from the computer and hand-held patient records:
- I have documented when and what was said in the discussions with Mr and Mrs J, the district nurses, the named GP and the consultant in elderly care
- each dated entry is therefore a mini-summary of what was discussed and concludes with the decisions I made with the information I obtained

- I have also outlined an action plan which states who will do what and by what time
- I have listed all relevant contact telephone numbers so that Mrs J or any member of the PHCT who looks at the notes will be able to contact individuals involved in the care

This, I think, will enable a seamless transfer of care.

What did you advise Mrs J to do if her husband deteriorated overnight?

What I advised Mrs J to do at the end of the consultation, was based on my knowledge of how she felt and what arrangements she already had in place.

- She had arranged with the district nurses and social services to have a sitter with her that night. I supported this because first, it looked as if Mr J may have another difficult night and would require someone with him, and secondly, Mrs Jones was very tired from being up for most of the previous night.
- The district nurse had arranged to show Mrs J how to give her husband the antibiotics without distressing him. Mrs J was happy to do this and said that if she ran into difficulty, she would contact the on-call district nurse whose telephone number she had.
- Mrs J believed that the antibiotics would ease her husband's breathing and he would start to improve. Her attitude was positive and pragmatic – if he deteriorated, she and the sitter would make him comfortable.
- She respected her husband's wishes not to be admitted to hospital and to die at home. She felt if he deteriorated, the sitter would call her. She would sit with him and talk to him to ease his distress.
- She wanted to be strong for her husband and felt capable of looking after him at home. With the support from her sons, with whom she had pre-arranged telephone calls for later that evening; her neighbours who were bringing her dinner; and the sitter, who would be with her for the night, she felt she had the resources to cope.

I was impressed by the arrangements Mrs J had made. I respected her decision to care for her husband at home, as per his wishes. I tried to convey my respect and empathy to her.

I told her that while I was not on call that night, a doctor could be contacted via the out-of-hours service. I explained that if Mr J died, a doctor was needed to certify death. I would telephone her first thing in the morning to review the situation and to arrange for another home visit, if needed. *The trainer could ask you whether you would give your telephone number or visit when you are not on call.*

What do you feel are your responsibilities to patients with regard to withholding and withdrawing life-prolonging treatment? How did you make sure you observed them?

My responsibility is to:

- give patients treatments for which they consent

- respect their wishes when they chose not to be treated
- give treatment in their best interest when patients lack the capacity to decide for themselves

To comply with these responsibilities, I read the GMC's advice – *Withholding and Withdrawing Life-prolonging Treatments: Good Practice in Decision-making* (GMC, 2002). This states that when adult patients cannot decide for themselves:

- any valid advance refusal of treatment should be respected. A living will made when the patient was competent and on the basis of adequate information about the implications of his/her choice is legally binding and must be respected where it is clearly applicable to the patient's present circumstances and where there is no reason to believe that the patient had changed his/her mind.
- an assessment of the benefits, burdens and risks, and the acceptability of proposed treatment must be made on their behalf by the doctor, taking account of their wishes, where they are known. Where a patient's wishes are not known it is the doctor's responsibility to decide what is in the patient's best interests. However, this cannot be done effectively without information about the patient which those close to the patient will be best placed to know. Doctors practising in Scotland need additionally to take account of the Scottish legal framework for making decisions on behalf of adults with incapacity.

I took the following steps to ensure I followed the above advice:

- I read the GMC statement and asked myself if I understood how the guidance applied to my case
- I found out what is meant by 'in the patient's best interests' by looking at the GMC's advice online: http://www.gmc-uk.org/guidance/current/library/consent.asp#best_interests
- I wanted to act in the Mr Jones' best interests. To do this, I had to decide:
  - is the treatment clinically indicated? In this case, pneumonia is a clear indication for giving antibiotics.
  - is there any evidence of an advance directive or did I know what the patient would have wanted? Unfortunately the living will in this case lacks sufficient information and is left open to interpretation. Therefore, I took into account Mrs J's view in her capacity as proxy and carer.
  - what are the views of the close family? Mrs J did not consider antibiotics to be 'life-saving' in the same way as CPR or ventilation in ITU. She considered giving antibiotics as treatment that would ease her husband's pain and make his breathing more comfortable, i.e. palliative.
  - if there are a few treatment options, to chose the option that least restricts the patient's future choices. In the case of Mr J, there are two reasonable options: to give or not to give antibiotics, but not to give is more likely to result in his death thus restricting his future choices.

I feel that in giving antibiotics, I respected Mr J's living will, as interpreted by his proxy and carer, and I gave treatment in his best interests.

Additional information

The GP trainer could ask *what qualities did you demonstrate in your role in treating Mr J? In other words, what made you a good doctor?*

A doctor can be considered to be 'good' by his patients, his profession, his colleagues and his family.

Professional qualities

A good doctor follows the profession's code of practice, as laid down by the GMC in *Good Medical Practice*. The doctor makes his patients his first concern and is respectful of the patient's primacy. The doctor is honest, trustworthy and ethical. He maintains his patient's confidentiality and establishes a relationship that is based on trust. He obtains appropriate informed consent and decides on treatments that are in his patient's best interests. The doctor does not abuse his position in society. He maintains his financial and personal integrity (probity). A good doctor is also a safe doctor – he recognizes the limits of his competence and does not put his patients at risk. He continues to improve his knowledge, skills, attitudes and professional values – he actively learns from his work and keeps up to date. He does not engage in unethical research.

Personal qualities

- Caritas – the Latin word 'caritas' describes the qualities of genuine caring that the doctor has for his patients. Good doctors are sensitive, empathetic, understanding, patient-centred and approachable.
- Self-awareness – a good doctor has insight into his own motives, needs and feelings. He is able to ask for help. He is able to challenge his assumptions and knowledge without being defensive and resistant to change.
- Good interpersonal skills – he is able to contribute to and appreciate the value of team work. He demonstrates leadership skills and is able to support other members of the group.
- He has good communication skills – he is able to listen and respond appropriately. He analyses well, marshals his facts, argues a case and establishes priorities.
- He has a good sense of humour, is conscientious, tolerant, flexible and affable.
- He is motivated, enthusiastic and committed to his work.
- He is able to achieve a good balance between his professional and private life. He is personally well organized and able to set good boundaries.

Leader and team player

He listens to and respects the views of all team members. He is skilled at motivating the quieter members of the team to contribute and skilfully moderates the more voluble. He is a skilled negotiator who provides a clear and detailed vision of what the team requires and encourages team members to work towards these goals.

What society expects
Society expects doctors to keep the patient at the focus of the consultation, to put the needs of the patient first, to be patient-centred. Doctors can achieve patient-centredness by:

- *reducing sapiential authority:* sapiential authority is possessed by virtue of the person's special knowledge, expertise and experience. Historically, the authority of doctors grew because they knew more about disease and treatments than their patients. Patients did not question the doctors and doctors rarely admitted that they did not know the answers. Doctors can reduce their sapiential authority by facilitating their patients' access to information, by explaining the treatment options in simple language and allowing patients to make the choice that suits them best.

- *reducing moral authority:* moral authority is possessed by virtue of the person's concern for the afflicted individual. Society expects doctors to work in the best interests of their patients. In the aftermath of the Bristol scandal and the Shipman murders, public confidence in the 'inherent good' of doctors has waned. Clinical governance, with its emphasis on transparency, accountability, and cultural openness is perhaps an attempt by the profession to show society that doctors are acting in the patients' best interests rather than in their own.

- *reducing charismatic authority:* charismatic authority is possessed by virtue of the afflicted person's faith that the doctor will be of help. A doctor was seen as having the healing power that was given by God to a chosen individual. There is a general social trend towards informality and openness. The priestly white coat has disappeared from general practice. Patients are more questioning of their doctors.

The GP trainer asks what calling the geriatric consultant for information tells you about your learning style.

Learning styles
Honey and Mumford (1989) describe learners as activists, reflectors, theorists or pragmatists based on their preferred learning style. They argue that if attention is paid to learning styles, then more effective learning can take place. Kolb (1984) describes a model of learning called experiential learning – the learner begins with an experience ('concrete experience') which is followed by reflection ('reflective observation'). The reflection is then assimilated into a theory ('abstract concepualization'). The theory is tested in new situations ('active experimentation') which in turn gives rise to more concrete experiences. A recurring cycle of learning occurs. Honey and Mumford built on Kolb's work by connecting a learning style to each stage of the learning cycle (as shown in the figure below). Depending on the preferred learning style, the learner will enter into the learning cycle at any of the four points.

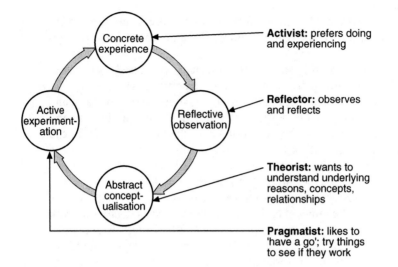

Typology of learners cycle.
Reproduced from http://www.learningandteaching.info/learning/experience.htm;
with permission.

Relevant literature

GMC (2002) *Withholding and Withdrawing Life-prolonging Treatments: Good Practice in Decision-making* (see http://www.gmc-uk.org/standards/whwd.htm).
GMC (2006) *The Duties of a Doctor* (see http://www.gmc-uk.org/guidance/good_medical_practice/duties_of_a_doctor.asp).
Honey P and Mumford A (1986) *The Learning Styles Questionnaire.* Peter Honey Publications Limited, Maidenhead.
Neighbour R. (1992) *The Inner Apprentice.* Kluwer Academic Publishers.
Kolb D (1984) *Experiential Learning: Experience as a Source of Learning and Development.* Prentice Hall, Englewood Cliff, NJ.
Tate P (2006) *The Doctor's Communication Handbook,* 6th edn. Radcliffe Publishing Ltd, Abingdon.
For information on working in teams, see:
http://www.bmjlearning.com/planrecord/servlet/ObligationsServlet?indObl=andnfsCategory=4#subcat_11
http://www.resourcefulpatient.org/ by Muir Gray and Harry Rutter
http://www.rcgp-curriculum.org.uk/PDF/curr_4_1_Management_in_Primary_Care.pdf
http://www.gmc-uk.org/guidance/current/library/consent.asp#best_interests

Euthanasia

Case summary

77-year-old Mr J with end-stage heart failure saw me eight months ago to draw up a living will stating that he did not want to be admitted to hospital or be given life-saving treatment in the event of irreversible deterioration. Two months ago he suffered a stroke and is now demented and bed-bound. Last week, his wife, who cares for him at home, requested a visit. After examining him, I suspected that he had pneumonia. Following consultation with his wife and the PHCT looking after him, I prescribed antibiotics. Unfortunately, he continued to deteriorate. Three days ago, the district nurse asked if she should start nasogastric feeds and fluids because Mr J has not eaten for the past four days. When I visited to make the assessment, I found his wife distressed by his loud, raspy breathing. She asked me to give him a large dose of morphine. I explained that euthanasia is illegal. After consultation with the family and PHCT, I decided against providing artificial nutrition and hydration.

Opening question:

What issues or challenges does this case raise for you, the trainee?
- Being asked to give Mr J a large dose of morphine made me uncomfortable.
- I am not sure if other doctors would have withheld artificial nutrition and hydration – I hope I did the right thing.

In this case, the trainer may decide to focus predominantly on two domains:
- **maintaining an ethical approach to practice** – the doctor shows integrity and a respect for diversity. He identifies the ethical aspects of clinical practice (prevention, diagnostics, therapy, factors that influence lifestyles), and understands how his own attitudes and feelings are important determinants of how he practises. He is able to justifying and clarify personal ethics.
- **managing medical complexity** – managing uncertainty and risk. The doctor tolerates uncertainty and makes effective and efficient use of therapeutic interventions.

To achieve sufficient depth of questioning in the above domains, the trainer may prepare the following questions:
- what consultation skills did you use to inform your understanding of the consultation with Mrs J?
- what ethical principles did you use to inform your decision-making?
- how did you feel about being asked to administer a large dose of morphine to Mr J?
- what issues did you consider when the district nurse asked if she should provide artificial nutrition and hydration?

What consultation skills did you use to inform your understanding of the consultation with Mrs J?

I used Berne's model of transactional analysis which addresses the roles that patients and doctors play within the consultation (Berne, 1964). Berne identifies three ego states:

- parent: may be critical or caring. In this mode, the doctor or patient commands, directs, prohibits, controls and/or nurtures the other party.
- adult: the doctor or patient sorts out information and works logically.
- child: the doctor or patient assumes the dependent role.

When I was asked to assist in Mr J's death, I tried to explore the reasons behind the request in an adult–adult fashion.

- What is Mrs J really asking for – is she indicating that she believes her husband to be in pain? Is better symptom control required?
- Is Mrs J indicating that she cannot cope with his care anymore and she would prefer that he be cared for in a hospice or hospital?
- Does Mrs J believe herself to be acting in accordance with her husband's wishes – did he hope to avoid a long, drawn-out death?
- Is Mrs J grief-stricken and depressed? Is she expressing her feelings of hopelessness?

By thinking through what the problem really is, both Mrs J and I sorted out the information logically within an adult–adult relationship. We came to a shared understanding of the problem and negotiated a course of action that was respectful of each other's views. I explained that in the UK, assisted suicide is currently illegal. However, by acknowledging the legitimacy of the request and expressing empathy for her situation, she felt better for being able to unburden her feelings to me.

The consultation was in danger of becoming a parent–child discussion had I acted in a critical manner 'How could you put me in this position?' or in a directive manner 'Let me call the palliative care services and we'll sort it out for you!'.

The consultation would have been in danger of becoming a child–parent discussion had I abandoned my professional judgement in an attempt to please Mrs J.

Talking to Mrs J was fundamental to understanding her concerns and providing support. Therefore, I was able to maintain a healthy doctor–patient relationship.

What ethical principles did you use to inform your decision-making?

I considered the following ethical concepts.

- *Relativism*: the idea that there are no absolute rights or wrongs – the morality of any action depends on the circumstances or culture. The culture of Western society is influenced chiefly by two principles: first, by religious teachings where the killing of innocent human beings is morally wrong, and secondly by a strong respect for autonomy where people believe that individuals should have the right to choose the manner and timing of their deaths, especially if it prevents people dying in pain and distress.

- *Doctrine of double-effect*: an action that has both good and bad effects may be justifiable. Doctors are legally bound not to assist suicide or take any action of which the primary purpose is to end life. However, a doctor can administer a dose of painkiller if the primary aim is to relieve pain, even if the secondary effect is to shorten the patient's life.
- *Ordinary and extraordinary means*: some treatments may not be justifiable because of the degree of intervention required. For example, the current system for treating terminally ill patients seeks to provide humane palliative care. Most forms of pain can be controlled, i.e. by ordinary means. Where alternatives exist, there is no need for euthanasia, i.e. extraordinary means.
- *Wants and needs*: patients want to die with dignity but society needs laws that protect the vulnerable. Changing the legislation may be dangerous because of the abuse that may occur. Elderly patients may become fearful of seeking medical attention in case their relatives and doctors choose euthanasia when they become incompetent. The cost of looking after terminally ill patients is increasing. On discharge from hospital, patients may need extensive care from the family or admission to a nursing home – this may place a financial burden on the family. People may feel pressurized into accepting euthanasia so as not to burden their relatives.

How did you feel about being asked to administer a large dose of morphine to Mr J?

I felt disturbed; my immediate reaction was that Mrs J was asking me to kill her husband, an act I would find difficult. This is not because I lack sympathy with the concept of euthanasia. After a few moments, I sensed that Mrs J was not asking me to kill her husband. Rather, she was expressing her sense of frustration with his suffering and wanted to do something to ease it. Once I said to her that it must be difficult to stand by, to be patient and to await events rather than to act, she felt I understood and empathized. Once she felt supported, we were able to discuss feelings more openly and make decisions more easily.

I felt relieved that I was able to make Mrs J aware of my principles without having to be blunt and confrontational. I was glad to be able to deal with my emotions quickly, that is, to house-keep efficiently. Neighbour (2004) called this dealing with 'present' stress, any unpleasant thoughts, and feelings that arise during the course of the consultation:

"In principle, the remedy for present stress is the ability, which can be readily acquired, to free the present moment from its unpleasant associations by focusing non-judgmental attention on the experience of the 'here and now'".

Neighbour's suggested techniques for focusing on the 'here and now' are to focus on the sensation of breathing and to unclench tense muscles. I tried this. It helped me to deal with my emotions quickly and to think about Mrs J's request with greater clarity. In retrospect, I feel pleased to have remembered and used a consultation technique during a challenging consultation, to good effect.

What issues did you consider when the district nurse asked if she should provide artificial nutrition and hydration?

Because Mr J's death seemed imminent, I needed to balance the benefits of starting artificial hydration or nutrition with the risks of intervention. Now that oral rehydration was not feasible, our options were nasogastric or subcutaneous fluids. Intravenous fluids would be too invasive. Inserting and maintaining a nasogastric tube or a subcutaneous catheter may be too burdensome in relation to its possible benefits. On the other hand, it may provide symptom relief. I asked Mrs J if she thought her husband was thirsty or hungry. Her view was that he seemed to be comforted by dampening his lips. Mrs J, the district nurse and I reached consensus that it would be better not to start artificial hydration or nutrition.

I acted on the ethical principle of futility – if an outcome is going to be poor anyway, any intervention or treatment needs to be judged in this light.

Additional information

You mention being pleased with your ability to housekeep during a challenging consultation. You described how you achieved good housekeeping. Tell me why is housekeeping important to you.

Housekeeping is concerned with stress prevention – with recognizing stress levels and doing something constructive about it because stress is bad for doctors and patients. Housekeeping is important for me because I want to avoid stress and burnout. By housekeeping, especially during challenging consultations, I am taking pro-active steps to maintain good mental health despite having quite a few of the risk factors for stress and burnout, such as high self-criticism, high discipline, and idealism.

Graske (2003) discussed the prevalence of any common mental disorder in doctors, which is thought to be as high as 28%, compared with 15% in the general population. However, these findings conflict with data from two other studies (described in Cunningham, 1994) which have shown mental illness in doctors to be no greater than in the general public and less than in the legal profession. Graske (2003) writes:

- depression occurs in 10% of doctors, compared with 5% of the general population
- suicide rates are worse too, with male doctors twice as likely and female doctors three to four times more likely to commit suicide than the general population
- the magnitude of addiction among medical professionals is largely unknown, but has been estimated at 1 in 15 doctors (BMA, 1998)

Certain personality types and learning styles are more susceptible to psychological difficulties in medicine. Common personality traits include perfectionism, high self-criticism, low flexibility, high discipline, idealism, and high empathy. When these traits are combined with over-commitment, social isolation, and poor coping strategies, mental distress often results.

Support services are emerging within and outside the NHS, such as the Doctors' Support Line and the National Counseling Service for Sick Doctors. Some trusts have implemented mentoring and peer support, and some medical students are receiving education regarding their own behaviour and health.

From **Stanton J and Caan W** (2003) How many doctors are sick? *BMJ Career Focus.* **326:** S97a-S97a.

This paper attempted to answer the above question by:
- **searching the literature:** one study (Newbury-Birch *et al.*, 2002) showed that 10% of all house officers were currently depressed
- **reviewing GMC data:** of the 201 doctors under GMC supervision at 31 December 2000, 199 were for alcohol, drug, and mental health related problems (GMC, March 2002)
- **analysing data from the BMA counselling service:** calls taken between January 2001 and January 2002 were analysed. Approximately 35% of the health-related calls are about depression and stress.

Burnout

Burnout is the end-stage of excessive stress. The stress can be intense, prolonged, or both. As the stress increases, productivity increases until it peaks. Beyond this, further loading on the individual leads to decreased performance (bell-shaped curve). It is characterized by four stages: overwork, frustration, resentment and depression. Christina Maslach, an American psychologist, drew up a scoring system to screen for burnout. She looked for features of:
- fatigue
- depersonalization (withdrawal from relationships; seeing people as problems/tasks)
- reduced levels of achievement

What factors may contribute to burn-out?
Intrinsic factors. A competitive, type A personality who is driven to constantly maintain high personal standards and may be reluctant to delegate work to others for fear of failure. Also displays a lack of external interests, for example, may have few hobbies.

Extrinsic factors. High patient expectation coupled with increasing litigation and patient complaints (increasing consumerism). Politically enforced changes: isolated (single-handed) practice, especially in areas where there are difficulties in recruiting and retaining doctors (inner city); the demands of the new contract; the high rate of change in the way doctors work, e.g. being inspected for QandO points by the PCT, which may be perceived as a loss of autonomy. Having conflict within the practice. Long working hours, including out-of-hours cover; lack of variety and little challenge (GPwSIs and those with diplomas and the MRCGP are less likely to suffer burnout).

Personal factors. Disenchantment with career; competing demands from family; difficulty maintaining a work/home balance.

What measures would you take to prevent burn-out?
Maintain a good work/home balance.
- *Work:* a varied work environment; good relationships, delegation; prioritization; support network (young principles group; Balint group; mentors). Work smart, not hard!
- *Home:* regular holidays; sport; hobbies; friends.

If your trainer asks you about treating respiratory secretions at the end of life, see http://cks.library.nhs.uk/palliative_cancer_care_secretions/view_whole_topic_review

If your trainer asks you about the guidance you consulted in making decisions about withholding treatments at the end of life, see: **GMC (2002)** *Withholding and Withdrawing Life-prolonging Treatments: Good Practice in Decision-making* http://www.gmc-uk.org/guidance/current/library/witholding_lifeprolonging_guidance.asp

Artificial nutrition and hydration

Where death is imminent, in judging the benefits, burdens or risks, it usually would not be appropriate to start either artificial hydration or nutrition, although artificial hydration provided by the less invasive measures may be appropriate where it is considered that this would be likely to provide symptom relief.

Where death is imminent and artificial hydration and/or nutrition are already in use, it may be appropriate to withdraw them if it is considered that the burdens outweigh the possible benefits to the patient.

Where death is not imminent, it will usually be appropriate to provide artificial nutrition or hydration. However, circumstances may arise where you judge that a patient's condition is so severe, and the prognosis so poor that providing artificial nutrition or hydration may cause suffering, or be too burdensome in relation to the possible benefits. In these circumstances, as well as consulting the health care team and those close to the patient, you must seek a second or expert opinion from a senior clinician (who might be from another discipline such as nursing) who has experience of the patient's condition and who is not already directly involved in the patient's care. This will ensure that, in a decision of such sensitivity, the patient's interests have been thoroughly considered, and will provide necessary reassurance to those close to the patient and to the wider public.

Relevant literature

Berne E (1964) *Games People Play*. Penguin, Harmondsworth.
Cunningham GM (1994) A treatment program for physicians impaired by alcohol and other drugs. *Ann R Coll Physicians Surg Can*, **27**: 219–221.
Graske J (2003) Improving the mental health of doctors. *BMJ Career Focus*, **327**: s188–s188.
Neighbour, R (2006) *The Inner Consultation*. Radcliffe Publishing, Oxford. See page 213 for helpful discussions.
Newbury-Birch D, Lowry RJ, Kamali F (2002) The changing patterns of drinking, illicit drug use, stress, anxiety and depression in dental students in a UK dental school: a longitudinal study. *British Dental Journal*, **192**: 646–649.

Teenagers and confidentiality

Case summary

15 year old patient TT attended the practice Young Person's Clinic (YPC) complaining of a wart on his penis. It transpires that he is having a relationship with his 32-year-old female teacher. I gave TT the option of treating the wart in YPC or at the Genito-Urinary Medicine (GUM) clinic. He chose to be treated at the GUM, where he would also get screening for further STDs and contact tracing.

I did some health promotion and took time to create a relationship with TT so that he would feel comfortable in consulting me again. However, early in the consultation, I informed TT that I am obliged to pass on any information that he volunteers if I strongly believe that he is at risk, i.e. I am obliged to contact social services if I felt he was being abused or coerced. During our discussion, I felt that TT is in a consensual adult relationship.

TT did not want to be referred; he left the consultation with GUM's contact details. I advised him to see me if he had difficulty accessing an appointment but I did not make any formal arrangements for follow-up.

Opening question:

What issues or challenges does this case raise for you, the trainee?
- If I inform the police or TT's school that a 32-year-old teacher is sleeping with her 15-year-old student, I will break the duty of confidentiality I owe to TT.

In this case, the trainer may decide to focus predominantly on two domains:
- **making diagnoses and decisions** – having a conscious, structured approach to decision making
- **community orientation** – to reconcile the health needs of individual patients and the health needs of the community in which they live, balancing these with available resources

To achieve sufficient depth of questioning in the above domains, the trainer may prepare the following questions:
- what were you particularly worried about in this case?
- what were your treatment options?
- which one did you choose? Why did you choose this option?
- did you consider the implications of your decision for the practice and for society?
- did you use any frameworks or models to help justify your decision?
- did you make the GUM appointment for TT or did you give him the GUM contact details? Do you have an approach to prioritizing referrals to GUM?

What were you particularly worried about in this case?
The consultation with TT presented me with an ethical and medico-legal dilemma. The conflicting issues here are:
- the patient's autonomy (the right to have sex with a consenting partner) versus beneficence (the doctor should be acting in the best interests of an underage and vulnerable child)
- the duty of confidentiality owed to the patient versus breaking confidentiality to preserve the public interest in protecting the vulnerable

Young people can legally consent to heterosexual and homosexual sex from the age of 16 years (Sexual Offences Amendment Act, 2000). However, one in four women and one in three men say they had sexual intercourse before the age of 16. The legal position does not mirror the social reality.
- In the above case, a sexual relationship between a 15 year old and a 32 year old is illegal because the minor is below the age of consent.
- In addition, the relationship between teacher and student is based on trust (similar to a relationship between a doctor and his patient). Turning a professional relationship into a sexual relationship violates the trust within the relationship. Even if both parties were consenting, the sexual relationship between teachers and their students can never be considered truly mutual and based on an equal footing; it would always be viewed to some extent as an abuse of the teacher's position of trust.
- If I maintain the patient's confidentiality, am I colluding with the teacher who is abusing her position of power and trust?
- If I break the patient's confidentiality, am I sending out a message to teenagers that doctors cannot be trusted to maintain their confidentiality? This message discourages teenagers from seeking medical advice, puts them at risk of teenage pregnancy and sexually transmitted disease, and discourages vulnerable patients from seeking support in the future. The trust within the patient–doctor relationship is lost.

What were your treatment options?
I had several options, each having implications.

Refer to GUM clinic
Advantages: the wart will be treated and screening for other sexually transmitted diseases will be offered. I would transfer responsibility for the ethical dilemma to clinicians who are better trained to deal with these issues – a better service is offered. The trust within the GP–patient relationship is maintained.

Disadvantages: transferring responsibility to the GUM clinic may be seen as 'passing the buck' or as a 'collusion of anonymity' (Balint, 1957). TT may feel daunted and stigmatized by the prospect of going to a GUM clinic. There may be practical difficulties in accessing the GUM clinic – it may be a bus-ride away.

Treat the wart without addressing the ethical issues
Advantages: TT's expectations of the consultation are met. I am seen as

approachable and non-judgmental and TT may feel more comfortable in returning to see me to discuss other sensitive issues. Doctor–patient trust is maintained.

Disadvantages: I am seen as potentially colluding with the teacher who is abusing her position of trust and breaking the law. I am possibly not fulfilling my moral and professional duty to society in protecting the interests of the socially vulnerable.

Treat the wart and advise TT to consider the legal and moral aspects of his behaviour
Advantages: I could assess whether TT, the minor, is being coerced within the relationship – if coercion (i.e. rape or sexual abuse) is occurring, then Child Protection procedures need to be followed. Social services need to be contacted.

If coercion is not occurring, is the minor competent – does TT understand the consequences of his actions? Does he understand that society has rules against teacher–student relationships to protect the student from being taken advantage of? By informing him of the wider implications of his actions, he can then decide on the moral course of action for himself – I am furthering his autonomy.

I could make a reasonable effort to persuade him against having a relationship (especially one that has already harmed his health) but I would reassure him that I would not break his confidentiality by approaching the school or his parents. I would stress that my door is always open and that he may return to discuss the issue further at a later date. I have respected his autonomy, I have maintained my doctor–patient relationship and I have not broken confidentiality, thus presenting general practice as a teenage-friendly service.

Disadvantages: by placing such emphasis on respecting the patient's autonomy, I could be accused of allowing a system of abuse to go unchallenged. My decision to keep quiet could be construed as not wanting to getting involved and not wanting to make waves.

Treat the wart and contact my medical defence union
Advantages: I would act once I have been advised about the correct medico-legal course of action.

Disadvantages: it may be difficult to contact TT once he has left the surgery and I may have missed my opportunity to act.

Treat the wart and inform social services/ TT's school/ his parents
Advantages: I would be discharging my responsibility to society by informing the relevant agencies so that an investigation of the teacher's alleged misconduct can occur.

Disadvantages: I have breached confidentiality and potentially damaged my relationship of trust with my patient. If TT's allegations were factually incorrect, I could potentially damage a teacher's position within her school and community and possibly blight her career. I would also send a message to young people that I would not always respect their confidentiality. Various surveys have estimated that at least 25% of teenagers do not believe that their consultation will be confidential.

Teenagers will be less likely to consult and this may have an adverse effect on teenage pregnancy and STD rates. Breaching confidentiality to stop potential abuse may have resulted in greater harm to teenage health in the long run.

Which option did you choose? Why did you choose this option?
In a case like this, I feel there is no morally right answer. I chose to:
- give TT the option of treating the wart in surgery or at the GUM clinic
- offer him screening for further STDs
- offer contact tracing
- inform him early in the consultation that I am obliged to pass on any information that he volunteers if I strongly believe that he is at risk, i.e. I am obliged to contact social services if I felt he was being abused or coerced. This informs TT of my legal and ethical responsibility and advises him that confidentiality can be broken under certain circumstances. If he then chooses to disclose information, he is aware that the information may be passed on.
- because I believed that he is in a consensual adult relationship, I advised him about his sexual health, his teacher's professional and legal obligations and asked him to pursue a course that he is morally comfortable with
- I contacted my medical defence union after the consultation and considered their advice
- because I felt this was not a Child Protection issue, I did not breach confidentiality because:
  - I thought I should respect the competent teenager's autonomy
  - I wanted to maintain a trusting doctor–patient relationship so that he would feel comfortable in consulting me at a future date.
  - I want to send out a message to other teenagers that I am a GP that can be trusted to respect their confidences and who will put their needs first. This will make me more effective in dealing with the issues of teenage pregnancy and the growing epidemic of teenage STDs.

Did you consider the implications of your decision for the practice and for society?
I have already discussed most of the implications (see above under implications of treatment options). In addition:
- hopefully, TT and other teenagers will continue to consult our practice, giving us the opportunity to provide family planning and sexual health advice. Refusal to supply contraception and provide sexual health treatment to minors is unlikely to deter those who want sexual intercourse. On this basis, a GP practice like ours that provides family planning and sexual health services to teenagers, with or without parental consent, is performing a duty to society.
- on the other hand, parents have a right to know what is happening to their children. Therefore, it serves society's interests for our practice to encourage teenagers, without breaking their confidentiality, to disclose their relationships and medical needs to their parents.

Did you use any framework or model to help justify your decision?

I used Simpson's (2004) decision-making model, which derives from a business model. This model breaks decision-making into eight stages.

- *Recognize the dilemma* – many of the problems require GPs to balance conflicting issues, for example, demand versus resources available, doing good as opposed to harm, the needs of the individual versus the needs of society.
- *Identify possible options and solutions* – understand the issues including the advantages and disadvantages of each solution.
- *Recognize the implications of these options* – each option carries its own potential consequences.
- *Prioritize and weigh each option.*
- *Choose an option* – make a plan of action.
- *Justify choice* – ensure that the plan of action is based on sound ethical and evidence-based reasoning.
- *Check that the option works and does not need further modification or reassessment* – be able to construct an evaluation plan that tells you, say in six months, that you have made the correct decision.
- *Reflect on what has been learnt from the experience.*

Did you make the GUM appointment for TT or did you give him the GUM contact details? Do you have an approach to prioritizing referrals to GUM?

I gave TT the GUM contact details because people with contagious diseases can self-refer. If I had called on his behalf, I would have passed on the same information as TT would give, and the health advisor making the appointment would not have prioritized differently.

There are advantages to me making the appointment: TT leaves the consultation with a definite GUM appointment and I have consciously delegated care. There are disadvantages to me making the appointment: it reduces TT's responsibility; it does not change his health-seeking behaviour; and we could have spent the limited time we had making the GUM appointment instead of addressing other important issues within the consultation. If TT makes the appointment himself, he can negotiate a time convenient to his schedule, which makes him more likely to attend.

It is important to prioritize referrals so that people with minor conditions, for example, those requesting pre-relationship STD screening, do not compromise the care of those with more serious conditions, such as PID. My approach to prioritizing depends on the service to which I refer. Patients with contagious diseases can usually self-refer to GUM and are prioritized in the same way as a GP referral. Patients who do not have contagious diseases, for example, those seeking treatment for dysparunia or impotence, need GP referral.

Some departments ask for GPs to prioritize the appointments. For example, GPs, using national or local guidelines, book two-week-wait appointments directly with the hospital. Other departments inform GPs, either by circular or on their website, what they consider to be:

- urgent/priority 1/(P1), e.g. acute PID
- semi-urgent/priority 2/(P2), e.g. genital warts
- routine/priority 3/(P3), e.g. STD screening.

In such cases, the GP referral letter, or the patient if they self-refer, needs to provide the clinical and social history needed to for the hospital staff to prioritize efficiently.

The medical defence union contacted for advice in the preparation of this case, advised that there is no right or wrong course of action; each case needs to be considered individually. Doctors are advised to contact their defence union if such a situation does arise to discuss the particulars of their case.

Additional information

If you had decided to inform the school or the police about the teacher's relationship with TT, you would have breached his confidentiality. Under what circumstances can confidentiality be breached?
The GMC does provide guidance about the disclosure of patient information, and their ethical standards largely reflect the legal standards. Exceptions to the duty of confidence exist in six main areas.

- **Consent:** the patient consents to the disclosure of information. Consent implies more than agreement, and takes into account competence, understanding and voluntary participation. Consent can be expressed (explicit) or implied (implicit). Implied consent means that the patient is aware of the practice of disclosure and has the option of opting out, as in HIV testing of pregnant women.
- **Public interest:** the public interest in maintaining confidence needs to be weighed up, or balanced, with the countervailing public interest favoring disclosure, such as protecting the public purse from people trying to defraud the health service, or protecting the public from dangerous people, such as psychotics wielding a knife or HIV-infected patients knowingly having unprotected sex with partners who are unaware of their HIV status.
- **Teaching, research and clinical audit:** patients have a choice (expressed as consent) in participating in research and medical student training. Research benefits society. The rights of patients not wanting to participate in research, such as inclusion within cancer registries, needed to be weighed against the necessity of medical research and its benefit to society – individual personal interest versus public interest.
- **Management and NHS administrative purposes:** there is a public interest in spending public money efficiently in the NHS, and financial auditors need access to some patient information to monitor NHS spending. The National Health Service Act 1977 provides the statutory backing for financial auditors to access patient information.
- **Genetics:** the information obtained from the genetic testing of an individual has consequences not only for that individual, but also for other family

members. The duty to the individual has to be balanced with a duty to other family members, and the possible impact of the genetic information on their health decisions (particularly with regard to exercising reproductive choice, or entering screening programmes).

- **Under particular statutes:**
  - The Abortion Regulations 1999
  - Public Health (Control of Disease) Act 1984
  - National Health Service (Venereal Diseases) Regulations 1974
  - Police and Criminal Evidence Act 1984
  - Health Act 1999
  - Health Service Commissioner Act 1993

Regarding the assessment of 'community orientation' in the above case, the GP trainer may go on to ask you *do you think that STD screening should be done in primary care; surely prevention is better than cure?*

Let us consider the issues raised by *Screening for Chlamydia in Primary Care – to screen or not to screen?* The issue could be analysed using Wilson's criteria for screening. Wilson's (1966) criteria define the requirements of a robust screening programme:

1. The condition being screened for must be:
   - Common: the national screening pilot found that
     - 14% of under 16 year olds
     - 11% of 16–19 year olds and
     - 7% of 20–24 year olds were infected.

Chlamydia is the commonest curable STD in the UK. The natural history of the disease should be known – chlamydia is a sexually transmitted, intracellular, gram-negative infection affecting the genital tract. 70% of infected women and 50% of infected men are asymptomatic (Chief Medical Officer's Report, 2004). Infection may result in severe complications.

   - Important: the complications of chlamydia are pelvic inflammatory disease, tubal infertility and ectopic pregnancies. 10–30% of infected women develop PID.
   - Diagnosed by acceptable methods: chlamydia can be diagnosed by two methods:
     - ELISA testing of endocervical +/– urethral swabs. These need to be taken by clinicians. Women find attending a Family Planning clinic less stigmatizing than attending a Genito-urinary medicine clinic.
     - Polymerase Chain Reaction (PCR) or Ligase Chain Reaction (LCR) on a sample of urine, a vaginal swab or a urethral swab. Studies show that urine sampling is more acceptable than self-taken swabs.

2. There must be a latent interval in which effective interventional treatment is possible. Screening in the USA has led to a 56% reduction in PID. A Swedish study in 1998 showed that ectopic pregnancies in 20–24 year olds were more likely to be associated with recent chlamydia infection. Therefore, screening for chlaymidia and treating it will reduce the incidence of PID and ectopics.

3. Screening must be:

- Cost-effective: the annual cost of chlamydia and its consequences in the UK are estimated to be more than £100 million. Studies from the USA and Sweden have shown that screening for chlamydia is cost-effective (Chief Medical Officer's Report, 2004). Screening can be performed at the time of doing a smear, doing a termination, or seeking gynaecological treatment thus reducing consultation rates. Postal screening will cost £21 per screening test and £38 per case identified.
- Continuous: the Chief Medical Officer's Report recommends opportunistic (as opposed to continuous) screening – the current programme is focussing on high risk groups, e.g. women under 25 years, those seeking termination and prior to insertion of IUDs. There is evidence from the countries which have introduced chlamydia screening that targeted screening of at-risk populations can reduce morbidity.
- Non-invasive and safe: screening is non-invasive and safe.
- Repeatable: it is relatively easy and cheap to repeat the test to confirm the diagnosis.
- Acceptable to patients: urine testing is largely far more acceptable than self-taken urethral or vaginal swabs.
- Highly sensitive (have few false negatives) and highly specific (have few false positives): For LCR, sensitivity is 90% versus 65% for ELISA. Liam Donaldson (CMO) highlighted the clinical governance issue of continuing to use suboptimal tests.
- Easy to interpret: PCR and LCR are relatively easy to interpret. Joint work with the Ministry of Defence intends to develop near patient testing (called NPTgold) which will give a result within one hour of testing.

What does the research show about screening for STDs in primary care?
From **Donym** S (2004) Sexual health entering primary care: is prevention better than cure? *The Journal of Family Planning and Reproductive Healthcare*, **30**: 267.

Over 10% of screening in the pilot programme was done in primary care. However, this depended on the goodwill of GPs. The new GMS contract does provide opportunities to remunerate GPs for opportunistic screening. However, there is debate as to whether sexual health services should be classified as 'essential' or 'enhanced'. Many GPs will argue that it is an enhanced service to ensure that they get paid for providing it. The paymasters will argue against this to contain costs. The obstacles to introducing chlamydia screening into primary care include:
- a lack of resources
- a lack of time
- the issues of contact tracing and partner notification
- the acceptability of the GP based service to patients. Patients may prefer the anonymity of a GUM clinic.
- if GUM clinics and GP practices both offer the service, it is in danger of becoming piecemeal and patients may 'slip through the net'. Who will take responsibility for providing the call and recall service?

Benefits of screening

Screening tests are relatively inexpensive when compared with the treatment of chronic disease or major operations.

A healthy person is screened – disease is picked up at a very early stage when effective, less invasive and life-saving intervention can be offered. Resources are invested to improve the health of the population as a whole – the service is proactive rather than reactive.

Harms of screening

The total expense of all screening programmes in the UK is considerable (£500 million per annum in 1995 according to Bandolier). A healthy person is invited to be screened – a test that has false positives causes anxiety in a healthy, asymptomatic person who, following the screening test, may be subjected to more invasive definitive testing.

Resources are limited – are screening programmes cost effective? Would it not be better to invest the money in treating symptomatic patients, such as stroke patients for example?

From **McNulty CAM, Freeman E** (2004) Barriers to opportunistic chlamydia testing in primary care. *British Journal of General Practice*, **54**: 508–514.

This qualitative study based in Herefordshire, Gloucestershire and Avon identified the greatest barriers to opportunistic chlamydia testing and screening in general practice as lack of knowledge of the benefits of testing, when and how to take specimens, lack of time, worries about discussing sexual health, and lack of guidance. Staff felt that any increased testing should be accompanied by clear, concise primary care trust guidance on when and how to test, including how to obtain informed consent and perform contact tracing. The study concluded that efforts to increase chlamydia screening in GP practices should be accompanied by clear guidance and education. Genito-urinary medicine clinics will need to be increased in parallel with testing in primary care to provide appropriate contact tracing and follow-up.

Relevant literature

Balint M (1957) *The Doctor, the Patient and the Illness*. Pitman, London.

General Medical Council (2000) *Protecting and Providing Information*. BMA, London. See paragraphs 34 and 35.

Mason JK (2000) The legal aspects and implications of risk assessment. *Medical Law Review*, **8(69)**: 106–116.

Neuberger J (2001) The educated patient: new challenges for the medical profession. *Journal of Internal Medicine*, **249**: 41–45.

Oakeshott P, Hay P, Pakianathan M (2004) Chlamydia screening in primary care. *British Journal of General Practice*, **54**: 491–493.

Sculpher et al. (2002) Shared treatment decision making in a collectively funded health care system: possible conflicts and some potential solutions. *Social Science and Medicine*, **54**: 1369–1377.

Simpson RG (2004) Preparing for the oral module. *The Practitioner*, **248**: 287–289.

Wareham NJ Griffin SJ (2001) Should we screen for type 2 diabetes? Evaluation against National Screening Committee criteria. *BMJ,* **322:** 986–988.

Wilson JMG and Jungner G (1966) *Principles and Practice of Screening for Disease.* WHO.

For a patient leaflet on genital warts, see: http://www.fpa.org.uk/attachments/published/146/PDF%20Genital%20warts%20October%202006.pdf

If the GP trainer had questioned you on the evidence base for the treatment of genital warts, refer to page 4: http://www.jr2.ox.ac.uk/bandolier/painres/download/Bando082.pdf

For the DoH (2004) report – The first steps: annual report for the National Screening Programme in England 2003 – 2004, see http://www.dh.gov.uk/assetRoot/04/09/30/91/04093091.pdf

For information on patient confidentiality, see DoH. (2001). The Health and Social Care Act 2001: Section 60 and 61. Background information.

Breast cancer reported for Significant Event Analysis

Case summary

Mrs FM, age 36, presented on 5 January with a two-day history of a left-sided breast lump, which she had noticed following an insect bite on the breast. She had made the appointment the previous day and had waited one day to see a female GP.

When examined, a discrete one-centimetre, hard lump was found in the 2 o'clock position of the left breast. There were no skin or nipple changes. There was no axillary lymphadenopathy. The right breast was entirely normal.

The Two Week Wait Clinic was contacted while the patient was still in surgery. An appointment at an outlying hospital was offered. The patient was happy to travel to this venue. If Mrs FM had not been happy with this venue, the appointments clerk would have offered her an appointment at the main hospital but this would have been at a later date.

The referral letter was faxed to the Two Week Wait appointment desk. However, there is no practice administration record of when it was faxed or who faxed it. Mrs FM was seen at the Breast Clinic on 10 January, eight days after discovering the lump. A fine needle aspiration biopsy showed invasive ductal carcinoma. Mrs FM was given the telephone number of the breast sister at the main branch of the hospital to contact for further information and support. Surgery was scheduled for 26 January.

Opening question:

What issues or challenges does this case raise for you, the trainee?

- My concerns are writing up and presenting this case at the practice Significant Event Analysis (SEA) meeting. I haven't presented at an SEA meeting before.

In this case, the trainer may decide to focus predominantly on two domains:

- **making diagnoses and decisions:** to selectively gather and interpret information from history-taking, physical examination and investigations; to intervene urgently when necessary; to manage conditions which may present early and in an undifferentiated way
- **primary care administration:** using information systems to effectively co-ordinate care, and to facilitate continuing learning and quality improvement

To achieve sufficient depth of questioning in the above domains, the trainer may prepare the following questions:

- which bits of the history and examination helped you to come to your final diagnosis?

- did you use any tools, guidelines or online information to help you?
- what were your treatment options? Which one did you choose? Why?
- do you think the information in your referral letter is adequate?
- what have you chosen to discuss at the SEA? Why have you selected these issues?

Which bits of the history and examination helped you to come to your final diagnosis?

History
Mrs FH has a few risk factors for breast cancer, namely:
- she is a woman
- she has not borne a child after the age of 30 – her daughter is 9
- she breastfed her daughter for three weeks; breastfeeding is protective
- she used combined oral contraception, which is a risk factor, from age 17 to 35

On the other hand, she does not have some of the risk factors for breast cancer, namely:
- her age – the risk increases with age: only 5% of cases present before age 40 and 2% before age 35
- she does not have a past history of breast cancer
- she does not have a significant family history of breast cancer or *BRCA1* or *BRCA2* genes
- she has not had radiation to the chest
- her alcohol intake is minimal

Examination
There were some features on examination to suggest breast cancer, namely:
- she had a discrete lump – 90% of women present with a lump
- the lump was hard, not cystic
- the overlying skin was affected – was this really an insect bite? Faye had not seen the insect bite her; she assumed an insect caused the skin changes. Skin ulceration, distortion or nodules are highly suggestive of cancer.
- the lump was in the 2 o'clock position – 45% of breast cancers are found in the upper outer quadrant

On the other hand, there were some reassuring features on examination, namely:
- there were no nipple changes, discharge or tenderness
- there were no palpable regional lymph nodes

I was suspicious of breast cancer because this 36 year old woman had a discrete, hard lump in the upper, outer quadrant.

Did you use any tools, guidelines or on-line information to help you?

I used *Referral Guidelines for Suspected Cancer* (NICE, 2005), which state that in a woman aged 30 years and older with a discrete lump that persists after her next period, or presents after menopause, an *urgent* referral should be made.

What were your treatment options? Which one did you chose? Why?

I could have:

- waited three weeks to see if the lump 'persists after her next period' before referring, as per the NICE guidelines
- I could have sought a second opinion from a colleague, that is, taken advice before making a decision
- I could have referred immediately, which I did, on a hunch

I am hard pressed to explain why I referred on a hunch. My referral was not triggered by past experience – I have not worked for a breast consultant and this is the first breast cancer I picked up in primary care. Referring on a hunch that something is wrong does not sound scientific. However, intuition or the 'art' of medicine has been the subject of much medical writing.

Greenhalgh (1999) wrote about the 'science' and 'art' of medicine. When I reflected on this case, I used her model of the communication between the doctor and patient, which she calls the 'diagnostic text' to analyse my reasoning. The diagnostic text has four secondary texts.

- The experiential text – the meaning the patient assigns to the various symptoms, deliberations, and lay consultations in the run up to the clinical encounter. This, to me, sounds like the patient's ideas. What were Mrs FM's ideas about her breast lump? Mrs FM was worried about breast cancer because 'it's in all the magazines' but she thought she was too young, so she hoped that the lump was the result of an insect bite
- The narrative text – what the doctor interprets to be 'the problem' from the story the patient tells – the traditional medical history. I thought this was a two-day history of lump in the left breast, perhaps with skin induration secondary to an insect bite.
- The physical or perceptual text – what the doctor gleans from the physical examination of the patient (using the ill-defined but recognizable set of skills that have been called 'practical reason'). The physical exam confirmed a hard lump in the left breast with some skin changes, but these were not typical of cellulitis or induration. In exploring the perceptual text, Greenhalgh describes:
  - comparing the patient's presenting illness script with the thousands of illness scripts for the same condition
  - feeling or perceiving that something in this patient's script does not fit. For example, an insect bite to the breast in the middle of the UK winter struck me as odd.
  - perhaps this dissonance is the hunch or 'art of medicine'

- The instrumental text – what the blood tests and X-rays 'say'. I had to refer the patient to breast clinic to get these texts. The fine needle aspiration biopsy confirmed cancer.

This experience does not encourage me to reject evidence-based guidelines in favour of anecdotal practice. Instead, I think that sound clinical judgment combines:

- the patient's individual and cultural perspective
- the doctor's own case-based experience
- the results of rigorous research

Do you think the information in your referral letter is adequate?
My referral letter:

- is dated
- contains the patient's administrative details
- clearly spells out the reason for the referral
- gives details of the examination I carried out
- includes relevant psychosocial details
- provides a list of drugs prescribed

The above criteria are drawn from the RCGP (Scotland) revalidation toolkit, which advises GPs to audit ten of their referral letters with respect to the above criteria. I learnt from the last practice audit on referral letters that I sometimes forget to include the findings of my examination. I was pleased to have included my findings in this letter. By the time the patient was seen in hospital, the skin appearance or regional lymphadenopathy might have changed. The changes may give valuable clinical detail.

What have you chosen to discuss at the SEA? Why have you selected these issues?
I have chosen to discuss this case as an example of positive practice and to highlight procedures that worked well. For example:

- our appointments system is working – the receptionists were able to give Mrs FM an appointment within 48 hours.
- the doctor was able to call the hospital to arrange an appointment while the patient was in surgery. If the surgery was overbooked, or if the practice did not have a robust system for storing important telephone numbers, then it would have been difficult to make these arrangements.
- the referral letter was typed and faxed on the day of the patient's presentation. Administrative support and prioritization was good.

I selected these issues because:

- it is as important for the PHCT to learn from positive incidents as well as adverse events
- research shows that SEA is effective because it uses emotional engagement to consolidate improvements in patient care. Diagnosing cancer in a 36 year old patient is an emotional experience – people are more likely to remember and learn from emotional experiences

This case gives us the opportunity to reflect on how important it is to have:

- an organized appointments system
- well trained receptionists
- clinics with minimal interruption
- good administrative support
- good communication with the local hospital
- cancer referral guidelines on desk-tops.

In addition, I also wanted the opportunity to discuss with the PHCT the lesson I learnt about combining the 'science' with the 'art' of medicine – the need to listen to our patients and heed our gut instincts.

Additional information

Significant event auditing

- SEA covers positive practice, adverse events and critical incidents. Some significant events are adverse events – when something has clearly gone wrong, such as a prescribing error or administering the incorrect vaccination. The team needs to establish what happened, what was preventable and how to respond.
- A critical incident is a half-way house – an event that may indicate sub-standard care, but which might also occur by chance, such as an allergic reaction to a drug or a teenage pregnancy. Critical incidents are theoretically avoidable and possible pointers to deficiencies in care.
- SEA needs a blame-free culture – it needs a willingness to honestly acknowledge genuine mistakes, reflect on them and improve practice, so reducing the potential for mistakes in the future.
- SEA is not an appropriate technique in cases where legal action is anticipated or where individual incompetence is suspected.
- As the aim is to be supportive of colleagues, feedback should be constructive, and should explore possible alternatives for the future. This links it to evidence-based practice, and the adoption of guidelines and best practice.

From **Westcott R** *et al.* (2000) Significant event audit in practice: a preliminary study. *Family Practice*, **17**: 173–179.

The aim of the study was to identify participants' perceptions of the benefits and problems associated with SEA in the context of primary care, and to derive suggestions which might improve the process of SEA. The study concluded that SEA is a powerful tool, which contributes to teambuilding, enhanced communication, and improvement in patient care. However, its implementation requires sensitive handling for optimal benefit, and to minimize difficulties.

Relevant literature

Greenhalgh T (1999) Narrative based medicine in an evidence based world. *BMJ*, **318:** 323–325.

NICE (2005) *Cancer Referral Guidelines:* http://www.nice.org.uk/pdf/cg027nice guideline.pdf

Auditing referral letters: http://www.rcgp.org.uk/pdf/Complete%20Revalidation%20Tool kit%20(Read%20Only)%20PDF.pdf

Breast lumps and breast examination: http://www.patient.co.uk/showdoc/40000260/

Clinical Governance and SEA: http://www.cgsupport.nhs.uk/Case_Study_Downloads/ Word/Primary_Care/Langbaurgh%20PCG.doc

Consultation models

This brief overview of the common consultation models is based on *The Consultation* by Pendleton *et al.* (2000).

What is a medical consultation?

The consultation is the medium through which medicine is frequently practised – it is the encounter between the patient and the doctor. Some encounters are satisfactory to both the patient and the doctor; others are unsatisfactory and dysfunctional to one or both parties. Researchers have studied these encounters from various perspectives:

- The medical perspective – this is concerned with diseases and diagnosis. The underlying assumption of the medical perspective is that illness and disease can be explained by changes to the structure or functioning of the body (pathophysiology). However, this rigorous scientific approach is limited – patients are not broken-down machines.
- The holistic perspective – this is concerned with placing the illness experience in physical, psychological and social contexts. The underlying assumption of the social perspective is that the understanding the patient has of what is happening to him as well as his emotional response to his illness define and determine the problem and its management. However, a danger with this model is that responsibility for the illness may be transferred to the doctor – the medicalisation of health.

In summary, 'disease' is the cause of sickness in terms of pathophysiology, whilst 'illness' is the patient's unique experience of sickness.

This chapter intends to present a brief overview of various consultation models. It will:

- describe the model
- discuss the assumptions made by the model
- discuss evidence (if any) to support or refute these assumptions
- discuss how the model has contributed to our understanding of the GP consultation.

The biomedical approach

Description

Take an accurate and relevant history – observation
Perform an accurate and relevant examination – observation
Make a provisional diagnosis – hypothesis
Order and interpret the results of appropriate investigations – hypothesis testing
Make a definitive diagnosis – deduction

Assumptions made
- Every illness is caused by a definable agent (Robert Koch's postulate).
- Once the diagnosis is made in terms of this definable agent, a rational treatment is applied.

Evidence

Hampton *et al.* (1975) studied 80 patients and found that taking a good history made the diagnosis in 66 patients. Physical examination was useful in 7 patients; investigations were useful in 7 patients. The biomedical model places too much emphasis on examination and investigation.

Elstein *et al.* (1978) showed that clinicians do not follow the model in a step-wise manner – they generate hypotheses early on in the consultation and direct the consultation towards testing these hypotheses in turn.

Contributions

Positive
- In any single consultation the doctor may form, test and discard a large number of diagnostic hypotheses based on the information or cues he receives from the patient.
- The biomedical model proposes a rigorous scientific approach to problem-solving – such disciplined thinking has been responsible for good quality research and is the cornerstone of evidence-based medicine (EBM).

Limitations of the model
- It is reductionist – patients are seen and treated in terms of signs, symptoms and diagnoses and labelled accordingly.
- It is doctor-centred – there is no mention of the patient's feelings, beliefs, and opinions, any sharing of information or agreement of a management plan.
- The biomedical model is of limited value when an objective physical disorder cannot be diagnosed. The model may actually encourage further investigation of the patient until a 'disorder' is unearthed.
- The biomedical model de-emphasizes the contribution of non-verbal communication.
- It omits the therapeutic use of the doctor–patient relationship.
- It fails to recognize that a consultation can be one of a series, as is often the case in general practice.

More modern consultation models have developed in response to these criticisms.

The anthropological approach

Description

This model was developed from studying man's illness behaviour in different cultures.

A healing ritual consists of:
- giving the problem a name (diagnosis)
- performing a therapeutic ritual (management)
- renaming the problem as cured or improved (cure)

Patients believe healers. Society has invested the healers with authority (called Aesculapean authority) which derives from:
- the doctors' greater knowledge or expertise – sapiential authority
- the doctors' desire or motivation to do good – moral authority
- the doctors' desire to see the practice of medicine as something of a mystery – charismatic authority

Assumptions made
In the healing process, doctors and patients have roles. The patient assumes the more passive, recipient role and doctors assume the pro-active, responsive role which in turn is the source of their authority.

Evidence
The model is based on anthropological research done by Kleinman (1980), Osmond (1980) and Waitzkin and Stoekle (1972).

Contributions

Positive
- The anthropological model highlights the 'sick role' and 'healing role' adopted by patients and doctors.
- By virtue of their healing role, society invests doctors with authority.

Limitations of the model
- The anthropological model tells us about the social interaction between doctors and patients. However, the model may be criticised for dealing with the wider social context and is limited in its application to the individual context.

The transactional analysis approach

Description
The human psyche consists of three ego states (Berne, 1964):
- the parent – commands, directs, prohibits, controls, nurtures
- the adult – sorts out information and works logically
- the child – intuition, creativity, spontaneity, enjoyment

At any point, each of us is in a state of mind where we think, feel, behave, react and have attitudes as if we were a parent (critical or caring), a logical adult or a child (spontaneous or dependent).

Assumptions

- Many general practice consultations are conducted between a parental doctor and a child-like patient. This interaction is not always in the best interests of either party.
- When transactions are repeated in a predictable way, for psychological benefit, they become games. One example is the 'yes but' game in which the patient produces reasons why a suggestion will not work, thereby relinquishing responsibility for the problem.

Evidence

The transactional model was based on the work of Berne (1964).

Contributions

Positive

- The transactional analysis model makes doctors aware of their patients' attempts to transfer responsibility to them.
- It also highlights the games people play and teaches doctors to break out of these cycles of behaviour.
- This model is particularly useful in analysing why communication breaks down during a consultation.

Limitations of the model

- Analysing the consultation in terms of Berne's model may be difficult and time-consuming.
- The transactional analysis model may make the doctor suspicious of his patients' motivation – consultations may be seen in terms of manipulative games.

Balint's approach to the consultation

Description

- Psychological problems are often manifested physically and even physical disease has its own psychological consequences which need particular attention.
- Doctors have feelings and those feelings have a function in the consultation.
- Specific training is needed to change the doctor's behaviour so that he can become more sensitive to the patient.
- The 'drug doctor' is a term that describes the doctor's therapeutic contribution to the consultation. It describes the degree of efficacy of the doctor as a therapeutic intervention, as well as the doctor's unforeseen negative outcomes (side effects).
- The 'flash technique' – the doctor becomes aware of his feelings in the consultation, and when he interprets this back to the patient, the patient gains some insight into his problems.

Evidence

Michael Balint based his writing (*The Doctor, his Patient and the Illness*, 1957) on his work with groups of doctors who regularly met to discuss their 'problem' cases.

Contributions

Positive
- The Balint model highlights the importance of treating bodies and minds simultaneously. It emphasizes the contribution of psychological factors to the presenting illness.
- Doctors are seen as active participants in the consultation. In particular, doctors are encouraged to acknowledge their feelings and to feed these back to the patient so that the patient may develop insight into his problem. This is the first consultation model to stress the importance of the doctor's feelings.

Limitations of the model
- Doctors may indiscriminately feed back their feelings to all their patients – 'to Balint'.
- A great deal of emphasis is placed on intuition – this should complement, not replace, logic and reasoning.

Byrne and Long (1976)

In 1976 Byrne and Long analysed approximately 2500 consultations from 71 GPs.

Description

Byrne and Long studied the verbal behaviour of doctors. They found that the doctor's consultation had 6 phases:
1. The doctor establishes a relationship with the patient.
2. The doctor attempts to discover or actually discovers the reasons for the patient's attendance.
3. The doctor conducts a verbal or physical examination or both.
4. The doctor and/or patient consider the condition.
5. The doctor and patient agree and detail further treatment or investigation if necessary.
6. The consultation is terminated (usually by the doctor).

The doctor's consultation style ranged from doctor-centred (based only on the doctor's knowledge) to patient-centred (incorporating the patient's experience). Dysfunctional consultations occurred when the doctor failed to discover the reason for the patient's attendance (2nd phase) or because the doctor did not tailor his explanation to his patient's beliefs (4th phase).

Assumptions
- The Byrne and Long (1976) model emphasizes the contribution of verbal communication and downplays the contribution of non-verbal

communication. The criticism here is that a picture is worth a thousand words – doctors often judge the severity of a patient's chest pain not only by the words he uses to describe the pain, but also by his appearance – his breathlessness, sweating and writhing.

- The Byrne and Long (1976) model assumes that the content of the conversation is all-important. It underestimates the importance of the communication process – the tone of voice, facial expression and warmth of the doctor.

Evidence
Byrne and Long conducted field research. Their work on non-verbal communication was expanded on by Bain (1976, 1977), Coope and Metcalfe (1979), Raynes (1980), Cartwright and Anderson (1981), Tuckett (1982) and Pendleton (1983).

Contributions

Positive
- Byrne and Long's model provides a practical approach to addressing individual dysfunctional consultations.
- They recommend that doctors be taught how to discover their patients' beliefs about their problems and to tailor their explanations of illness to incorporate these beliefs.

Limitations of the model
- Verbal communication is disproportionately emphasized. Attention must also be paid to the process of communication, including non-verbal communication.

Pendleton *et al.* (2003)

In *The Consultation* (2003), Pendleton *et al.* propose a task-based approach to effective consulting. These tasks are derived from the needs of the patient, the aims of the doctor, the desired outcomes and the evidence that links them.

Description
The seven tasks of the GP consultation.
1. To understand the reasons for the patient's attendance, including:
   - the patient's problem: its nature, history, aetiology and effects
   - the patient's perspective: their personal and social circumstances; ideas and values about health; their ideas about the problem, its causes and its management; their concerns about the problem and its implications; their expectations for information, involvement and care.
2. Taking into account the patient's perspective, to achieve a shared understanding:
   - about the problem
   - about the evidence and options for management

3. To enable the patient to choose an appropriate action for each problem:
   - consider options and implications
   - choose the most appropriate course of action
4. To enable the patient to manage the problem:
   - discuss the patient's ability to take appropriate actions
   - agree doctor and patient actions and responsibilities
   - agree targets, monitoring and follow-up
5. To consider other problems:
   - not yet presented
   - continuing problems
   - at-risk factors
6. To use time appropriately:
   - in the consultation
   - in the longer term
7. To establish or maintain a relationship with the patient that helps to achieve the other tasks.

Assumptions

- The Pendleton model assumes that consulting is effective if it is patient-centred. There are two main problems with this assumption. First, how do we measure effectiveness – patient satisfaction, disease-based outcome criteria, doctor satisfaction, or fewer follow-up appointments? Secondly, does 'patient-centredness' actually improve the doctor's effectiveness?

Mead and Bower (2000) defined patient-centredness as:
1. understanding the biopsychosocial context in which the problem presents
2. appreciating the individual patient's experience of the illness
3. sharing the power within the relationship to maintain joint responsibility
4. recognizing the effect of the relationship on the illness and maximizing the benefits of the therapeutic alliance
5. recognizing the doctor as a person and appreciating the impact of the doctor as an individual on the relationship.

Evidence

The task model is based on an analysis of the relevant literature, field research and the practical experience of the authors.

Contributions

Positive
- The recommendation for each of the seven tasks is evidence-based.
- The model is easy to teach and easy to use. A doctor can analyse the effectiveness of his consulting by reviewing his consultations against the suggested criteria. He is then able to identify the reasons for the dysfunctional consultation and take steps to improve his consulting technique – the model is practical.

- By focusing on the tasks, the feelings of the patient and the doctor can be relatively neglected.
- By reducing the complex behaviour of consulting into the completion of 7 tasks, the doctor's consultation is in danger of being converted into a tick-box exercise.
- The doctor is expected to complete each task proficiently, sensitively and smoothly within the allocated time – a rather daunting task in itself!
- Doctors have a set of beliefs that underpin their core values. If their fundamental beliefs about patients and medicine do not change, it is quite likely that task-based changes to their consulting behaviour will remain superficial and short-lived.

Neighbour (1987)

In *The Inner Consultation* (1987), Neighbour proposed that there are five important checkpoints along the consultation journey.

Description
The five checkpoints are:
- connecting
- summarizing
- handing over
- safety netting
- housekeeping

Connecting refers to establishing and maintaining a non-threatening relationship with the patient to achieve a level of rapport.

Summarizing refers to taking a comprehensive history and reflecting this back to the patient. This ensures that both doctor and patient have reached a common, shared understanding of the presenting complaint – the physical problem as well as the patient's ideas, concerns and expectations of the illness and its management.

Handing over refers to the transfer of responsibility for management back to the patient. The doctor and the patient may well have different objectives for the consultation; the negotiation and handing over the consultation may involve some degree of compromise on both sides.

Safety netting refers to providing the patient with information on what to expect and what to do if they do not improve. General practice has been described as the art of managing the uncertain and provision needs to be made within the consultation for this. Patients will feel more secure if they have a clear outline of what to expect from their treatment and under what circumstances to re-consult.

Housekeeping refers to the doctor attending his own feelings, particularly those brought about by a consultation. If the emotions engendered by the consultation are not acknowledged and dealt with, they may spill over into the next.

Sometimes, acknowledging these concerns may be all that is required. Occasionally, the doctor needs to reflect on a consultation and possibly consider how to handle things differently in the future. In this way, the doctor learns from his practice.

Assumptions

The Neighbour model assumes that through good communication, it is possible for the doctor and patient to reach a shared understanding of the presenting problem. The counter argument is that you can bring a horse to water but you can't make it drink. Reaching a shared understanding is a two way process – the patient must have some understanding, insight and a willingness to modify his health beliefs. It is the doctor's responsibility to enter into the negotiation and to do so in language the patient understands. However, the overall responsibility for reaching a 'shared understanding' cannot be the doctor's alone. To assume sole responsibility invites 'medicalisation' of social problems.

Evidence

The Neighbour model is a theory on consultation and communication based on the practical experience of the author and informed by his reading of the medical, educational and philosophical literature.

Contributions

Positive

Other consultation models have already discussed ways of integrating the medical and holistic perspectives. Neighbour introduced the concepts of safety netting and housekeeping. Housekeeping is built on Balint's concept of the doctor's emotions having a useful purpose in the consultation. Where Balint advised doctors to reflect these feelings back to their patients to develop the patients' insight into the problem, Neighbour advises doctors to reflect on their feelings to develop their own insight into their strengths and weaknesses as doctors. By developing self-awareness, doctors can improve as clinicians – they can, in the words of Neighbour, 'develop an effective and intuitive learning style'.

Limitations of the model
- When safety netting, doctors are in danger of slipping into a prescriptive consultation style if they assume a parent–child approach.
- Sometimes, because of the doctor's fears and insecurities over medico-legal concerns, safety netting transforms from a tool to manage uncertainty into a technique for practising defensive medicine.

Learning points

For doctors to consult effectively, they need the requisite 'tools of the trade':
- Personal qualities: clinical ability, warmth, *caritas*, empathy
- Skills: active listening, negotiating, influencing, explaining
- Attitudes: self-awareness, flexibility, an appreciation of diversity

In addition, GPs must want to do their best for their patients. Tate (2003) wrote, 'For GPs to be effective they must be interested in people and not diseases. This means an intensely personal form of doctoring'.

References

Bain JD (1976) Doctor–patient communication in general practice consultations. *Medical Education*, **10**: 125–131.

Bain JD (1977) Patient knowledge and the content of the consultation in general practice. *Medical Education*, **11**: 347–350.

Balint M (1957) *The Doctor, his Patient and the Illness*. Pitman, London.

Berne E (1964) *Games People Play*. Penguin, Harmondsworth.

Byrne PS, Long BEL (1976) *Doctors Talking to Patients*. HMSO, London.

Cartwright A, Anderson R (1981) *General Practice Revisited*. Tavistock, London.

Coope J, Metcalfe D (1979) How much do patients know? *Journal of Royal College of General Practitioners*, **29**: 482–488.

Elstein AS, Shulman LS, Sprafha SA (1978) *Medical Problem Solving: an analysis of clinical reasoning*. Harvard University Press, Cambridge, MA.

Hampton JR, Harrison MJE, Mitchell JRA, Pritchard JS, Seymour C (1975) Relative contributions of history taking, physical examination and laboratory investigation to diagnosis and management of medical outpatients. *BMJ*, **ii**: 486–489.

Kleinman A (1980) *Patients and Healers in the Context of Culture*. University of California Press, Berkeley.

Mead N, Bower P (2000) Patient centredness: a conceptual framework and review of the empirical literature. *Soc. Sci. Med.*, **51**: 1087–1110.

Neighbour R (1987) *The Inner Consultation: how to develop an effective and intuitive consulting style*. MTP Press, Lancaster.

Osmond H (1980) God and the doctor. *New England Journal of Medicine*, **302**: 555–558.

Pendleton DA (1983) Doctor–patient communication: a review. In: *Doctor–Patient Communication* (eds Pendleton DA and Haslar JC). Academic Press, London

Pendleton D, Schofield T, Tate P, Havelock P (2000) *The Consultation: an approach to learning and teaching*. Oxford University Press, Oxford.

Pendleton D, Schofield T, Tate P, Havelock P (2003) *The New Consultation: developing doctor–patient communication*. Oxford University Press, Oxford.

Raynes NV (1980) A preliminary study of search procedures and patient management techniques in general practice. *Journal of Royal College of General Practitioners*, **13**: 166–172.

Silverman J, Kurtz S, Draper J (1998) *Skills for Communicating with Patients*. Radcliffe Medical Press, Oxford.

Stott NCH, Davis RH (1979) The exceptional potential in each primary care consultation. *Journal of the Royal College of General Practitioners*, **29**: 201–205.

Tate P (2003) *The Doctor's Communication Handbook*, 4th Edition. Radcliffe Medical Press, Oxford.

Tuckett D (ed) (1976) *An Introduction to Medical Sociology*. Tavistock, London.

Waitzkin H, Stoekle JD (1972) The communication of information about illness: clinical, social and methodological considerations. *Advances in Psychosomatic Medicine*, **8:** 180–215.

Additional information

Freeman GK, Horder JP, Howie JGR, Hungin AP, Hill AP, Shah NC, and Wilson A (2002) Evolving general practice consultation in Britain: issues of length and context. *BMJ*, **324:** 880–882.

Kravitz RL and Melnikow J (2001) Engaging patients in medical decision making. *BMJ*, **323:** 584–585.

Little P, Everitt H, Williamson I, Warner G, Moore M, Gould C, Ferrier K, and Payne S (2001) Observational study of effect of patient centredness and positive approach on outcomes of general practice consultations. *BMJ*, **323:** 908–911.

Little P, Everitt H, Williamson I, Warner G, Moore M, Gould C, Ferrier K, and Payne S (2001) Preferences of patients for patient centred approach to consultation in primary care: observational study. *BMJ*, **322:** 468.

McKinstry B (2000) Do patients wish to be involved in decision making in the consultation? A cross sectional survey with video vignettes. *BMJ*, **321:** 867–871.

Stewart M (2001) Towards a global definition of patient centred care. *BMJ*, **322:** 444–445.

Walter J and Bayat A (2003) Neurolinguistic programming: verbal communication. *BMJ*, **326:** 83.

Clinical governance

Clinical governance (CG) is unlikely to be asked as a direct question. However, an understanding of CG is needed to answer questions regarding the quality of care in the NHS. Questions such as 'What do you understand by quality assurance and accountability in the NHS?' and 'How could GPs improve their delivery of care to patients?' all link up with the concept of CG.

CG is a complex concept. This chapter tries to explain the concept simply; a comprehensive discussion would take an entire book! Complicated questions can be answered using a simple format called the '**5 Ws and 1 H**': what, when, why, where, who and how.

What is CG?

'A framework through which NHS organisations are accountable for continuously improving the *quality* of their services and safeguarding high standards of care by creating an environment in which excellence in clinical care will flourish'
A first class service (DoH, 1998)

The DoH defined *quality* as doing the right things, to the right people, at the right time.

CG aims to evaluate the quality of medical practice against agreed standards and to remedy any gaps identified in routine practice.

'Putting quality at the top of the NHS agenda will ensure fair access to effective, prompt, high quality care wherever a patient is treated in the NHS'
A first class service (DoH, 1998)

When was CG introduced?

The NHS introduced the concept of clinical governance in 1998.

Where will CG be introduced?

Improvements are needed at every level of the NHS, from GP surgeries to national structures (hence the introduction of NSFs, NICE, and the Modernisation Agency).

What needs improving?

Improvements can be made to:
- the physical components of the NHS – the surgery buildings, practice equipment, patient records and the practice team.

- the care given to patients and carers – are we following best practice?
- the outcomes of the treatment given – are we improving morbidity and mortality?

A criteria-based approach is a good objective way of measuring and achieving quality. The RCGP Quality Practice Award (QPA) and the new GMS contract provide a ready-made set of criteria that can be used locally.

Why is improvement needed?

- The public has lost faith in the health service following the Bristol, Alder Hay and Shipman scandals.
- There is increased consumerism – people demand high quality care.
- The government spends a large proportion of the budget on health – it wants an accountable NHS.

The public and government both want a high quality, accountable and transparent health service. Within the context of general practice, CG is about *assuring quality*:
- reducing the variation in the delivery of care by different GPs,
- setting agreed targets for improvement,
- systematically meeting targets.

CG in primary care is also about *assuring accountability* – demonstrating to patients, members of the PHCT, the PCT and the government that standards are satisfactory and are being achieved.

How will we make these improvements?

Improvements within the practice will take place by:
- practising evidence-based medicine – assessing clinical information on the internet from desktops; making clinical guidelines available electronically.
- disseminating good practice – copying letters to patients, sharing clinical 'titbits' with colleagues electronically and at meetings.
- adopting quality improvement processes – undertaking audits regularly, updating the practice drug formulary, participating in primary care collaborative projects.
- using data appropriately – auditing chronic disease management, analysing prescribing data, working with local pharmacists to review patients on regular medication.
- reducing clinical risk – by having regular significant event meetings.
- learning lessons from complaints – holding multidisciplinary meetings to reflect on and learn from complaints.
- tackling poor performance – undertaking annual resuscitation training, lengthening the appointment times for doctors who regularly over-run.
- continuing professional development – using staff PDPs, staff appraisal and 360 degree feedback.

- developing leadership – defining the roles of the CG partner and nursing representative.

These initiatives are known as the Ten Commandments of CG (Van Zwanenberg and Harrison, 2003).

Does CG work? What do we evaluate?

There is currently little published evidence that clinical governance makes any measurable difference.

When Degeling *et al.* (2004) reviewed CG in practice, they thought that CG should be a bottom-up (not top-down) activity – there should be less emphasis on inspection and performance management. The top-down model is flawed and should be replaced by a model that asks the following questions:
- **Are we doing the right things?** Given assessed health needs and existing resource constraints, are we delivering value for money? For common conditions, how appropriate and effective are the services we offer?
- **Are we doing things right?** Are we managing clinical performance according to national codes of clinical practice? For common conditions, how systematised are our care processes and how are we performing on risk, safety, quality, patient evaluation and clinical outcomes?
- **Are we keeping up with new developments** and what are we doing to extend our capacity to undertake clinical work in these areas? What strategies are in place for service and professional development for each condition? What are we doing about clinical mentoring, leadership development and staff appraisals?

How will we deliver and support the cultural changes needed?

A number of NHS and DoH organizations are working to improve quality in the NHS. Dr Tim Wilson, writing for the National Electronic Library for Health, identifies the following agencies:
- *National Patient Safety Agency* – making the NHS safer for patients
- *National Institute for Health and Clinical Excellence* – telling us what to do (and sometimes what not to do)
- *Commission for Health Improvement* – the independent watchdog that reports to Parliament on the performance of Trusts in England and Wales
- *National Clinical Assessment Authority* – helps local organizations with the assessment of doctors whose performance gives concern
- *Modernisation Agency* – the body charged with modernising care across the NHS. Within the Mod Agency (as it is known) are a number of teams including
  - *Clinical Governance Support Team* – doing just that

- *National Primary Care Development Team* – working on a number of large improvement projects nationally and regionally to improve amongst other things, access and coronary heart disease care
- *Leadership Centre* – helping to create more leaders in the NHS
- *National PCT Development team* (known as NatPaCT) – helping to build the capabilities of Primary Care Trusts
- *Changing workforce programme*
- *Service Improvement* (formerly NPAT)

Who are the key players?

The Labour Government discussed CG in '*A first class service: quality in the new NHS*'. Liam Donaldson wrote a key paper about the introduction of CG to the NHS (*BMJ*, 1998) and Neville Goodman (speaking for many doctors) wrote a critique of this paper.

CG appears in Annex B of the new contract (number 21) as a statutory and contractual requirement. This states that:
- all practices should have a system of CG to enable quality assurance, quality improvement and enhanced patient safety.
- there should be a nominated clinical governance lead in each practice.
- CG should be embedded in all the structures underpinning practice.

Learning points

- Assuring quality and accountability
- The Ten Commandments of CG
- Evaluation: doing the right things, doing things right, keeping up to date?
- *A first class service: quality in the new NHS*
- Annex B of the new contract (number 21)

Additional information

Goodman NW (1998). Clinical Governance. Sacred cows: to the abattoir. *BMJ*, **317**: 1725–1727. Neville Goodman writes:

'I have read "Clinical governance and the drive for quality improvement in the new NHS in England" carefully, word by word, and some parts several times. I have tried to understand why they needed over four pages to impart the commonsense message that we must all strive after quality in practising medicine; I have retained little beyond that it is our statutory duty now to provide quality in our medical care. The essay is all thought and no action, an epitome of hope over expectation, a high sounding clarion call of wonderful things just over the horizon. Most depressing of all, the authors seem to recognise the real difficulties but ignore just how obdurate these difficulties are. The result is an essay full of the "what" but short on the "how."'"

Marshall M *et al.* (2002) A qualitative study of cultural changes in PCOs needed to implement clinical governance. *British Journal of General Practice*, **52:**, 641–645.

The aim of this qualitative study was to investigate the importance of culture and cultural change for the implementation of clinical governance in general practice by PCGs / PCTs, to identify perceived desirable and undesirable cultural facilitators and barriers to changing culture. Results: The most desirable cultural traits were the value placed on a commitment to public accountability by the practices, their willingness to work together and learn from each other, and the ability to be self-critical and learn from mistakes. The main barriers to cultural change were the high level of autonomy of practices and the perceived pressure to deliver rapid measurable changes in general practice.

Campbell S (2001) Improving the quality of care through clinical governance. *BMJ*, **322:** 1580–1582.

Primary care groups and trusts are responsible for implementing clinical governance, including monitoring and improving the quality of care. In their first two years they have concentrated on educating and supporting health professionals and encouraging shared learning. Information about the quality of care provided in general practice is shared between practices and with the public, offered in a form that permits practices to be identified. Many groups and trusts are offering incentives to practices to promote improvement in the quality of care. Sanctions and disciplinary action are rarely used when dealing with poor performance. Limited resources and the pace of change are potential obstacles to future success in improving the quality of care.

Pringle M (2000) Participating in clinical governance. *BMJ*, **321:** 737–740.

Clinical governance is intended to improve standards of care and at the same time to protect the public from unacceptable care. The move from continuing medical education for doctors to continuing professional development for the whole primary care team presents new challenges for multidisciplinary learning and performance monitoring. To deal with poor performance, clinical governance leaders will need skills to assess the nature of the problem, educational resources to deal with it, and managerial resources to facilitate the process.

Allen P (2000) Accountability for clinical governance: developing collective responsibility for quality in primary care. *BMJ*, **321:** 608–611.

Clinical governance in primary care is aimed at enhancing the collective responsibility and accountability of professionals in primary care trusts. It is mainly concerned with increasing accountability of primary care professionals to local communities (downwards accountability), the NHS hierarchy (upwards accountability), and their peers (horizontal accountability). Limited resources are likely to ensure that upwards accountability is given priority.

Rosen R (2000) Improving quality in the changing world of primary care. *BMJ*, **321**: 551–554.

Clinical governance in primary care must focus on individual patients and whole populations; this creates tensions between a view of good practice based on individual rights and a population approach focused on the distribution of services.

Relevant literature

Journal articles
Pringle M, Bradley C, Carmichael CM et al. (1995) Significant event auditing: a study of the feasibility and potential of case based auditing in primary medical care. *Occasional paper no. 70.* RCGP Publications, London.
Scally G, Donaldson LJ. (1998) Looking forward: clinical governance and the drive for quality improvement in the new NHS in England. *BMJ*, **317**: 61–65.

Books
Van Zwanenberg T, Harrison J (eds) (2003) *Clinical Governance in Primary Care*, 2nd edition. Radcliffe Medical Press, Oxford.

Internet
- http://www.nelh.nhs.uk/quality/
- http://www.doh.gov.uk/clinicalgovernance
- http://www.rsm.ac.uk/pub/cgb.htm
- **Roland M, Baker R** (1999) *Clinical Governance: a practical guide for primary care teams*.: National Primary Care Research and Development, Manchester. http://www.npcrdc.man.ac.uk/publications/handbook%20clinical%20governance.pdf
- Secretary of State for Health. (1998) *A first class service. Quality in the new NHS.* NHS Executive, Leeds. www.nhshistory.net/a_first_class_service.htm

Patient safety

Why do I need to know about patient safety for the nMRCGP exam?

Patient safety is an important component of the Clinical Governance (CG) agenda. CG has changed the way in which we deliver care to patients. The aim is to give safe, high quality care. A question on patient safety may appear in many guises, for example, the discussion in case presentations and significant event audits may focus on issues such as:

- the referral letter was sent to the incorrect hospital department. What mechanisms should GP practices have in place to reduce mistakes?
- you prescribed an incorrect dose of medication. How did you manage this situation?
- you say that you had failed to refer this patient with retinal detachment early. What steps will you take to prevent this from happening again in the future?

Why is patient safety important in general practice?

- Non-maleficence is a key component of our professional ethics.
- Society expects good quality, safe care.
- Patient safety is an integral part of the CG agenda.
- Doctors are remunerated for having systems in place to reduce the risk of harm to their patients and to learn lessons from mistakes that were made. For example, four Q and O points are given if the practice undertakes six significant event reviews in the past three years.

How are patients harmed by healthcare professionals?

1. **Unavoidable risks** in medicine (some adverse events are inevitable)
   - Risks of medication (risk of a seizure with anti-malarials) or
   - Risks of treatment (risk of uterine perforation with the insertion of an IUD).

   Patients need to be warned about the possible harms and benefits of treatments in order to make informed choices. Good record-keeping is also important.

2. **Avoidable risks**

   These usually occur as a result of genuine mistakes. Research has suggested that around 10 per cent of patients admitted to UK acute hospitals suffer some kind of patient safety incident. Up to half of these mistakes may have been preventable. Systems should be designed to minimise such mistakes. For example, analysis of reported incidents involving intrathecal chemotherapy injections resulted in changes to the design of the delivery system.

3. **Criminal doctors**

   This constitutes a very small proportion of patient harm. Unfortunately Shipman will be remembered for a long time by the public.

4. Underperforming doctors

Doctors have a professional duty to maintain good medical practice and to keep up to date. Doctors may be underperforming because:

- they become deskilled (some GPs who became deskilled at providing intra-partum care withdrew these services)
- doctors fail to provide up-to-date treatments which evidence-based research has shown to be effective. For example, failure to treat hypertension aggressively results in increased morbidity.
- some doctors have poor diagnostic skills and behaviour (poor prescribing and referral patterns).

Addressing avoidable risk

The NHS intends to learn from the airline industry. The National Patient Safety Agency (NPSA) was formed following the publication of two reports on patient safety:

- *An organisation with a memory* (DoH, 2000), and its follow-up
- *Building a safer NHS for patients* (DoH, 2001).

The NPSA was tasked with developing:

- A **blame-free culture** – this will encourage doctors to openly discuss mistakes – theirs, their colleagues' and those due to the system in which they work. Staff who find themselves in a dysfunctional or repressive organization will continue to be protected by whistleblowing legislation.
- A **national mechanism** for reporting and analysing risk. This aims to tackle the root cause of the risk. The NPSA is developing the National Reporting and Learning System (NRLS).
- Summary:

Government Papers
↓
National Patient Safety Agency
↓
National Reporting and Learning System
↓
Reports back to National Patient Safety Agency
↓
Changes made to working practices and devices to reduce risk

Mechanisms for reporting risk

NHS staff, patients and their carers will be able to report any patient safety incidents or near misses to the NRLS electronically. The NRLS has been designed to complement local systems, such as significant event reporting. The information they provide will be fed to the National Patient Safety Agency. The NPSA will:

- *collect and analyse* information on adverse events;
- *assimilate* other safety-related information from a variety of existing reporting systems and other sources in the UK and abroad;
- *learn lessons* and ensure that they are fed back into practice,
- where risks are identified, produce *solutions to prevent harm and specify national goals*.

Responding to the harm

At present, when there has been a failure of the service, a range of responses occurs. In future there will be two ways of responding – an independent investigation commissioned by either the Department of Health or by the Commission for Health Improvement.

What can be done locally to reduce patient harm?

The National Patient Safety Agency has issued a guide to NHS staff – *Seven steps to patient safety* (2003). It sets out the seven steps that NHS organizations should take to improve patient safety.
- Build a safety culture – create a culture that is open and fair.
- Lead and support your staff – establish a clear and strong focus on patient safety throughout your organization.
- Integrate your risk management activity – develop systems and processes to manage your risks and identify and assess things that could go wrong.
- Promote reporting – ensure your staff can easily report incidents locally and nationally.
- Involve and communicate with patients and the public – develop ways to communicate openly with patients.
- Learn and share safety lessons – encourage staff to use root cause analysis to learn how and why adverse incidents occurred.
- Implement solutions to prevent harm.

Risk management in general practice

Clinical risk management aims to identify, assess and then reduce risk to patients. The most common errors in general practice are due to administrative failures, such as errors in taking and passing on messages (31%). Treatment failures account for 23% of errors.

How do general practices reduce their risk?

Practice equipment – a named individual should be responsible for regularly monitoring, maintaining and calibrating equipment. Drugs and vaccinations should be stored at the correct temperature.

Staff training – good induction and regular training should occur in manual handling, confidentiality issues, filing results and dealing with violent patients.

Health and safety – the practice should have a policy in place to deal with fire drills, the disposal of sharps, sterilising equipment and vaccination against hepatitis B.

Record-keeping – good notes are essential: they may form the GP's defence against a complaint.

Clinical guidelines – evidence-based guidelines should be easily available (preferably on desktops) and should be regularly updated.

Confidentiality and consent – practice staff must be made aware of the strict rules governing confidentiality. Patients should not be able to view the notes or overhear discussions about other patients. Practices should have appropriate consent forms for minor surgery, immunizations and other procedures.

Complaints – the practice should have an agreed procedure for handling patients' complaints. This should comply with the NHS procedures, and should be outlined in the practice leaflet.

Audit and significant event analysis – lessons learnt should improve patient care.

Adverse incident reporting – practices should have a mechanism for identifying and reporting adverse or significant events to the NPSA.

Learning points

- Patients are harmed by avoidable errors, unavoidable errors, criminal doctors and underperforming doctors
- National Patient Safety Agency was formed to develop a blame-free culture and a national mechanism for reporting risk
- *Seven steps to patient safety* (2003)
- Audit and significant event analysis – learning lessons and improving care

---

Additional information

Quality indicators in the new GMS contract – a few examples are listed below.

4 points	There is a record of all practice-employed clinical staff having attended training / updating in basic life-support skills in the preceding 18 months
3 points	All new staff receive induction training
4 points	The practice has undertaken a minimum of 12 SEAs in the past three years which include (if these have occurred): • Any deaths occurring in the practice premises • Two new cancer diagnoses • Two deaths where terminal care has taken place at home • One patient complaint • One suicide • One section under the Mental Health Act
3 points	The practice has systems in place to ensure regular and appropriate inspection, calibration, maintenance and replacement of equipment including: • A defined responsible person • Clear recording • Systematic pre-planned schedules • Reporting of faults

Relevant literature

The complaint's procedure is available at: http://www.dh.gov.uk/en/Policyandguidance/Organisationpolicy/Complaintspolicy/NHScomplaintsprocedure/index.htm

Confidentiality regulations and guidance are at: http://www.dh.gov.uk/en/Policyandguidance/Informationpolicy/Patientconfidentialityandcaldicottguardians/index.htm

Consent: http://www.dh.gov.uk/en/Policyandguidance/Healthandsocialcaretopics/Consent/index.htm

Data protection help is available at: http://www.dh.gov.uk/en/Policyandguidance/Organisationpolicy/Recordsmanagement/DH_4000489

The Health and Safety Executive website is found at: www.hse.gov.uk.

Evidence-based medicine

Why do I need to know about evidence-based medicine for the nMRCGP exam?

The nMRCGP tests the doctor's ability to obtain and understand the best available evidence, integrate this into current practice, communicate it effectively to patients to enhance or facilitate our patients' decision-making. A question on EBM may appear as:
- you said you would prescribe topical non-steroid gel to a patient with osteoarthritis of the knee. Is this evidence-based management? Where did you obtain your evidence?
- how do you communicate the results of the research into the use of antibiotics in the treatment of earache to the parent?
- do you think that EBM has improved the quality of the care you delivered to the angina patient?

Why is EBM important in general practice?

Practice could be improved if practitioners were more familiar with the results of research. Doctors need to be able to access the literature, appraise papers for their validity and value and then convert their learning into practice that benefits their patients.

What is EBM?

EMB is a systematic approach to clinical decision-making. It involves:
- framing a focused question
- searching thoroughly for research-derived evidence
- appraising the evidence for its validity and relevance
- seeking and incorporating the user's values and preferences
- evaluating effectiveness through planned review against agreed success criteria.

It is based on similar principles to audit and performance review.

1. Framing a focused question:
Use the SMART principle to focus the question. The question must cover four areas:
- the patient or problem,
- the intervention being considered,
- the alternative intervention where appropriate and
- the outcome.

For example, in the question 'Do broad-spectrum antibiotics reduce the duration of pain and fever in acute, purulent OM in children aged 2 to 12 years?' the patient is a child between the ages of 2 and 12; the intervention is a broad-spectrum antibiotic; the alternative is treatment without antibiotics; the outcomes are duration of pain and fever.

2. Searching for the evidence

Searches can be done manually by trawling through textbooks and journals but these sources rapidly become outdated. Electronic databases are a reliable alternative. A good starting point is Medline and the Cochrane library. Other useful online databases include Bandolier, Best Evidence and General Practice Notebook (www.gpnotebook.co.uk). Searches can be done by the practitioner or by a medical librarian.

3. Appraising the evidence

Doctors apply their critical reading principles to understand the research. On first glance, doctors need to ascertain:
- whether the trial is valid,
- what the results are,
- whether the results are applicable locally.

To make these decisions, doctors need to understand, amongst other things, the concepts of P-values, confidence intervals, bias, confounding factors, intention to treat analysis, numbers needed to treat (NNT) and numbers needed to harm (NTH).

4. Incorporating the user's values

Using the example of otitis media, the research will not be applied to every child irrespective of their circumstances. Professional judgement is exercised in the application of research findings to clinical practice.

> 'Focusing too much on the rational and quantitative aspects of clinical problems – an inherent danger in EBM – can have a negative influence on the doctor–patient relationship and can erode the caregivers' role in providing care in fullest and most human way possible . . . Evidence is not enough: we need to communicate with our patients, listen to their concerns, elicit their values, be involved, really care about them. We also need to integrate the evidence with patients' values and preferences.'   (Hunink, 2004)

5. Evaluating the effectiveness against agreed success criteria

EBM is about incorporating research evidence into clinical practice. How will doctors know if the changes they introduced improved the health of their patients? The final step involves assessing the usefulness of the intervention. For example, did the reduction in antibiotic prescribing in OM lead to more follow-up consultations, greater use of the out of hours service, or result in a higher complication rate? Did many patients complain about the new practice?

Evidence is classified according to the strength of the study design.

Grade 1	Strong evidence from at least one published meta-analysis / systematic review of multiple well-designed randomized controlled trials (RCT)
Grade 2	Strong evidence from at least one RCT of appropriate size and in an appropriate clinical setting
Grade 3	Evidence from published well-designed trials without randomization, single group pre-post, cohort, time series or matched case-controlled studies
Grade 4	Evidence from well-designed non-experimental studies from more than one centre or research group
Grade 5	Opinions of respected authorities, based on clinical evidence, descriptive studies or reports of expert consensus committees

The hierarchy of EBM may be misleading. Hunink (2004) writes that a systematic review of a few small, poorly-conducted trials is clearly not better than one large, well-done, double-blind trial. Randomization is not always ethically justifiable. Some information such as the treatment of fractures with plaster casts comes from observational data (grade 5 evidence).

What do GPs think about EBM?

Most GPs believe that EBM will improve their practice but many do not know how to conduct a search. In a 1998 survey of 450 Wessex GPs, fewer than half were aware of the Cochrane Database of Systematic Reviews and less than a quarter had access to Medline at their surgeries (McColl *et al.*, 1998).

However, the current consensus is that it is unrealistic to expect GPs to search for and critically appraise primary evidence. GPs are being advised not use internet search engines, such as Google or Medline, when seeking advice, particularly on what to prescribe. Instead they are advised to 'stick to 'premier' information sources, such as the National Institute for Health and Clinical Excellence (NICE), the Cochrane Collaboration, or national service frameworks because 'this would eliminate waste and improve patient care' (Day, 2006).

How often do GPs need to look for further information?

It has been estimated that GPs experience areas of uncertainty that raise questions about their practice at least once every 15 patients (Ely *et al.*, 1992).

Additional information

If you wanted to know whether antibiotics could be prescribed for earache in a 6 year old child, you could:

● Access Medline. However, to get good quality information, you would need to structure your search question properly and have the critical reading skills to analyse the research.

● Access the Cochrane library for systematic reviews of the primary evidence.

● Access synopses or journal abstracts, such as *bmjupdates*, which provides a cumulative, searchable database of recent journal article citations. However, to search this database, you must register.

● Access summaries, such as Prodigy.

● Access computerized decision support systems, such as http://www.library. nhs.uk/.

The information in the latter sources is of better quality and has been pre-appraised. Therefore, if you are looking for evidence to support your decision-making, then it is entirely acceptable to first search the NHS library or Prodigy for guidance.

Relevant literature

BMJ (30 October 2004; volume 329) is a themed issue dealing with EBM.

Day M (2006) GPs should use "premier" information sources when prescribing. *BMJ*, **333:** 1239.

Ely JW, et al. (2002) Obstacles to answering doctors' questions about patient care with evidence: qualitative study. *BMJ*; **324:** 710.

Ely JW, Burch RJ, Vinson DC. (1992) The information needs of family physicians: case-specific clinical questions. *J Fam Pract*, **35:** 265–269.

Fowkes FGR, Fulton PM. (1991) Critical appraisal of published research: introductory guidelines. *BMJ*, **302:** 1136–1140.

Hunink MGM. (2004) Does evidence based medicine do more good than harm? *BMJ*, **329:** 1051.

McColl A, Smith H, White P, Field J. (1998) General practitioner's perceptions of the route to evidence based medicine: a questionnaire survey. *BMJ*, **316:** 361–365.

Internet
See: http://www.jr2.ox.ac.uk/bandolier/booth/booths/trials.html

See: http://www.clinicalevidence.com/ceweb/resources/index.jsp. You can use the *Resources* section of the site for useful materials and tools, including the *EBM introductory workshop* intended to help beginners with the following questions:

- What is EBM and how does it relate to me?
- What problems can it help me solve?
- What are the basic principles underlying EBM and how might I apply them to my own work?
- Where can I go for more information?

Giving feedback

Feedback is given to colleagues, employers and students. In the exam, a question about giving a colleague feedback tests your communication skills. Doctors often use Pendleton's rules to structure their feedback (see below). The SET–GO method (see Additional information section) has become increasingly popular.

What is good feedback?

Feedback must enable change. Feedback is about telling people about specific aspects of their behaviour in a way that facilitates their adoption of more effective behaviours. These can be about their consulting behaviour or the way they interact with staff or the way in which they teach. It is about getting people to improve and also about motivating them so that they feel these improvements are not out of their reach. For feedback to do this, it needs to be:

- Specific: 'When you discussed the hospital referral with your patient, she looked surprised.' This is more specific than, 'Your consultation was awful. The poor woman left in tears.'
- Selective: address one or two key issues rather than too many at once.
- Honest: Don't be dishonestly kind. Tackle ethical and attitudinal issues. 'When you spoke to the receptionist, you sounded patronising.' This is different to, 'You are patronising and sarcastic.' You have distinguished between the behaviour that needs changing and the personality of the individual. Keep feedback directed to behaviour that can be changed.
- Helpful: offer alternatives. 'I wonder if you had tried ...'; or 'Sometimes I find it helpful...' or 'Have you considered..' The person needs to identify and address the behaviour that needs changing.
- Sensitive: nobody likes to be told that their behaviour was lacking, and that changes are recommended. They respond by attacking the bearer of the news, or feeling deflated ('I tried my best and it still isn't good enough'), or by becoming defensive. Their effort needs to be acknowledged and appreciated so that they feel heard and understood. Only then will they feel motivated to continue.

Effective feedback requires a combination of qualities, skills and some structure. A person's performance is boosted by providing challenge with an appropriate level of support. The key skills are to listen and to ask, not to 'show and tell.'

Why use Pendleton's rules?

Pendleton recognized that people have insight into their strengths and weaknesses. By allowing them to discuss their insights, you are harnessing their intrinsic motivation to improve. By discussing the positive aspects of their behaviour, you are acknowledging their effort and contribution. By then tackling the areas for improvement, you are identifying specific behaviours that need to change and suggesting ideas for improvement.

What are Pendleton's rules?

1. The recipients of the feedback go first and describe what went well and which of their strengths they demonstrated.
2. The person giving feedback goes next and also discusses their strengths. This acknowledges the other person's effort – it is encouraging. It also allays their anxiety.
3. The recipients then discuss how things may be done differently.
4. The person giving feedback then makes suggestions. For the suggestions to effect a change in behaviour, they have to be specific, honest, helpful and sensitive.

Advantages of Pendleton's rules

- With increasing familiarity, the rules provide a useful tool by which to structure feedback.
- The recipients are left with a clear summary of their strengths and an action plan for their improvement.
- Destructive criticism is minimised. The feedback concentrates on the person's behaviour and does not degenerate into an unhelpful attack on his personality.
- The recipients develop insight and a realistic understanding of the strengths and weaknesses of the performance.

Disadvantages of Pendleton's rules

- The feedback can be disjointed. People tend to remember events chronologically and may find it difficult to analyse the event in terms of 'things that went well' and 'areas for improvement'.
- The recipients and appraiser may disagree. If the parties disagree about the behaviour being a strength or a weakness, a confrontation develops. It is difficult to facilitate change in a confrontational environment.

Receiving feedback

- The recipient should listen to the feedback with an open mind and assume that it is constructive. However, it is difficult not to be defensive. The more time spent on convincing someone of the need to change, the less time available for discussing how to change.
- If the recipient did not understand what was said, he should ask for examples and clarify the advice. The person giving the feedback may be very experienced, or in a rush, or embarrassed and may say things quickly, using jargon. If the recipient wants to improve, he needs to understand exactly what needs changing and discuss ideas for improvement.
- The recipient should thank the person for their time and the thought they put into helping him develop.

Learning points

Effective feedback requires a combination of:
- **qualities:** someone who is sensitive, honest, helpful, tactful and insightful
- **skills:** skills of communication – asking a balance of open, reflective, facilitating and closed questions; challenging and summarizing
- **structure:** Pendleton's model

Additional information

SET–GO
The SET–GO method of descriptive feedback is adapted from Kurtz *et al.* (1998). Feedback is given under the following headings:
- **what I Saw** – the person giving feedback describes the event in a detailed and non-judgmental manner
- **what Else did you see?** – in addition to what the facilitator saw, can the person receiving the feedback describe in further detail what has happened?
- **what do you Think?** – the person receiving feedback is given the opportunity to problem-solve, with input from the facilitator
- **can we clarify what Goal you would like to achieve?** – the person receiving feedback is encouraged to draw up goals or outcomes that he would like to achieve
- **any Offers of how you should get there?** – the person receiving feedback and the facilitator make suggestions about how the goals can be achieved

Relevant literature

Articles
King J. (1999) Giving feedback. *BMJ Classified*, **26:** 2–3.
Parikh A, McReelis K, Hodges B. (2001) Student feedback in problem based learning: a survey of 103 final year students across five Ontario medical schools. *Medical Education*, **35:** 632–636.
Ward D. (2003) Self-esteem and audit feedback. *Nursing Standard*, **17:** 33–36.

Books
Kurtz SM, Silverman JD, Draper J. (1998) *Teaching and Learning Communication Skills in Medicine*. Radcliffe Medical Press, Oxford.

Internet
For further information on feedback, see http://www.skillscascade.com/.

Reflective learning and mentoring

Definition

Reflection is the process of deliberately and methodically considering past actions and learning lessons on what worked and what didn't and arriving at a plan of what to do next.

Reflective learning is seen as one of many tools for self-directed learning and development. The aim of reflective learning is for the doctor to develop self-awareness, to confirm his strengths and to identify his areas for improvement. As a result of developing self-awareness, the doctor's practice should improve.

Types of reflection

Reflection can be formal or informal; facilitated or self-conducted. In medicine, doctors are becoming increasingly familiar with mentorship or appraisal. Here the doctor's reflection is facilitated by a colleague. Formal facilitated reflection is a relatively new concept in medicine, whereas it is deeply embedded in nursing practice where it is called clinical supervision. There are many models of clinical supervision – Driscoll's 'What?' model (2000) being one.

The framework of Driscoll's 'What?' model comprises:
- 'What?': A description of the events. What happened?
- 'So what?': An analysis of the event. What resulted from these events? How did people feel?
- 'Now what?': Proposed actions following the event. What can you do now and should this occur again, what can you do differently?

Driscoll's trigger questions are:
1. A description of the event: **What?**
   - What is the purpose of returning to the situation?
   - What happened?
   - What did I see / do?
   - What was my reaction to it?
   - What did other people that were involved in this do?
2. An analysis of the event: **So what?**
   - How did I feel at the time of the event?
   - Were those feelings I had any different from those of other people who were also involved at the time?
   - Are my feelings now, after the event, any different from those I experienced at the time?
   - Do I still feel troubled? If so, in what way?
   - What were the effects of what I did (or did not do)?
   - What positive aspects emerge for me from the event?
   - What have I noticed about my behaviour in practice by taking a more measured look at it?

- What observations does any person helping me to reflect on my practice make about the way I acted at the time?
3. Proposed actions following the event: **Now what?**
   - What are the implications for me and others in clinical practice based on what I have described and analysed?
   - What difference does it make if I choose to do nothing?
   - Where can I get more information to face a similar situation again?
   - How can I modify my practice if a similar situation were to happen again?
   - What help do I need to help me 'action' the results of my reflections?
   - Which aspect should be tackled first?
   - How will I notice that I am any different in clinical practice?
   - What is the main learning that I take from reflecting on my practice in this way?

The benefits of facilitated reflection

The facilitator provides a supportive, non-judgemental environment. However, within this supportive climate, challenging questions are asked. Challenging the doctor within a supportive environment is ideal for a doctor's growth and development – challenge without support is seen as an attack whereas support with no challenge is seen as molly coddling.

A facilitator does not say, 'You are bad at explaining things to patients!' A facilitator will ask the doctor questions: 'Why did your patient became angry? Could you do it differently next time? How would you do it differently?' By asking these questions, the doctor will hopefully become aware of his deficiencies and will hence gain insight into the problem. Hopefully he will correct the problem without the facilitator's prompting and will be more insightful of his behaviours in the future.

Facilitated reflection is useful for exposing blind spots – see Johari's window figure opposite. Johari's window is a pictorial representation of the facilitator's knowledge (Y axis) and doctor's knowledge (X axis). The aim of facilitated reflection is to reduce the 'blind-spot' by the facilitator 'feeding back' what he knows about the doctor to him. The facilitator challenges the doctor's deeply held assumptions (his blind-spots) and encourages him to question the validity of these assumptions. By making the doctor overtly conscious of his assumptions, the doctor becomes aware of how others perceive him. This increased self-awareness can be directed towards making effective adaptations to his behaviour.

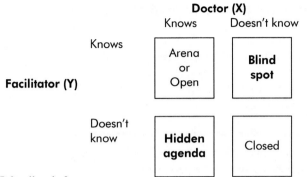

Johari's window.

Mentoring in general practice

Mentoring is defined as:

'an experienced highly regarded empathic person (the mentor) guides another individual (the mentee) in the development and re-examination of his or her own ideas, learning, personal, and professional developments. This is achieved by listening and talking in confidence.'

Standing Committee on Postgraduate Medical and Dental Education (1999)

Responsibilities of mentor and mentee

Mentors facilitate the process of constructive reflection. The mentees set the agenda – they determine the topics or incidents they wish to reflect upon. The meeting usually takes place at the surgery – the content of the meeting is often confidential, making public venues unsuitable (Alliot, 1996). Meetings usually last between 60 and 90 minutes. For mentoring to be successful, a caring and trusting relationship must develop between mentor and mentee.

Grainger (2002) identified the three most common instances when people find the mentorship useful:

- Mentees who are new to an organization.
- Mentees who are concerned with their career development.
- Mentees who are being developed for future leadership positions.

Mentoring dos and don'ts

Adapted from Grainger (2002).

Dos

- Listen carefully and watch for non-verbal cues
- Facilitate the mentee's development – do not expect your mentee to do what you would do
- Help with networking

- Be honest with feedback – be direct, constructive, and kind when making suggestions
- Maintain confidentiality
- Make notes if these help maintain the focus of your discussions from one meeting to the next
- Discuss in advance with your mentee what the two of you would do in emotionally stressful discussions – safety net

Don'ts
- Don't shy away from giving 'negative' feedback, but avoid being unnecessarily critical. Describe the behaviour, not the personality.
- Don't abuse your authority as a mentor. Recognize that a power differential exists.
- Don't expect your mentee to defer to you.
- Don't use your mentee's achievements to further your own agenda.

Cued modelling

Cued modelling is a process of highlighting examples of good practice. It is the result of deliberate analysis by the facilitator and the doctor – what was it that made a particular behaviour successful or less successful? How did the doctor feel when this behaviour occurred and why? The motivations and consequences of the doctor's actions are discussed to develop awareness of his own behaviours. For example, a doctor may pick up that a patient is depressed and based on his intuition, he may sensitively probe the issue. The facilitator, in analysing this piece of behaviour, asks the doctor how he picked up the depressive symptoms and why he chose the questions he used. The doctor then becomes consciously aware of his good consulting behaviours – his ability to use his intuition, his ability to time his questions well and to use silence to allow the patient space in which to explore her feelings. In facilitation, the doctor develops self-awareness – he gains insight into his good (and less good) consulting techniques.

Unconditioned positive regard

Facilitators need to be sensitive to the effort that the doctor has put into his work and to value his contribution before attempting to address his deficiencies. Rogers (1983) called this 'unconditioned positive regard'. If a warm and understanding atmosphere is created, then deficits in knowledge, attitudes and skills may be explored without these being interpreted as a negative comment on the doctor personally. Balanced feedback is important: the doctor must come to an understanding of what he needs to improve but he must leave feeling motivated to make these changes.

Role play

In facilitated reflection, role play can be used to try out new ways of doing things. A doctor may role play a situation to gain a greater understanding of the dynamics.

Learning points

- Considering past actions to develop self-awareness
- Models of structured reflection, e.g. Driscoll's 'What?' model
- Johari's window – revealing the 'blind-spots'
- Cued modelling
- Unconditioned positive regard

Additional information

ROGER (Reciprocal Observation, Guidance, Education, and Reflection) is a newly developed teaching tool that offers opportunities for reflection (Williams and Bache, 2004).

The ROGER process has five essential elements:

- It is a *Reciprocal* process. One professional acts as the appraiser and the other acts as the appraisee. They then reverse roles and repeat the process.
- *Observation* of the normal practice of the appraisee is undertaken by the appraiser, normally without interruption.
- The appraiser then offers *Guidance* to the appraisee. This guidance may be clinical or related to other aspects of the consultation – for example, communication skills.
- An opportunity exists for *Education* through observation of good practice, feedback on the consultation, and discussion of clinical topics. Education is usually clinical – for example, interpretation of electrocardiograms, radiological interpretation, pharmacological options, management options.
- Finally, there is opportunity for *Reflection*. What was done well? Could the consultation have been improved? Was treatment appropriate? Could communication have been better? What was learnt today?

Relevant literature

Alliott R. (1996) Facilitating mentoring in general practice. *BMJ Career Focus,* **313**(7060).

Butterworth T et al. (2001) *Clinical Supervision and Mentorship in Nursing.* Stanley Thornes Ltd, Cheltenham.

Casement P. (1985) *On Learning from the Patient.* Routledge, London.

Cottrell D et al. (2002) What is effective supervision and how does it happen? A critical incident study. *Medical Education,* **36:** 1042–1049.

Cowan L. (2000) Lessons from experience: working with students in community midwifery practice. In: *Successful Supervision in Health Care Practice*, pp 50–57 (Spouse J and Redfern L, eds). Blackwell Science Ltd, Oxford.

Driscoll J. (2000) *Practising Clinical Supervision: A reflective approach*. Balliere Tindall, Edinburgh.

Grainger C. 2002. Mentoring: supporting doctors at work and at play. *BMJ*, **324:** S203.

Grant J. et al. (1999) *The Good CPD guide*. Reed Healthcare Publishing, Sutton.

Havelock P. et al. (1995) *Professional Education for General Practice*. Oxford University Press, Oxford.

Wilkinson TJ, et al. (2002) The use of portfolios for assessment for practice of the competence and performance of doctors in practice. *Medical Education*, **36:** 918–924.

Williams P, Bache J. (2004) Learning with ROGER. *BMJ Career Focus*, **329:** 58–59.

Winstanley J, White E. (2003) Clinical supervision: models, measures and best practice. *Nurse Researcher*, **10**(4), 7–38.

Van Zwanenberg T, Harrison J. (eds) (2003) *Clinical Governance for Primary Care*. Radcliffe Medical Press, Oxford.

Managing change

Questions on managing change appear in many guises, such as:
- You said that better communication with the triage nurses is needed. How would you improve communication?
- You said that the practice could deliver information to patients via a website. Discuss the issues in undertaking this project.
- You want the practice to use computer-based decision-making support systems to improve the clinical management of common ailments. Before you propose the plan to the practice, what issues do you need to consider?

Just as there are models for breaking bad news, negotiating a difficult consultation or giving feedback, there are models for managing change. A comprehensive discussion of all the change models is beyond this chapter. The following models will be discussed:
- Model for Improvement
- RAID model
- Kaufman's discrepancy model
- Lewin's force-field analysis

Model for improvement

The NHS Modernisation Agency uses the Model for Improvement. Its framework includes:

- **Asking three key questions**
  What are we trying to accomplish?
  How will we know that a change is an improvement?
  What changes can we make that will result in improvement?

- **It uses a process for testing change ideas:** Plan, Do, Study, Act (PDSA) cycles.

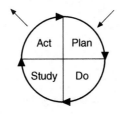

The PDSA cycle:
- Plan: plan the change to be tested or implemented
- Do: carry out the test or change
- Study: study data before and after the change and reflect on what was learnt
- Act: plan the next change cycle or plan implementation

Features of the model for improvement
- Ideas are tested on a small scale first
  - Less disruptive to employees / patients
  - Each cycle builds on the previous learning – incremental, structured, less threatening change occurs
  - Different people are involved in many small changes – higher chance of success
- Small changes involve less time, money and risk
- Some changes do not work – people learn from these before new changes are made
- The ideas and changes are 'owned' by the team – there is less resistance to change

RAID model

RAID is the model for change currently used by the Clinical Governance Support Team of the Modernisation Agency. RAID stands for:
- Review: look at the current situation and prepare the organization for change
- Agree: ensure staff are signed up to the proposed changes
- Implement: put in place the proposed changes
- Demonstrate: show that the changes have made improvements

Kaufman's discrepancy model

- Where are we now? To answer this question, identify what we have and what we lack, i.e. do a needs analysis, using a SWOT analysis or a Manchester rating scale.
- Where do we want to get to? These outcomes must be SMART (specific, measurable, achievable, realistic, time-bound).

Lewin's force-field analysis

- Where are we now?
- Where do we want to be?
- What are factors resisting change?
- What are the drivers encouraging change?

This model recognizes that change is achieved by tackling the resisting factors. If the drivers are increased in the face of opposition, resistance simply increases. For change to occur, the resisting factors should be reduced.

Developing a learning organization

Managing change locally (at practice level) and managing change more widely (at PCT and NHS level) have many things in common – the same change management models can be used. In addition, the correct organizational culture needs to be developed. An organization that fosters a culture that supports learning is called a 'learning organization.' Learning organizations create an atmosphere of sharing their experience to keep up with changes; these organizations do not reinvent the wheel.

Peter Senge, a professor of management, wrote about the five disciplines of a learning organization. These are: systems thinking, personal mastery, mental models, shared vision, and team learning.

- Systems thinking: See the whole picture and recognize the patterns and interactions within the system. Success depends on reinforcing or changing the underlying patterns, not just completing a series of tasks.
- Personal mastery: Three important elements are personal vision, creative tension and commitment to truth.
  - Personal vision: This is about what you want (your goal) and why you want it (your purpose).
  - Creative tension: There are unavoidable gaps between one's vision and current reality. Gaps are a source of creative energy. There are only two ways to resolve the tension between reality and the vision. Either vision pulls reality toward it, or reality pulls vision downward.
  - Commitment to truth: Be honest about the limiting factors. The underlying structures need to be changed to produce results.
- Mental models: Our understanding of the world is based on our assumptions. New ideas rarely get put into practice because they conflict with deeply held assumptions. To improve, current mental models must be questioned and challenged.
- Shared vision: Everybody within the organization needs to have a clear idea of what they want to create – shared visions create focus and energy. They give a sense of purpose and coherence to all the activities the organization carries out.
- Team learning: Each member is committed and shares a vision of greatness. The team's collective competence is far greater than any individual's.

Learning points

- Model for Improvement; RAID model; Kaufman's discrepancy model; Lewin's force-field analysis
- Plan, Do, Study, Act (PDSA) cycles
- For change to occur, the resisting factors (obstacles) should be reduced.
- Senge – the five disciplines of a learning organization

Additional information

Consider the move away from PGEA to PDPs – this was an organizational change in the funding and delivery of continuing professional development to GPs.

The old system of GP education was based on PGEA.

Criticisms levelled at PGEA:
- the top-down didactic approach (mainly lecture-based)
- its non-inclusiveness (addressed the talkers' interests and rarely considered the learners' learning needs)
- not involving learners (in what, how and when the learning was delivered)
- failing to influence working behaviour (education was responsible for only one third of the changes seen in clinical practice)
- has been open to abuse and yielded little professional satisfaction – 'bums on seats'.

What was the vision for GP education?
The vision was to provide an effective education that met the needs of the patient, the NHS and the practitioner, including GPs with special interests. Educationalists wanted a more 'adult-learning' orientated system. The GMC wanted a system that met the requirements for appraisal and revalidation.

How was this new vision going to be delivered?
The Chief Medical Officer (Calman, 1998) advocated the use of Personal Development Plans (PDPs). Drivers for change included the drive for multi-professional education, inter-professional education and the focus on outcome-based education (results-orientated thinking). A credit based system of education (as used in Australia and South Africa) could have been introduced, however reviews evaluating credit based educational schemes show that these do not lead to changes in behaviour or organizational improvements.

It was proposed that PDPs would bring medical education into the realms of adult education principles. However, PDPs have met with great resistance, with pressure of work and lack of protected time being quoted as reasons for resisting uptake. Also the introduction of PDPs is seen as being a top-down process. Despite these arguments, PDPs were introduced.

The system will need evaluation. What outcomes do we evaluate? It is not the provision of educational opportunities which improves patient care, it is the reflection and application of the learning. Therefore outcomes to be measured need to show the effectiveness of the education – changes in practice not numbers of doctors participating.

The change in GP education can be reviewed as:
- Plan: change from PGEA
- Do: set up a new system. Reject credit based education in favour of PDPs
- Study: reflect on whether these changes have delivered our vision (evaluate)
- Act: make changes to the PDP system to make the process more robust, or change to a new system.

Did the NHS use Senge's principles:

- Systems thinking: Yes. The entire system of funding, organizing and delivering GP education changed.
- Personal mastery: PDPs were a top-down approach – educationalists wanted it; the GMC revalidation procedures needed it; the Government's agenda in *A first class service* liked it. There wasn't much of a shared vision amongst grass-roots GPs.
- Mental models: The model of education as 'chalk and talk' was questioned and replaced by a model of adult education or 'learner-centred learning.'
- Shared vision: Not really!
- Team learning: Once the system was introduced, ideas on PDPs were shared in the medical literature and by the local deaneries.

Relevant literature

Articles
Calman K. (1998) *A review of continuing professional development in general practice.* DoH, London. http://open.gov.uk/doh/cme/cmoh.htm
Davies HTO, Nutley SM. (2000) *Developing learning organizations in the new NHS.* BMJ, **320:** 998–1001.

Internet
http://www.jr2.ox.ac.uk/bandolier/ImpAct/imp01/BACKPAGE.html
http://www.library.nhs.uk/
http://www.infed.org/thinkers/senge.htm

Ethical frameworks

Doctors are most familiar with the four ethical principles of:
- **Autonomy:** People of sound mind should have the right to determine what happens to them (literally, self-rule). Respect for patient autonomy requires doctors to help patients come to their own decisions, for example by providing important information in a way they can understand. Doctors should respect their patients and follow their decisions even when they believe that the patient is wrong. The doctor has a duty to respect the rights and dignity of the person, to promote their well-being, and to be truthful, honest and sincere.
- **Beneficence:** Doctors should do good and promote what is best for their patients. The principle of autonomy captures the patient's views; the principle of beneficence captures the doctors' views of the patient's best interests. The two principles conflict when competent patients choose a course of action that is not in their best interests (Piccoli *et al.*, 2004). The doctor has a duty to inform and educate the person, enhancing his capability to continue care for himself.
- **Non-maleficence:** First do no harm. The potential good and harm of a therapeutic intervention need to be weighed up to decide what, overall, is in the patient's best interests.
- **Justice:** When doctors make decisions, their actions should be fair not only to the patient, but also to others. Doctors must try to distribute limited resources (time, money, expensive treatments) fairly. The doctor has a duty to avoid discrimination, abuse or exploitation of people on grounds of race, age, class, gender or religion.

Why are ethical theories important?

Ethical theories can help you to consider various aspects of a situation so that you can weigh up the pros and cons of each course of action. Ethical theories don't tell you which course of action to follow. Different people have different values, so their actions will be different, but they may need to justify why they have chosen a particular course of action. Ethical theories provide the basis for justifying specific ethical decisions.

Consider the following scenario. You go Christmas shopping with your teenage niece. She chooses a bright orange and purple coat. She smiles excitedly and says to you, 'Does this look cool?' You are faced with a moral dilemma. You can take a step back and apply a few ethical frameworks to the dilemma to weigh up the pros and cons of each possible course of action.

Ethical theories

Four ethical theories can be applied to the above scenario:
- **Duty based ethics** (deontology) – These state that an action is right if it is in accord with a moral rule or principle. Certain acts are wrong in themselves, independent of their foreseeable consequences.

With regard to the scenario, lying is wrong, so you should tell your niece the truth irrespective of the hurt you cause. When applying deontology principles, two questions should be asked. First, could you accept a world in which everybody did that? In the above scenario, could you accept a world in which everybody who wanted to be considerate or avoid confrontation lied? Secondly, is the person to whom the principle is being applied being treated as a means to an end? In the above scenario, if you wanted to finish the trip early (the end), then lying to your niece to meet this end, implies that you have treated her as a means to your end. People should be treated as 'means', never just as 'ends'.

Deontology impacts on how we practice as doctors. The GMC produced *The duties of a doctor* – a code of practice that considers the doctors' duties and the patients' rights. Beneficence (doing good) and non-maleficence (not doing harm) are principally about the duty that doctors have to patients.

- **Utilitarianism ethics, particularly consequentialism** – These principles state that an action is right if it promotes the best consequences – the greatest good or happiness for the greatest number. Those actions that promote, or intend to promote, more happiness are better than those that promote less happiness. A weakness of this theory is that it is not possible to measure happiness.

  With regard to the scenario, lying to your niece now may make her happy, but on your return home, her mother may be unhappy with the choice of coat and disallow its wearing. Your niece would be unhappy and so would you for being instrumental in the conflict.

- **Virtue ethics** – These state that an action is right if it is what a virtuous agent would do in the circumstances. The central focus is the moral character of the person, e.g. kind, generous, and empathetic. A weakness of this theory is that it is tied to cultural norms – a virtuous doctor half a century ago may have been one who was paternalistic with little consideration for patient autonomy.

  With regard to the scenario, you could spend a bit more time looking and find a present that pleases both of you and would have the approval of her mother. You would be generous with your time, considerate of your niece's (and her mother's) feelings.

- **Principlism** – There are four important principles: autonomy, non-maleficence, beneficence, and justice. First, you should respect the autonomy of other people. In this case, your niece should be allowed to make her own fashion choices, no matter how different or eccentric these seem to you. A person should be allowed to make her own choices because she knows what is best for her. Your niece may know that bright colours suit her colouring and express her personality. Secondly, the action taken should not cause net harm. Allowing your niece to buy a coat on a whim, which she later regrets, of which her mother disapproves and which you dislike as a gift causes net harm. Thirdly, you should produce net benefit to certain people. Allowing your niece to choose her own coat may help her develop her own sense of fashion and identity. Finally, you should be fair in offering your help, treat people equally, and not discriminate. You should pay as much attention to your niece's feelings as you would to her mother's even though her mother may be more capable of expressing her disapproval to you.

The law

Consent is the expression, in law, of the ethical principle of autonomy. In seeking consent from a patient, a doctor has the duty to ensure that:
1. The consenting patient has capacity.
2. The consenting patient is appropriately informed before making a decision.
3. The consent is given voluntarily.

Patients are presumed **competent** unless they are shown to lack decision-making capacity.

The current test of competence was set by Judge J. Thorpe in the case known as Re C.

To meet the test of competence, the patient must:
1. comprehend and retain the necessary information,
2. believe it,
3. weigh the information, balancing risks and needs, to arrive at a true choice.

The law differs slightly in its treatment of adults and minors.

Learning points

- Deontology, utilitarianism and virtue ethics
- Consent
- Competence

Additional information

The treatment of an adult
The treatment of the adult depends on whether she is competent, or not.
- If the adult is incompetent, she can be treated in her best interests.
- If the adult is competent, she has the right to refuse medical treatment, even if the treatment is life-saving or life-sustaining.

But a patient, competent or incompetent, can be detained under sections 2 or 3 of the Mental Health Act (MHA) 1983 if she meets the criteria for detention. If she is detained, even if she is competent, she can be treated without her consent, under section 63 of the MHA 1983.

The treatment of a minor
A minor aged sixteen or seventeen can be treated in the same way as an adult, and competence assessed using the adult test of competence.

If the patient is *under the age of sixteen*, competence will be tested using the Fraser guidelines. Judge Fraser formulated these guidelines in the Gillick case. Consent for treatment may be obtained from a minor if:

- The implications of the treatment are understood
- Seeking of parental advice is encouraged
- Without treatment, the minor is still likely to pursue the course of action
- The minor's health needs and best interests are met by giving the treatment.

Therefore, a Gillick competent child may give consent to medical treatment, although refusal of consent may be overridden.

The GMC guidance in assessing the patient's best interests
In deciding what options may be reasonably considered as being in the best interests of a patient who lacks capacity to decide, you should take into account:

- options for treatment or investigation which are clinically indicated;
- any evidence of the patient's previously expressed preferences, including an advance statement; your own and the health care team's knowledge of the patient's background, such as cultural, religious, or employment considerations;
- views about the patient's preferences given by a third party who may have other knowledge of the patient, for example the patient's partner, family, carer, tutor-dative (Scotland), or a person with parental responsibility;
- which option least restricts the patient's future choices, where more than one option (including non-treatment) seems reasonable in the patient's best interest.

There are conditions which must be satisfied under section 63 of the Mental Health Act before the patient can be treated:

1. The patient must be detained under the Act.
2. The treatment proposed must count as 'medical treatment'.
3. The treatment proposed must constitute treatment for the mental disorder.

If the detained patient is competent, it is best practice to obtain her consent to treatment. If she does not consent, the doctor may proceed with treatment in the patient's best interests, as is therapeutically necessary. If the patient resists the treatment, the doctor can use such restraint as is clinically necessary.

Relevant literature

Journal articles
Greenhalgh T, Kostopoulou O, Harries C (2004) Making decisions about benefits and harms of medicines. *BMJ*, **329**: 47–50
Parker MJ (2004) Getting ethics into practice. *BMJ*, **329**: 126.
Piccoli GB, Mezza E, Grassi G, Burdese M, Todros T (2004) Interactive case report. A 35 year old woman with diabetic nephropathy who wants a baby: case outcome. *BMJ*, **329**: 900–903.

Pollard JP, Savullescu J (2004) Ethics in practice: eligibility of overseas visitors and people of uncertain residential status for NHS treatment. *BMJ*, **329:** 346–349.
Sokol DK Bergson G (2006) Ethics made easy. *StudentBMJ*, **14:** 397–440.

Books
Orme-Smith A, Spicer J (2001) *Ethics in General Practice*. Radcliffe Medical Press, Oxford.
Kennedy I, Grubb A (2000) *Medical Law*, 3rd edition. Butterworths, Oxford.

Internet
For a very good overview of ethics, see
http://www.uq.edu.au/oppe/PDFS/Ethics_primer.pdf

Professionalism

Why do I need to know about professionalism for the nMRCGP exam?

Professionalism can be incorporated into any question regarding doctors' professional values and professional growth. A question on professional values may appear in many guises, such as:
- you said that keep a log of PUNs and DENs within your appraisal folder. Do you think that appraisal improves the care patients receive?
- you said that you found communicating with the cardiology registrar difficult because he was sarcastic on the telephone. How do you deal with sarcastic colleagues?

Why is professionalism important in general practice?

- As doctors we are expected to follow a code of ethics. The public have certain expectations of us and we have certain responsibilities to them.
- Since the introduction of appraisal and revalidation, doctors are expected to demonstrate evidence of their professional development.

The doctors' code of ethics incorporates the attitudes, values and beliefs that the profession and the public have agreed on. These are stated in the GMC's *Good Medical Practice* as:
- make the care of your patient your first concern;
- treat every patient politely and considerately;
- respect patients' dignity and privacy;
- listen to patients and respect their views;
- give patients information in a way they can understand;
- respect the rights of patients to be fully involved in decisions about their care;
- keep your professional knowledge and skills up to date;
- recognize the limits of your professional competence;
- be honest and trustworthy;
- respect and protect confidential information;
- make sure that your personal beliefs do not prejudice your patients' care;
- act quickly to protect patients from risk if you have good reason to believe that you or a colleague may not be fit to practice;
- avoid abusing your position as a doctor; and
- work with colleagues in the ways that best serve patients' interests.

In all these matters doctors must never discriminate unfairly against their patients or colleagues and they must always be prepared to justify their actions to them.

Characteristics of professionalism

Central to the concept of professionalism are four attributes:

1. **Putting patients' interests first** – Rationing and payment for medical treatment may conflict with this principle.
2. **Ethical behaviour** – doctors should not breach confidence or take advantage of their position or abuse drugs to which they have access.
3. **Being responsive to society** – doctors need to adapt to a changing society, e.g. a move away from the paternalism of the 1950s to increased patient choice and a respect for patients' autonomy.
4. **Being humane** – behaving with empathy, integrity, altruism and trustworthiness.

(Swick, 1999)

What defines the medical profession?

1. The medical profession holds specialized knowledge and is responsible for imparting this knowledge to its students.
2. This knowledge is used to improve the lives of patients.
3. The profession is self-regulating. It establishes and maintains its own standards of practice.
4. The profession is responsible for its research.

The contract with society was renegotiated recently following several high profile scandals (Shipman, Alder Hay and Bristol). Following the Bristol scandal, there was a confidential inquiry which highlighted deficiencies in the professional conduct of some doctors. The GMC heeded these recommendations and changed its licensing procedures accordingly. If these changes had not been made, the profession was in danger of losing its self-regulatory powers. These changes have been called 'New Professionalism'.

Learning points

- Doctors' code of ethics and professionalism – GMC's *Good Medical Practice*
- The four attributes of professionalism (Swick, 1999)
- 'New Professionalism' (Stacey, 1992)
- Bristol Royal Infirmary Inquiry (1996) highlighted the cultural changes that need to occur to improve the professionalism of doctors
- Emphasis on greater lay involvement, peer appraisal, accountability, quality assurance and transparency within the NHS

Additional information

The Bristol Royal Infirmary Inquiry
In 1996 parents of children undergoing routine cardiac operations wrote to the GMC asking for an investigation into the practice of three doctors (Mr

Dhasmana who had 20 deaths following 38 arterial switch operations; Mr Wisheart who had 9 deaths following 15 atrio-ventricular septal defect operations; and Dr Roylance who was the chief executive of the United Bristol Healthcare NHS Trust).

After a consultant anaesthetist reported his concerns, an independent review investigated. In 1998, the GMC found all three doctors guilty of serious professional misconduct. In a landmark decision, Dr Roylance, in his administrative, not clinical capacity, was found guilty due to his failure to *act upon concerns*. This was seen as an act of collusion with poorly performing doctors at the expense of society.

In June 1998, Professor Ian Kennedy, a law professor, was appointed to conduct an inquiry. The aim of the inquiry, the biggest in the history of the NHS, was to uncover all aspects of what went wrong.

The King's Fund report summarized the findings and recommendations of the inquiry as follows:

Events similar to Bristol are unlikely to happen again for three reasons:
- Professional bodies and NHS managers will regularly audit outcomes of treatment and will need to explain variations in performance against peers.
- The attitude and accountability of professionals is undergoing change, and it is now a professional requirement to report concerns about the performance of colleagues – 'whistleblowing'.
- The public and media are holding the health service to account, and asking for data on performance measures, such as league tables.

Changes to the culture that allowed the events at Bristol to happen, have occurred:
- There is greater public involvement in professional regulation.
- A formal process of local, peer appraisal and regular GMC revalidation has been rolled out.
- There are attempts to change the culture of the NHS to a more open, less blaming culture. Cultural change is recognized as a difficult task.

The public expressed concerns with the following aspects of medical professionalism:

1. Deficiencies in self-regulation and quality of care
(i) The public felt that the medical profession turned a blind eye to poorly performing doctors who potentially harmed patients.

'Medicine has been excessively paternalistic, too tolerant of poor practice, and lacking in openness about clinical ability.' (Irvine, 2001)

But in attempting to maintain its self-regulation, the pendulum may have swung too far.

'..the arm of self-regulation in medicine can be seen as attempting to convince those concerned that registration represents more than competence and professional probity but a conscience beyond reproach; a superhuman paragon of virtue'.

Such was Case's (2003) comment in her legal analysis of GMC hearings following the 1995 reforms. She goes even further:

'protecting the dignity of the profession is borne out of self interest and therefore might undermine the GMC's efforts to protect the broader public interest'.

(ii) With the move away from individual doctoring to team doctoring, a blame culture needs to be replaced by a culture of openness and a willingness to acknowledge and learn from our mistakes.

In trying to develop a blame-free, responsible and robust culture, Liam Donaldson proposed a systems approach to error. This involves looking at the technical, organizational, social, and communication factors that predispose to human error.

'The recognition that human error is inevitable in a highly complex and technical field like medicine is a first step in promoting greater self awareness of the importance of systems failure in the causation of accidents.'

(Donaldson, 2002)

2. Conflict between the doctor's advocacy role and his gatekeeper role

The doctor is the patient's advocate. He needs to put his patients' interests first. However, he has a duty to distribute limited healthcare resources efficiently. For example, a doctor may want to prescribe beta-interferon to his multiple sclerosis patients, but if all doctors did this, the health service would soon be bankrupted! His relationship with the patient is strained by his duty to the wider public.

Due to this increasing conflict, NICE was established in April 1999. NICE reviews the evidence with regard to the cost-effectiveness and clinical effectiveness of new and existing therapies with a view to issuing guidelines to the NHS. Some people argue that NICE is a rationing organization. However, NICE's advice still puts doctors in difficult positions with the patient. As in the above example of MS, NICE does not recommend the use of beta-interferon on the grounds that it is neither curative nor cost-effective. The doctor knows that beta-interferon will help to reduce the debilitating symptoms experienced by MS sufferers, and in not prescribing it he is not acting in the patient's best interests.

3. Less altruistic behaviour on the part of some doctors

There are concerns about poorly performing doctors and the tendency of the profession to close ranks. The GMC needs to be seen as an organization that polices its doctors. The GMC needs to identify and deal with the poorly performing doctors. In response, revalidation has been developed. However, there is scepticism that revalidation will successfully identify poor performance and poor professionalism – those who need revalidation most are unlikely to be recognised by this system. Would it have identified Harold Shipman?

The GMC's response: New professionalism

'New professionalism' was a term coined by Stacey (1992) to describe the qualities of good doctoring that the public and the medical profession together agree upon and the means of delivering them effectively. The Bristol inquiry spurred on the GMC reforms and

> 'resulted in the construction of a new government framework for the regulation of medicine, putting the safety of patients treated by the NHS first... However good the systems and institutions are that govern medicine, they will only work properly if doctors are clinically competent, honest, and want to provide a consistently good standard of practice and care.' (Irvine, 2001)

And so revalidation was born. Irvine recognized that changing the rules, structures and processes was easy; changing the attitudes of the medical profession would be far more difficult. New professionalism was the key to change.

The early changes were:
- Public involvement in medical regulation increased, with the doubling of the lay proportion on the Privy Council between 1995 and 2000.
- The GMC was restructured into a more proactive, quality-orientated organization, assuring clinicians' fitness to practice.
- '*Good Medical Practice* is an explicit statement of duties, responsibilities, values, and standards for doctors, based on a strong public and professional consensus about the qualities that are important' (Irvine, 2001). The new standards for the profession were agreed, explicitly stated and policed.
- Compliance with the principles of *Good Medical Practice* will be secured by the changes to the medical curriculum, and by revalidation. Doctors who breach *Good Medical Practice* will be supported until they reach an acceptable level of practice.

> 'To ensure patient safety, the new professionalism requires professional leadership with greater public input to medical regulation, a modern GMC, and a closer fit between the licensure of doctors and the quality assurance of the organisations in which they work.' (Irvine, 2001)

The King's Fund has published a report – *On being a doctor: redefining medical professionalism* – which argues that while individual doctors remain highly trusted, confidence in the profession as a whole is being undermined. It highlights challenges, including growing public expectations of health care and government demands for more responsive public services.

Relevant literature

Case P. (2003) Confidence matters: the rise and fall of informational autonomy in medical law. *Medical Law Review*, **11**: 208–229.

Cruess RL et al. (1999) Renewing professionalism: an opportunity for medicine, *Acad Med*, **74**: 878–884.

Cruess RL et al. (2000) Professionalism: an ideal to be sustained. *Lancet*, **356**: 156–159.

Donaldson L. (2002) An organisation with a memory. *Clinical Medicine*. **2**: 452–457.

Epstein, RM, Hundert EM. (2002) Defining and assessing professional competence. *JAMA*, **287**: 226–235.

Horton R. (2002) The doctor's role in advocacy. *Lancet*, **359:** 458.

Hunter DJ. (2000) Managing the NHS. *Health Care UK*, 69–76.

Irvine D. (2001) Doctors in the UK: their professionalism and its regulatory framework. *Lancet*, **58:** 1807–1810.

Kennedy I, Grubb A. (2000) *Medical Law*, 3rd edition. Butterworths, Oxford.

King's Fund background briefing to the Bristol Royal Infirmary Inquiry. (2003) King's Fund, London.

Neuberger J. (2001) The educated patient: new challenges for the medical profession. *Journal of Internal Medicine*, **249:** 41–45.

Sculpher M, Gafni A, Watt I. (2002) Shared treatment decision making in a collectively funded health care system: possible conflicts and some potential solutions. *Social Science and Medicine*, **54:** 1369–1377.

Smith R. (2001) Why are doctors so unhappy? *BMJ*, **322:** 1073–1074.

Spencer J. (2003) Teaching about professionalism. *Medical Education*, **37:** 288–289.

Stacey M. (1992) *Regulating British medicine: the general medical council*. Wiley, Chichester.

Swick HL *et al.* (1999) Teaching professionalism in undergraduate medical education. *JAMA*, **282:** 830–832.

Answers to 'Test your knowledge' questions

Answers to Case 1 – Back pain

1. False – back pain is the commonest cause of long-term sickness absence
2. True
3. False – urinary retention, not frequency, is a symptom of cauda equina syndrome
4. True
5. False – in a patient >50 years, severe unremitting night pain that gets worse on lying down is suggestive of cancer

For further information see:
- www.cks.library.nhs.uk/back_pain_lower/in_depth/management_issues
- **Khot A, Polmear A** (2006) *Practical General Practice*, 5th edition, p. 198. Butterworth-Heinemann, Oxford.

Answers to Case 2 – Injectable contraception

1. True
2. False – 50% are amenorrheic at 12 months
3. False – low serum estradiol is not a useful proxy indicator for bone mineral density – bone densitometry is the test of choice
4. True
5. True

For further information see:
- www.cks.library.nhs.uk/contraception/in_depth/management_issues
- **Khot A, Polmear A** (2006) *Practical General Practice*, 5th edition, p. 288. Butterworth-Heinemann, Oxford.

Answers to Case 3 – Blacked out / neurology

1. consciousness
2. thirty
3. ten
4. midazolam
5. lorazepam

For further information, consult:
- the SIGN guidelines on the diagnosis and management of epilepsy in adults (April, 2003) on www.sign.ac.uk/guidelines/fulltext/70/section3.html
- www.cks.library.nhs.uk/epilepsy/view_whole_guidance

Answers to Case 4 – Menorrhagia

1. progestogen-containing IUD
2. anti-fibrinolytics
3. danazol
4. anti-fibrinolytics
5. NSAIDs

For further information, consult:
- www.cks.library.nhs.uk/menorrhagia/in_depth/management_issues

Answers to Case 5 – Knee injury / acute joint injuries

1. True
2. False – the 'Ottawa Knee Rule' states that an X-ray should be performed if, after the knee injury, the patient is unable to transfer weight twice on to each leg.
3. True
4. False – the 'Ottawa Ankle Rule' is better at eliminating patients who do not need an X-ray (high sensitivity) than identifying those who have a fracture (low specificity).
5. True

For further information, see:
- www.gp-training.net/rheum/ottawa.htm
- www.cks.library.nhs.uk/sprains_and_strains/view_whole_guidance

Answers to Case 6 – Pins and needles in hands

1. median
2. abductor pollicis brevis
3. ninety
4. sixty
5. radial
6. median

For further information, see:
- www.arc.org.uk (CTS, June 2004)
- www.arc.org.uk/arthinfo/medpubs/6523/6523.asp

Answers to Case 7 – Smoking cessation

1. C
2. D
3. A

4. C

5. B
- NRT gum is available in 2 mg or 4 mg dosages
- Nicorette make a 16-hour patch in either 15 mg or 10 mg or 5 mg per 16 hours
- Bupropion should not be prescribed to patients with a past history of head trauma or eating disorders, or to those under 18 years, or to women who are breastfeeding

For further information, see:
- www.cks.library.nhs.uk/smoking_cessation/in_depth/management_issues

Answers to Case 8 – Termination of pregnancy

1. False – in a typical abortion service, up to 5% of women require in-patient care
2. True
3. True
4. True
5. True – note that an intra-uterine contraception can be inserted immediately following a first or second trimester TOP
6. False – following a TOP, the incidence of placenta praevia and infertility is not known to be increased

For further information, see:
- www.rcog.org.uk/resources/Public/pdf/abortion_summary.pdf
- **Khot A, Polmear A** (2006) *Practical General Practice*, 5th edition. Butterworth-Heinemann, Oxford.

Answers to Case 9 – Sore throat

1. False – there is no evidence that bacterial sore throats are more severe than viral ones or that the duration of the illness is significantly different in either case
2. False – paracetamol is the drug of choice for analgesia in sore throat, taking account of **the increased risks of** gastrointestinal bleeding, nausea, vomiting, abdominal pain, and diarrhoea **with NSAIDs**
3. True
4. False – the incidence of rheumatic fever in the UK is extremely low and there is no support in the literature for the routine treatment of sore throat with penicillin to prevent the development of rheumatic fever
5. True

For further information, see:
- www.sign.ac.uk/guidelines/fulltext/34/index.html (Jan. 1999)

Answers to Case 10 – Struggling to cope with a baby

1. False – current evidence does not support routine screening
2. True
3. False – it doubles the recovery rate
4. False – TCAs, with the exception of doxepin, appear safe in lactation
5. True

For further information, see:
- **Khot A, Polmear A** (2006) *Practical General Practice*, 5th edition. Butterworth-Heinemann, Oxford.

Answers to Case 11 – Painful shoulder

1. False – pain in the mid-range of shoulder abduction suggests a rotator cuff injury
2. False – pain at the end of shoulder abduction suggests acromioclavicular arthritis
3. True
4. False – when testing passive movement, a true assessment of glenohumeral abduction involves pressing firmly top of the shoulder with one hand while moving the patient's arm with the other hand
5. False – the long thoracic nerve is C5, 6, 7
6. True
7. False – power in the deltoid muscle is tested by asking the patient to move his hand sideways to point to the ceiling, against resistance

For further information, see:
- **Apley GA, Soloman L** (1994) *Concise System of Orthopaedics and Fractures*, 2nd edition. Butterworth-Heinemann, Oxford.

Answers to Case 12 – Forearm in plaster cast

1. False – heavy cannabis use causes short-term memory impairment
2. True
3. False – irritability, sweating and anxiety are symptoms of withdrawal from long-term cannabis use; euphoria and altered perception of passing time are symptoms of the cannabis high
4. True
5. False – historically, delirium tremens has had a death rate of about 20%
6. False – cognitive behaviour therapy, motivational interviewing and twelve-step programmes are equally effective for people with alcohol dependence

For further information, see:
- www.nzgg.org.nz/guidelines/0040/full_guideline.pdf – this is an excellent reference, particularly page 15 which lists examples of open questions when assessing cannabis and alcohol use in primary care

Answers to Case 13 – Haematuria

1. False – in men treated for a lower urinary tract infection, arrange for a mid-stream urine (MSU) before, and 7 days after finishing, antibiotics
2. False – in men with a lower urinary tract infection, an ultrasound scan (USS) and abdominal X-ray of the urinary tract detect any underlying pathology as reliably as intravenous pyelogram (IVP)
3. False – 90% of patients with small renal stones (<5 mm) pass the stones spontaneously
4. True
5. False – patients with oxalate renal stones are advised to avoid spinach and tea
6. False – patients with calcium renal stones are advised to reduce their dairy intake

For further information, see:
- **Khot A, Polmear A** (2006) *Practical General Practice*, 5th edition. Butterworth-Heinemann, Oxford.

Answers to Case 14 – Erectile dysfunction

1. True
2. True
3. False – GPs provide Meningitis A and C immunisation for holiday travel at a charge to their NHS patients
4. False – medication for malaria prophylaxis may not be reimbursed under the NHS, as per Department of Health guidance, FHSL(95)7
5. False – patients <16 years and 60 years or over are eligible for free NHS prescriptions
6. True – only diabetics on oral hypoglycaemics or on insulin are eligible for free NHS prescriptions
7. True

For further information, see:
- www.burypct.nhs.uk/fileadmin/user_upload/clinical_governance/MM/BuryversionNon-nhspresc.doc

Answers to Case 15 – Hypothyroidism

1. False – if TSH is raised and thyroxine is normal, he has sub-clinical hypothyroidism
2. False – if TSH is raised and thyroxine is normal, his thyroid peroxidase antibodies should be measured
3. True

4. True
5. True

For further information, see:
- **Weetman AP** (1997) Hypothyroidism: screening and subclinical disease. *BMJ*, **314**: 1175–1178.

Answers to Case 16 – Hyperthyroidism

1. False – symptoms include heat intolerance, palpitations, anxiety, fatigue, weight loss, muscle weakness, and, in women, irregular menses
2. False – clinical findings may include tremor, tachycardia, lid lag, and warm moist skin
3. False – due to Graves' disease, protrusion of the eyes and diplopia is clinically evident in 30% of patients
4. True
5. False – in a patient with a normal to elevated radioactive iodine uptake (as in Graves' disease), treatment options include antithyroid drugs, radioactive iodine therapy, and thyroidectomy; a low radioactive iodine uptake suggests thyroiditis

For further information, see:
- **Pearce EN** (2006) Diagnosis and management of thyrotoxicosis. *BMJ*, **332**: 1368–1373.

Answers to Case 17 – Hypertension

1. True
2. True
3. False – if hypertensive therapy is needed, the first choice should be an angiotensin-converting enzyme (ACE) inhibitor
4. False – suspect phaeochromocytoma if he has headache, palpitations, and pallor
5. False – suspect malignant hypertension if BP is more than 180/110 mmHg with signs of papilloedema and/or retinal haemorrhage

For further information, see:
- **NICE** (2006) Hypertension

Answers to Case 18 – Grief

1. False – if results vary when rechecking her fasting lipids, use the average to decide whether treatment for hypercholesterolaemia is required
2. True – illness can depress the cholesterol

3. False – levonorgestrel could raise her cholesterol
4. True – a person who stopped smoking in the last 5 years after considerably more years as a smoker should be assessed as a smoker
5. False – if she has premature menopause, multiply her CVD risk by 1.5
6. False – a triglyceride >5.0 mmol/l requires referral to a lipid clinic for consideration of fibrate therapy

For further information, see:
- **Khot A, Polmear A** (2006) *Practical General Practice*, 5th edition. Butterworth-Heinemann, Oxford.

Answers to Case 19 – Obsessive compulsive disorder

1. True
2. False – if a selective serotonin re-uptake inhibitor (SSRI) is prescribed for the treatment of OCD, expect to continue it for at least 1 year
3. False – if a tricyclic antidepressant (TCA) is prescribed for the treatment of OCD, the best evidence is for clomipramine
4. True
5. False – it is appropriate to prescribe benzodiazepines for 2–4 weeks in a generalised anxiety crisis but not in panic disorder

For further information, see:
- **Khot A, Polmear A** (2006) *Practical General Practice*, 5th edition. Butterworth-Heinemann, Oxford.

Answers to Case 20 – Tinea pedis

Regarding retinal screening for diabetics:
1. False – direct ophthalmoscopy is not acceptable
2. True
3. False – it should occur at least annually

UKPDS has:
1. True
2. False – in diabetics who are overweight (body mass index >25 kg/m^2) metformin may be particularly advantageous
3. False – observed the progressive nature of Type 2 diabetes, for example, for people taking tablets it is often necessary to increase the dose, add other tablets or eventually to commence insulin treatment
4. False – shown that the additional cost of medication to improve blood pressure levels was directly recouped by a reduced cost of hospital admissions

For further information, see:
- www.diabetes.org.uk/

Answers to Case 21 – Migraine

1. False – five attacks of the headache described in the question, with nausea, vomiting, photophobia or phonophobia meet the diagnostic criteria for migraine without aura
2. False – if she describes blurred vision or 'spots' preceding the development of the headache, this is not diagnostic of migraine with aura
3. True
4. False – if she describes motor weakness in one arm preceding the development of the headache, this requires referral to a specialist for exclusion of other disease, such as familial hemiplegic migraine
5. True

For further information, see:
- www.bash.org.uk/

Answers to Case 22 – Non-accidental overdose

1. False – the physical severity of the self-harm is not a good indicator of suicidal intent because adolescents are often unaware of the relative toxicity of supposedly harmless substances such as paracetamol
2. True
3. False – teaching problem-solving techniques and rehearsing coping strategies are helpful
4. True
5. False – problem-solving therapy starts with identifying and deciding what problem(s) to tackle first

For further information, see:
- **Hawton K, James A** (2005) Suicide and deliberate self harm in young people. *BMJ*, **330**: 891–894.

Answers to Case 23 – Hernia

1. False – if asymptomatic, bilateral and bluish in appearance, they are most likely hydroceles
2. False – inguinal hernias are virtually all indirect and often complete (that is, the sac comes all the way to the scrotum)
3. True
4. False – if the lump becomes tender, the infant starts to vomit and refuses to feed, this is a surgical emergency
5. False – if hydroceles persist beyond infancy, they require an operation for the processus to be ligated

For further information, see:
- **Davenport M** (1996) ABC of general paediatric surgery. *BMJ*, **312**: 564–567.

Answers to Case 24 – Osteoarthritis

1. True
2. False – in patients with osteoarthritis of the knee, controlled studies have shown that regular telephone contact from a healthcare worker produces significant improvement in functional status
3. False – the two main approaches used by physiotherapists are muscle strengthening programmes specific for certain joints and general aerobic conditioning
4. True
5. False – trials that have compared random needling with acupuncture have failed to show measurable benefit for true acupuncture
6. False – capsaicin, a naturally occurring compound, has significantly greater analgesic effects than placebo

For further information, see:
- **Walker-Bone K, Javaid K, Arden N, Cooper C** (2000) Medical management of osteoarthritis. *BMJ,* **321**: 936–940.

Answers to Case 25 – Request for cosmetic surgery

1. True
2. False – routine radiography of the **nasal** bones in a suspected simple **nasal** bone fracture is unnecessary
3. True
4. False – plain radiographs cannot exclude nasoethmoid fractures
5. True

For further information, see:
- **Hodgkinson DW, Lloyd RE, Driscoll PA, Nicholson DA** (1994) ABC of emergency radiology: maxillofacial radiographs. *BMJ,* **308**: 46–50.

Answers to Case 26 – Insomnia

1. False – it arises from incomplete emotional processing of the trauma
2. False – hypervigilance, increased startle reaction, and insomnia are symptoms and signs of hyperarousal
3. True
4. False – it is associated with increased secretion of corticotrophin-releasing factor and hypocortisolaemia
5. True

For further information, see:
- **Lyons D, McLoughlin D** (2001) Recent advances: psychiatry. *BMJ,* **323**: 1228–1231.

Answers to Case 27 – Emergency contraception

1. True
2. False – if started on day 1–5 of her period, extra precautions are not needed (provided she does not have a short, i.e. less than 23 day, cycle)
3. False – if one or two 30 μg pills are missed at any time, emergency contraception is not required
4. False – if one or two 30 μg pills are missed at any time, emergency contraception is not required
5. True

For further information, see:
- Contraception – combined pill – your guide (fpa) available online: www.cks.library.nhs.uk/patient_information_leaflet/contraception_combined_pill_your_guide_fpa/how_do_i_start_the_first_pack_of_pills
- Contraception – combined pill – your guide (fpa) available online: www.cks.library.nhs.uk/patient_information_leaflet/contraception_combined_pill_your_guide_fpa/how_many_pills_have_you_missed

Answers to Case 28 – Bariatric surgery

1. True
2. False – the receptionist should refer Mrs FW to the complaints administrator (usually the practice manager)
3. False – the written complaint should normally be acknowledged within 2 working days
4. False – an explanation should normally be provided within 10 working days
5. True
6. False – a record should not be kept in the patient's medical records
7. False – the complaints administrator should support the practice nurse
8. True

For further information, see:
- DoH (1996) Practice-based complaints procedures: guidance for general practices, available online: www.dh.gov.uk/en/Publicationsandstatistics/Publications/PublicationsPolicyAndGuidance/DH_4005491

Answers to Case 29 – Multiple sclerosis

1. False – being female is associated with a better prognosis
2. True
3. True
4. False – there is no evidence that steroids shorten the long-term course of MS
5. False – baclofen, a muscle relaxant, should be reduced over several weeks because abrupt withdrawal may provoke seizures

6. False – neuropathic pain may be treated with gabapentin, amitriptyline or carbamazepine

For further information, see:
- **Khot A, Polmear A** (2006) *Practical General Practice*, 5th edition. Butterworth-Heinemann, Oxford.

Answers to Case 30 – Balance problems

1. False – a sudden onset of decreased vision and soreness when moving the eye suggests optic neuritis
2. False – in a 70-year-old, presentation with a sudden, severe loss of central vision suggests central vein occlusion
3. True
4. True
5. True

For further information, see:
- www.stlukeseye.com/Conditions/Default.asp

Answers to Case 31 – Tonsillitis

1. True
2. False – even if the sore throat persists, a throat swab to identify group A beta-haemolytic streptococcus (GABHS) may not be helpful, as the poor specificity and sensitivity of throat swabs limit their usefulness
3. False – although antibiotic therapy has been shown to alleviate symptoms even in sore throats not caused by bacteria, the superiority of antibiotics over simple analgesics is marginal in reducing duration or severity
4. True
5. False – in children under 16 years, emergency re-admissions within 4 weeks of discharge after tonsillectomy occur in 1.3% of cases

For further information, see:
- SIGN (1999): www.sign.ac.uk/guidelines/fulltext/34/index.html

Answers to Case 32 – Menstrual problems

1. True
2. Women with PCOS at high risk of diabetes include:
   - False – women with a body mass index greater than 30 kg/m^2
   - True
   - False – women who have a waist circumference greater than 80 cm
   - True

3. True
4. False – there is no evidence to suggest an increased risk of ovarian cancer when clomifene is used for less than 12 cycles
5. True
6. False – women with PCOS, in middle age, have a 10–20% risk of developing type 2 diabetes
7. False – women with PCOS have risk factors for cardiovascular disease (CVD), namely obesity, hypertension, hyperandrogenism and hyperinsulinaemia
8. False – in women diagnosed as having PCOS before pregnancy, metformin taken throughout pregnancy reduces their chances of developing gestational diabetes
9. True

For further information, see:
- RCOG Green Guidelines (2003) available online: www.rcog.org.uk/resources/Public/pdf/Polys_Ovary_Syndrome_No33.pdf
- www.cks.library.nhs.uk/polycystic_ovary_syndrome/in_summary

Answers to Case 33 – Irregular heart beats

1. True
2. False – the ECG findings of atrial flutter are saw-tooth flutter waves with 2:1 or 3:1 conduction
3. False – third-degree block, where atrial impulses are not conducted to ventricles, presents with bradycardia
4. True
5. False – where potassium is increased in Addison's disease, the ECG shows PR and QT interval prolongation
6. False – Wolff–Parkinson–White is suspected in a young man presenting with palpitations and light-headedness whose ECG shows broad, bizarre complex tachycardias

For further information, see:
- **Goodacre S, Irons R** (2002) ABC of clinical electrocardiography: atrial arrhythmias. *BMJ,* **324**: 594–597.

Answers to Case 34 – Psoriasis

1. False – a tar-based cream treats localised plaque psoriasis such as on the elbows or knees; methotrexate is useful in acute, generalised, pustular psoriasis, psoriatic erythroderma, psoriatic arthritis, and for extensive chronic plaque psoriasis in patients who are inadequately controlled by topical therapy alone
2. True

3. False – when there is significant scaling, use a keratolytic agent such as 5% salicylic acid in emulsifying ointment first or other treatments will fail
4. True
5. False – if the patient developed psoriasis soon after starting on NSAIDs and paracetamol, the provocative agent is likely to be the NSAID

For further information, see:
- Joint BAD/PCDS guideline, available online: www.bad.org.uk/healthcare/guidelines/psorrecommend.asp

Answers to Case 35 – Onychomycosis

1. True
2. True
3. True
4. True
5. False – eradication of fungus in onychomycosis does not always render the nail normal in appearance

For further information, see:
- www.bad.org.uk/healthcare/guidelines/Onychomycosis.pdf

Answers to Case 36 – Transient ischaemic attack

1. True
2. False – TIA patients, irrespective of whether or not they have a history of hypertension, should have their BPs reduced by 10/5 mmHg
3. False – thiazide diuretics, beta-blockers, ACE-Is and ARBs are beneficial in reducing cardiovascular events and stroke incidence in patients with diabetes
4. True
5. False – for patients with recent TIA and ipsilateral carotid artery stenosis, there is no indication for carotid endarterectomy if the degree of stenosis is <50%

For further information, see:
- AHA Guidelines (2006) http://stroke.ahajournals.org/cgi/content/full/37/2/577

Answers to Case 37 – Newly diagnosed diabetes mellitus

1. True
2. False – type 2 diabetes is one-and-a-half times more prevalent in the most deprived one-fifth of the population
3. True
4. True

5. False – diabetic ketoacidosis (DKA) is precipitated by insulin omission, severe illness (e.g. myocardial infarction) or infection (e.g. pneumonia)

For further information, see:
- NSF for diabetes (2001), available on-line: www.dh.gov.uk/en/Publications andstatistics/Publications/PublicationsPolicyAndGuidance/DH_4002951

Answers to Case 38 – Cognitive impairment

1. False – reversible causes of dementia, such as those due to hypothyroidism or vitamin B12 deficiency, are rare (<1%)
2. True
3. False – bright light therapy is not recommended for the treatment of cognitive impairment
4. True
5. False – a Cochrane systematic review suggests that *Gingko biloba* is less potent in establishing cognitive improvement than cholinesterase inhibitors
6. True
7. False – anti-inflammatories are not recommended for treatment of cognitive decline in patients with Alzheimer's disease

For further information, see:
- SIGN (2006) www.sign.ac.uk/pdf/sign86.pdf

Answers to Case 39 – Gout

1. True
2. False – anti-inflammatory drug therapy should be commenced immediately and continued for 1–2 weeks
3. False – colchicine, an effective alternative, should be used in doses of 500 μg bd–qds
4. False – patients already established on allopurinol should continue to take their allopurinol
5. True
6. True

For further information, see:
- Guideline for the management of gout (2007), available online at: http://rheumatology.oxfordjournals.org/cgi/content/full/kem056av1

Answers to Case 40 – Renal colic

1. True
2. False – if diclofenac gives inadequate pain relief, give diamorphine 5–10 mg by intramuscular or subcutaneous injection

3. True
4. True
5. False – the absence of haematuria makes the diagnosis of renal colic less likely (but does not exclude the diagnosis)
6. False – advise people to filter their urine to capture the stone (using a nylon stocking or a tea strainer)

For further information, see:
- Guideline summary: www.cks.library.nhs.uk/renal_colic_acute/in_summary

Answers to Case 41 – Neck of femur fracture

1. True
2. False – alendronate and risedronate reduce the incidence of both vertebral and non-vertebral fractures; etidronate reduces the incidence of vertebral fractures but there is less evidence that it reduces non-vertebral fractures, and it is likely to be less effective than alendronate and risedronate for these fractures
3. True
4. False – an active or past history of venous thrombosis precludes the use of raloxifene and strontium ranelate
5. False – when investigating osteoporosis, if the ESR is raised, then serum and urine electrophoresis are indicated to exclude multiple myeloma
6. True

For further information, see:
- Guideline summary: www.cks.library.nhs.uk/osteoporosis_treatment/ in_summary/scenario_postmenopausal_women

Answers to Case 42 – Drug use

1. False – 20% of people will fight the infection and naturally clear it from their bodies within 2–6 months
2. True
3. True
4. False – interferon and ribavirin can clear the virus in approximately half those treated
5. False – if hepatitis C is cleared with treatment, patients are not immune to future infections of hepatitis C

For further information, see:
- www.cks.library.nhs.uk/patient_information_leaflet/hepatitis_c